Bottom Line's
HEALTH
2019
BREAKTHROUGHS

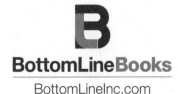

BottomLineBooks

BottomLineInc.com

ISBN 0-88723-809-2

Bottom Line Books® publishes the advice of expert authorities in many fields. These opinions may at times conflict as there are often different approaches to solving problems. The use of this material is no substitute for health, legal, accounting or other professional services. Consult competent professionals for answers to your specific questions.

Telephone numbers, addresses, prices, offers and websites listed in this book are accurate at the time of publication, but they are subject to frequent change.

Bottom Line Books® is a registered trademark of Bottom Line Inc.
3 Landmark Square, Suite 201, Stamford, Connecticut 06901

BottomLineInc.com

Bottom Line Books is an imprint of Bottom Line Inc., publisher of print periodicals, e-letters and books. We are dedicated to bringing you the best information from the most knowledgeable sources in the world. Our goal is to help you gain greater wealth, better health, more wisdom, extra time and increased happiness.

Printed in the United States of America

Contents

Contents

Contents

Contents

Preface

We are proud to bring you the all-new *Bottom Line's Health Breakthroughs 2019*. This collection represents a year's worth of the latest health news and scientific discoveries in a broad spectrum of fields.

When you choose a Bottom Line book, you are turning to a stellar group of experts in a wide range of specialties—medical doctors, alternative practitioners, renowned nutrition experts, research scientists and consumer-health advocates, to name a few.

We go to great lengths to interview the foremost health experts. Whether it's cancer prevention, breakthrough arthritis treatments or cutting-edge nutritional advice, our editors talk to the true innovators in health care.

How do we find all these top-notch professionals? Over the past 40 years, we have built a network of leading physicians in both alternative and conventional medicine. They are affiliated with the world's premier medical institutions. We follow the medical research and bring the latest information to our readers. We also regularly talk with our advisers in teaching hospitals, private practices and government health agencies.

Bottom Line's Health Breakthroughs 2019 is a result of our ongoing research and contact with these experts, and is a distillation of their latest findings and advice. We hope that you will enjoy the presentation and glean helpful information about the health topics that concern you and your family.

As a reader of a Bottom Line book, please be assured that you are receiving reliable and well-researched information from a trusted source. But, please use prudence in health matters. Always speak to your physician before taking vitamins, supplements or over-the-counter medication…changing your diet…or beginning an exercise program. If you experience side effects from any regimen, contact your doctor immediately.

The Editors, Bottom Line Books, Stamford, Connecticut.

CHAPTER 1

Allergies and Lung Health

Natural Treatments for a Difficult Allergy Season

If your nose is stuffed up and your eyes are watering, you're not alone. What's an allergy sufferer to do—especially when the usual remedies for allergies (whether conventional medications or natural remedies) don't seem to be helping? We asked Holly Lucille, ND, RN, who practices naturopathic medicine in Los Angeles, how she helps her allergy patients when pollen, mold and other allergies are at their worst. *Here's her advice…*

CONVENTIONAL VS. NATURAL REMEDIES

One of the problems with taking conventional medications such as Claritin, Zyrtec or Allegra is that they offer only temporary relief for allergy symptoms and can produce uncomfortable side effects, such as fatigue, headache and dry mouth, among others. In addition, when an allergy season lasts many weeks or even months, you may be on these medications for longer than you want or longer than feels good.

Here's where the benefit of natural remedies comes into play. Natural treatments generally are much easier on the body—which means that you can take them for longer periods of time.

There are many natural treatments available in supplement form that work to control allergies. They often work in different ways. *For symptom relief, try the following combination…*

A detoxifier…

• **Milk thistle** (*Silybum marianum*), a flavonoid that helps the liver process toxins more efficiently, thereby helping to clear out potential allergens.

A remedy for symptom relief…

Try one of the four remedies below. If it doesn't help your allergy symptoms within two weeks, try the next one on the list…

Holly Lucille, ND, RN, is a nationally recognized naturopathic doctor, author and educator practicing in Los Angeles. DrHollyLucille.com

• **Quercetin,** a flavonoid antioxidant, reduces the inflammation caused by allergens.

• **Stinging Nettle** (*Urtica dioica*), a plant that has been found to reduce the amount of histamine created in response to an allergen.

• **Butterbur** (*Petasites hybridus*), an herb that prevents the release of chemicals that cause inflammation in the nasal passages.

Caution: Butterbur is related to ragweed, so if you have a ragweed allergy, taking butterbur can make your symptoms worse. Also, some butterbur preparations contain *pyrrolizidine alkaloids* (PAs), which can damage the liver. Use only butterbur products that are certified and labeled "PA-free."

And an immune booster...

• **A probiotic.** These are "good bacteria" in supplement form that boost health and the immune system. They are especially helpful for people fighting allergies because they improve immune function and reduce inflammation associated with allergies. There are specific types of probiotic species that help specific ailments. When it comes to boosting the immune system, one combination to consider is *Lactobacillus acidophilus* and *Bifidobacterium*. Taking a probiotic can help the immune system year-round, not just during allergy season.

All of these remedies, which are available online and in health-food stores, are safe for adults. Follow label instructions. Pregnant women should not use these supplements—and should speak to a physician before taking probiotics.

COMBINING NATURAL AND CONVENTIONAL REMEDIES

What about taking both conventional medications and natural remedies? While the goal is to avoid drugs, it's OK to add a drug to your natural therapies when symptoms are very severe. It's best to do this for the shortest possible time—for example, only a few days. Conversely, for allergy sufferers who rely on drugs, adding one or two natural treatments may eventually enable them to lower the dosage or even wean themselves off of the drugs altogether.

GETTING TO THE ROOT OF THE PROBLEM

In addition to helping patients find the remedies that work best for them, holistic doctors believe in getting to the root cause of a patient's allergy problem. Often, a diet high in sugar, processed foods or mucus-producing foods such as dairy can make a patient more susceptible to allergies. Stress and lack of sleep can depress the immune system—and contribute to allergies. If your allergies are particularly stubborn during a specific season, consult a holistic doctor who can help you get to the root of your problem.

Common Seasonal-Allergy Mistakes

Clifford Bassett, MD, founder and medical director, Allergy and Asthma Care of New York, quoted at Live Science.com.

Common seasonal-allergy mistakes and what to do instead...

Mistake: Opening windows, which lets pollen in.

Better: Run the air conditioner, and use high-efficiency filters to trap pollen.

Mistake: Not taking regular antipollen steps.

Better: Wash hair at the end of every day, keep pets clean, avoid hanging laundry outdoors.

Mistake: Neglecting your eyes, through which pollen often enters the body.

Better: Wear sunglasses and a brimmed hat when outdoors, and use eye rinses regularly.

Mistake: Waiting too long to start on allergy medicines.

Better: Take them at the start of pollen season instead of waiting for symptoms to get worse.

Mistake: Overusing nasal sprays.

Better: Use them for no more than five days in a row to avoid irritating sinuses and the lining of the nose.

4 Surprising Facts About Mucus

Neil L. Kao, MD, a board-certified specialist in internal medicine, allergies and immunology and an attending physician at Greenville Health System and Spartanburg Regional Medical Center, both in South Carolina. He regularly blogs about allergy and asthma issues at KaoAllergyAsthma.blogspot.com.

Mucus. It's hard to even say the word without curling a lip in disgust. But this much-maligned secretion is really a superhero in disguise—a stoic defender of the unprotected parts of your body. Sound like too much horn-blowing for such a yucky substance? Not so.

Few people understand the important role that mucus plays in keeping us healthy…and how to keep one's supply of this gooey substance functioning optimally. *What you need to know…*

WHAT MUCUS DOES

Mucus is a watery, slick secretion that forms a physical and chemical barrier on many of the body's internal surfaces. Mucus protects the entire respiratory tract—that is, your nose, sinuses, mouth, throat, trachea, bronchial tubes and lungs—against foreign invaders such as bacteria and viruses. Mucus lubricates the surface and prevents excessive dryness.

The entire gastrointestinal tract, from mouth to colon to anus, as well as the genital tract in both males and females, produces mucus to perform these same functions. The principle of producing secretions like mucus is also present elsewhere in the body. For example, your eyes constantly produce a protective film of secretions that function just like mucus. We call them tears.

YOUR PROTECTOR

When your body senses danger, mucus is part of a defense system that kicks into gear. All mucus contains disease-fighting enzymes, chemicals and sometimes white blood cells called neutrophils. They work together to trap, inactivate or kill the foreign substances.

One purpose of mucus is to prevent these substances from entering the body. Having lots of mucus helps to wash away any offensive microorganisms and particles, such as bacteria and pollen. We blow our noses to eliminate mucus from our bodies. The remaining mucus is swallowed, digested and reabsorbed by the intestines. Stomach acid or enzymes from the pancreas should inactivate and destroy any disease-causing substances.

What you may not know: *Any* perceived attack—not only viruses, bacteria or allergens (such as pollen or pet dander) but also chemicals—can increase mucus production.

When this occurs, your mucus-making machinery can get busy when you least expect it. For example, the chemical compound *capsaicin*, which is found in chili peppers, will temporarily ramp up mucus production in the nose (making the nose "run") in an effort to clear the irritant from the body.

And what about dairy products? Studies have not shown that dairy increases mucus production. When the question was investigated, researchers found only that milk causes phlegm (a sticky form of mucus) to thicken. However, in my practice, I've observed that mucus does increase in some patients—perhaps due to the individual's reaction to the proteins in milk.

My advice: If you feel that dairy increases your mucus production, you may be more comfortable if you cut back or eliminate your dairy intake.

A COLOR CHANGE

Healthy mucus is usually clear and thin. Sometimes, however, nasal mucus may change from clear to a deep yellow-green. This color change is due to the heavy presence of *neutrophils*. They are naturally light green in color, even though they're considered "white" blood cells.

Anytime there is a greater concentration of neutrophils, secretions may appear green. This can happen, for instance, during a respiratory infection when extra neutrophils are dispatched to fight the infection…or if your mucus dries out due to dehydration.

What you may not know: Contrary to popular belief, greenish-yellow mucus does *not* always mean that you have a bacterial infection. You may have a viral infection. Yet many people make that faulty assumption and demand antibiotics from their doctors. Antibiotics, as most people know, do nothing to eliminate a viral infection.

A nasal or throat swab or sputum test can be performed to tell whether your infection is caused by bacteria (which may necessitate antibiotic treatment) or a virus (which you'll have to live with until it passes).

DANGER SIGNS

In rare instances, mucus can signal a serious health problem.

What you may not know: If your nasal mucus turns brownish-black, it may be caused by a fungal infection (*aspergillosis*) of the lining of the nose. Aspergillus is a common mold found on dead leaves, rotting vegetation and in some heating and air-conditioning systems. When aspergillus particles are inhaled, an infection can develop in people with weakened immunity or lung disease. The infection also causes shortness of breath, fever and fatigue. Aspergillosis requires prompt treatment with steroids and antifungal medication or it can become fatal.

When your eye is the target of disease or irritation, mucus can alert you to a potential danger. With conjunctivitis (pink eye), the eye usually produces a watery discharge or white or light yellow mucus.

While most cases of pink eye are benign, some may progress and cause permanent damage to your vision. To prevent such damage, see a doctor promptly if you have green or yellow mucus coming from your eye or if you wake up with eyes sealed shut from dry, crusty mucus.

WHEN THE BODY AGES

As we get older, we lose our ability to control how much mucus we produce, leaving mucus-containing organs more prone to disease-causing organisms.

For example, decreased mucus production results in an increased risk for ear, nose, sinus, throat and lung infections, including pneumonia, because the body is less able to efficiently kill and clear away bacteria and viruses. To help maintain the full function of mucus-producing cells, it's important to treat allergies and not smoke or snort products.

What you may not know: Mucus protects the sensors in the nose that are responsible for smell and taste. If the body does not make enough mucus to keep the inside of the nose moist, sensors in the nasal passages don't function well and food tastes bland. One way to help retain these senses is with regular nasal washes (see below). *Note:* If the inside of your nose feels dry, it can also be a sign that you are dehydrated and need to drink more fluids.

A ONE-TWO PUNCH

Nasal irrigation may sound like a messy proposition, but it's a healthy habit for most people. Irrigation can remoisten dry nasal passages if there's not enough mucus...or it can help remove excess mucus when you have a bad cold or congested sinuses.

How nasal irrigation can help: If you have a runny nose with thick mucus, it's a good idea to perform a nasal wash *at least* once a day. It helps remove excess mucus and whatever elements may be causing this excess, such as viruses, bacteria, allergens (such as pollen and molds) and irritant particles such as the chemicals in smoke. Also, don't worry about leaving yourself "dried out"—the body simply produces more mucus.

A worthwhile daily habit: Even for those who are not battling an overabundance of mucus, a daily nasal wash can assist breathing and promote healthy nasal passages.*

You can use a bottled nasal irrigation product or saline solution. Such products include Ayr, Ocean, Simply Saline and drugstore brands. But this approach can become expensive with daily washes.

Many people prefer to use a teapot-shaped device called a neti pot. They're available at drugstores and online for around $15. Follow label instructions.

To avoid infection, the FDA advises against using tap water, which may contain low levels of organisms such as bacteria and protozoa. Instead, the agency recommends using bottled distilled or sterile water...boiled and cooled tap water (boiled for three to five minutes, cooled to lukewarm and used within 24 hours)...or water

*If your immune system is compromised for any reason or if you've had recent nasal or sinus surgery or have a structural abnormality such as a deviated septum, consult your doctor before practicing nasal irrigation.

passed through a filter designed to trap potentially infectious organisms.

Important: Make sure to wash your neti pot with hot water and soap after each use, rinse thoroughly and dry with a paper towel or let it air-dry to keep it free of mold, bacteria or other contaminants.

Natural Cough Remedies That Work Better Than OTC Drugs

Gustavo Ferrer, MD, a pulmonologist in private practice in Weston, Florida. He is the author of *Cough Cures: The Complete Guide to the Best Natural Remedies and Over-the-Counter Drugs for Acute and Chronic Coughs.* Dr. Ferrer grew up in Cuba, a culture that effectively utilizes herbal teas and folk remedies for coughs and colds.

It's enough to make you dizzy—hundreds of boxes and bottles lining the drugstore shelves, all promising to eradicate your cough...and perhaps also chest congestion, postnasal drip, sneezing and other related symptoms. Americans spend billions a year on over-the-counter (OTC) respiratory medications—including cough suppressants, decongestants and antihistamines. Coughs are also one of the top reasons why we see a doctor.

Here's a surprise...most of the time, it's all unnecessary. Why? Most acute coughs brought on by a cold or the flu go away on their own within a few days and don't require a doctor's care. Sometimes, though, a cough can linger as long as two or three weeks, so you want to take something for relief.

Here's the real bombshell: Most OTC cough remedies just don't work! Back in 2006, the American College of Chest Physicians concluded that there's no strong evidence of effectiveness for the vast majority of drugstore cough medications. In 2014, a Cochrane review of 29 clinical trials involving nearly 5,000 people reached the same conclusion. But they are heavily advertised, so people still buy them.

But don't despair. There is real help out there. Some OTC remedies really do relieve coughs—though not in the way you'd expect. Even better

are natural cough remedies, using readily found ingredients, which are both effective and safe.

THESE OTC PRODUCTS MAY HELP

Nine times out of 10, acute cough symptoms are triggered by post-nasal drip—that annoying mucus trickling down the back of your throat. *These OTCs decrease secretions to ease post-nasal drip...*

•**Antihistamines.** *Loratadine* (Claritin), *fexofenadine* (Allegra), *cetirizine* (Zyrtec) and *diphenhydramine* (Benadryl) block histamine, a naturally occurring chemical that provokes mucus production. They dry up mucus and decrease nasal secretions—even if you don't have an allergy.

Caution: They can cause water retention as a side effect. Avoid if you have glaucoma or prostate enlargement or are taking diuretics. Also, because these old-fashioned antihistamines can make you drowsy, you can become dependent on them to fall asleep.

My advice: Take half the recommended dose, for no more than a week.

•**Saline nasal spray.** Salt plus water—it doesn't get much more natural than that! The simple act of spraying this combination into nasal passages usually alleviates the stuffiness that can trigger constant hacking. Try versions that contain only these two active ingredients, such as Ocean Nasal Spray, Ayr Saline Nasal Mist or Little Remedies Saline Spray/Drops.

Caution: Avoid sprays containing *oxymetazoline* (Afrin), *phenylephrine* (Sudafed) or *xylometazoline* (Triaminic), which lead to "rebound congestion" when they wear off.

NATURAL REMEDIES FOR THE WIN

These natural cough relief remedies are your best bet for cough relief. They calm throat irritations, dry up mucus and boost the immune system—safely. *My top picks...*

•**Warm lemon and manukah honey "tea."** Everyone knows about the lemon/honey combo, which calms a cough while cutting mucus. But you can make it even more effective with manukah honey, a special kind from New Zealand that has strong antimicrobial properties, so it protects against the underlying cold virus.

Regular raw honey also has antimicrobial properties. Blend a tablespoonful of honey with the juice from half a lemon in a cup of just-boiled water. For optimal benefit, drink it just before bedtime, when coughs typically rev up…and again in the morning.

•**Dark chocolate.** Most people have no idea that one of their favorite treats is also a natural cough suppressant—thanks to *theobromine*, a chemical component in chocolate. The darker the chocolate, the more theobromine, so aim for versions containing more than 65% cocoa. Eat a small square—about one-half to one ounce— two or three times a day.

Caution: Chocolate has caffeine, so don't eat it in the evening.

•**Beet and/or pineapple juice.** Both beet and pineapple juices have long been standbys for coughs due to bronchitis. Both help open bronchial passages and make it easier for your body to bring up excess mucus. Whichever you choose, a half cup (four ounces) is enough. It's fine to drink it two or three times a day. (*Note:* If you've been told to limit nitrates, avoid beet juice.)

•**Elderberry syrup.** Elderberry syrup, readily available in health-food stores, is a traditional remedy for colds, coughs and the flu. It acts as an expectorant and also has anti-viral and anti-flu properties. Take as directed on the package, up to three times a day. Dilute in water if that makes it easier to take.

Important: If your cough lasts beyond three weeks—or includes symptoms such as coughing up blood, significant shortness of breath, chest pain or persistent fever—see a doctor.

AVOID THESE OTC COUGH PRODUCTS

•**Cough suppressants.** A common ingredient is *dextromethorphan* (DXM), first introduced 60 years ago. It's found in popular brands including NyQuil, Coricidin HBP Cough & Cold, Delsym and Dimetapp DM. Not only is there no evidence that it works, it can provoke a narcotic-like "high" when taken in large amounts, leading to potential for abuse.

•**Cough expectorants.** *Guaifenesin*, the active ingredient in Mucinex, Robitussin, Tussin and Guaifenesin LA, doesn't have the narcotic-like downside of DXM, but there's no evidence that it works, either.

•**Combination products.** Most OTC remedies combine ingredients in the same product to treat a variety of symptoms.

Example: DXM, guaifenesin, an antihistamine, plus acetaminophen. This kitchen-sink approach is a bad idea—you're treating symptoms you don't have with drugs you don't need. The biggest pitfall? You might be taking acetaminophen for a headache or fever and don't realize that it's also in your combo cough remedy…so you may exceed the safe daily limit, which increases the risk for liver damage.

Oxygen for Asthma? No!

George M. Boyer MD, FACP, FCCP, chairman, department of medicine, Mercy Medical Center, Baltimore.

Sessions at oxygen bars—where you pay to inhale highly concentrated oxygen through tubes placed in your nose—have been touted as relieving stress, alleviating hangovers and providing other benefits. However, there have been no long-term studies backing up these claims. For a person with asthma, a visit could trigger an attack due to the scent, or "flavoring," that some bars add to the oxygen (such as lavender to "relax").

When experiencing asthma symptoms, use an inhaled bronchodilator or anti-inflammatory agent (such as an inhaled corticosteroid) to open your airways. Oxygen does not relax the bronchial tubes or prevent inflammation in this way.

How to Have a Safe Vacation If You Have Asthma

Melanie Carver, vice president of digital strategy and community services, Asthma and Allergy Foundation of America, Landover, Maryland.

Spending your long-anticipated time off laid low with asthma symptoms isn't anyone's idea of a fun vacation.

So the first thing to keep in mind when you're poring over glossy brochures of dream locales is to know and recognize your asthma triggers. For example, if hot, humid air makes you breathless and wheezy, a week on the Gulf coast is a riskier getaway for you. Or if cold, windy air brings on symptoms, then you'd be better off skipping the sites in locales with those kinds of climate.

But besides your specific triggers, anyone with asthma should avoid exposure to bad air quality and pollution. In fact, when air quality is very poor, people with asthma are advised to stay indoors with their windows closed—most likely not exactly the vacation itinerary you had in mind.

If your asthma is triggered by pollen, it's a good idea to check out the pollen count where you're traveling on AccuWeather.com and Pollen.com. If you have to drive in an area that has a high count for the particular pollen that triggers your symptoms and/or bad air quality, keep your car windows rolled up and the air-conditioning on.

To find places that you might particularly want to avoid, check the list of Asthma Capitals on the Asthma and Allergy Foundation of America (AAFA) site. The list ranks the 100 largest cities in the US according to how challenging they are for people with asthma. AAFA looks at 13 factors, including air quality, pollen counts and smoking laws. The most recent Asthma Capitals report names Memphis, Richmond (Virginia), Philadelphia, Detroit and Oklahoma City as the five worst US cities for asthma sufferers.

Be prepared: Before heading off on your vacation, be sure to follow your treatment plan so your asthma is under control before you go. If you take medications, bring enough to last at least the length of your trip—and, ideally, a bit longer in the event that your return home is delayed. Also, keep emergency medications (such as rescue inhalers) on you at all times. If you depend on an inhaler, bring an extra in case one runs out...or you leave it behind in a hotel room or restaurant. If you're flying or traveling by train, pack some sanitizing wipes to wipe down tray tables and armrests to remove pet dander.

Note: Even if there is no pet on board, pet dander is always present on planes and trains because the dander travels on people's clothing. AAFA has more tips for traveling safely with asthma.

Lung Disease Can Strike Anyone...Even Nonsmokers!

David M. Mannino, MD, the Kurt W. Deuschle endowed chair in preventive medicine and environmental health at the University of Kentucky, Lexington, where he directs the Pulmonary Epidemiology Research Laboratory and the Southeast Center for Agricultural Health and Injury Prevention. He is chief scientific officer of the COPD Foundation, COPDFoundation.org.

You notice that you're feeling tired all the time, short of breath and can't get rid of a nagging mucus-filled cough. These all could be symptoms of chronic obstructive pulmonary disease (COPD). But you've never smoked a cigarette in your life and that's a smoker's disease, right? Yes...but not always.

What few people realize: About 25% of people who show signs of lung disease and airway obstruction don't smoke and never have... and about 10% of people formally diagnosed with COPD have never smoked.

Since most never-smokers are unaware that they could be at risk, they tend to blame early COPD symptoms on ailments such as allergies, asthma or lingering colds. Even doctors may fail to consider COPD in never-smokers. As a result, many patients with early—and mild—COPD aren't taking the necessary steps to protect their lungs. That's a problem because undiagnosed COPD not only can affect one's quality of life, it also can lead to flare-ups, hospitalizations and even early death. *What you need to know...*

A MAJOR THREAT

COPD is the third-leading cause of death in the US, and it affects 15 million adults—more if you count those with impaired lung function that has gone undetected.

COPD is a broad term that's used to describe a number of lung diseases, including emphysema (damage to the alveoli, small air sacs in the lungs)…chronic bronchitis (inflammation of the large bronchial tubes)…and some cases of severe asthma that do not completely reverse between flare-ups or exacerbations. COPD is a progressive disease—it develops slowly (often over decades), and the symptoms always worsen over time.

RISKS FOR NONSMOKERS

Giving up cigarettes is the best way for smokers to guard against COPD. For nonsmokers, many common COPD risk factors are tricky (or impossible) to avoid. *For example…*

•**Asthma.** Roughly 40% of COPD patients have a history of chronic obstructive asthma, and many of them have never smoked.

•**Pneumonia or other severe respiratory infections.** People who have these illnesses in childhood experience lung damage that increases their risk for COPD.

•**Genetics.** Among nonsmokers with COPD, 1% to 3% have alpha-1 antitrypsin (AAT) deficiency, a genetic defect that can lead to damaged alveoli and emphysema. Anyone who has a first degree relative with COPD is at increased risk for this genetic defect.

•**Environmental factors.** These can include smoke (for firefighters)…dust (agricultural workers and miners)…chemical fumes (mani-

Don't Clean with This

Regular use of bleach is linked to lung disease. Nurses who used disinfectants such as bleach…glutaraldehyde, a strong disinfectant for medical instruments…hydrogen peroxide…or cleaning alcohol at least weekly were 22% more likely to develop chronic obstructive pulmonary disease (COPD) over an eight-year period than ones who did not use disinfectants. The preliminary, unpublished study showed association but not cause and effect.

Study of 55,185 working nurses by researchers at the French National Institute of Health and Medical Research, presented at a recent meeting of the European Respiratory Society International Congress.

curists and janitors)…and air pollution (everyone). Scented products, such as candles or air fresheners, can irritate the lungs, too. Anything that chronically irritates your lungs, such as secondhand smoke, can increase risk for COPD.

SHOULD YOU GET TESTED?

If you have any of the symptoms described earlier, you should ask your doctor to test you for COPD. Past-smokers and those who work in high-risk industries—coal miners, for example—might want to get tested even if they don't have symptoms. Anyone with asthma should be tested for pulmonary function at least once every five years.

Red flag: It takes you longer than expected to recover from colds, the flu or other respiratory illnesses. Someone who's healthy will generally start feeling better—with less coughing and shortness of breath—within a week or two. In my practice, I've noticed that those with early COPD take several weeks or even months before they're fully recovered. Other symptoms include a nagging cough, wheezing and tightness in the chest.

The most common lung test is called spirometry. With this test, you blow into a tube that's connected to a machine that measures both your lung capacity and how quickly you're able to exhale air. The test takes only a few minutes, and it can detect early COPD even when you don't have symptoms.

If spirometry shows your lung function to be normal, you won't need other tests unless your doctor feels there's a strong chance that you have COPD based on your symptoms. In that case, he/she might recommend other lung-function or imaging tests (such as a chest X-ray or CT scan).

Exception: If your lung function is impaired but you don't have any obvious COPD risk factors, your doctor will want to know if there's a genetic cause. A blood test for AAT deficiency is done routinely for those who test positive for impaired lung function, as well as for those who develop COPD symptoms at an early age or have a family history of the disease.

WHAT CAN YOU DO?

Most patients with COPD will need to use treatments such as bronchodilators and inhaled steroids—and perhaps use supplemental oxygen when the disease advances.

Patients with AAT deficiency can take a synthetic form of the missing protein, given weekly in IV infusions. Some studies have shown that the treatments help protect the lungs…others have been less conclusive.

To keep your lungs healthier…

•**Try to breathe clean air.** If you have a smoky fireplace, clean the chimney, or don't use the fireplace at all. Wear a dust mask or respirator (see below) if you're tilling a field or working in a woodshop. Do your best never to breathe secondhand smoke.

Helpful: Check the Air Quality Index (AQI) in your area by going to the EPA website AirNow.gov. People with COPD or other lung diseases may be advised to stay indoors on days when the AQI is elevated.

If you're moving: Go to Lung.org, search "State of the Air" and plug in possible zip codes to see where the air is cleanest—and where it's not.

•**Avoid toxic fumes.** This includes fumes from oven cleaners, drain cleaners, paint, etc.

If it makes you cough or burns your nose, you shouldn't be breathing it.

If you must use such products, wear a respirator. A respirator labeled N95 will protect you from particulate matter (such as dust or sawdust), while respirators that contain chemical cartridges will protect you against fumes from cleaning supplies and similar products.

If you have COPD, also eat a healthy diet, with lots of fruits and vegetables, and exercise if you can. Doing so can reduce symptoms and add to your quality of life.

Statins and COPD

Larry Lynd, PhD, is professor of pharmaceutical sciences at University of British Columbia, Vancouver, Canada.

People with COPD live longer with statin drugs.

Recent study: Patients with chronic obstructive pulmonary disease (COPD) who used statins were 45% less likely to die from lung-related issues than other COPD patients and had a 21% lower risk of dying from any cause.

Possible reason: Statins, used to reduce cholesterol levels, have anti-inflammatory properties that may benefit certain people with COPD.

E-Cigarettes Can Help You Quit

Jeffrey Drope, PhD, is vice president of economic and health policy research at the American Cancer Society, Atlanta.

It still is best to quit all nicotine-containing products, including e-cigarettes, using FDA-approved smoking-cessation aids (such as nicotine gums and patches) to wean yourself off nicotine addiction. But e-cigarettes are less harmful than cigarettes, according to the American Cancer Society's review of evidence—and research suggests that e-cigarettes may help some smokers quit all nicotine products.

Try This CPAP Trick

Mark Aloia, PhD, associate professor, department of medicine, National Jewish Health, Denver.

Most people with sleep apnea (a disorder that causes breathing to be interrupted during sleep) know that using a continuous positive airway pressure (CPAP) machine can help them breathe easier…sleep better…and avoid dangers associated with the condition, such as heart disease. Yet more than half choose not to use the machines.

Recent study: Sleep apnea sufferers shown a video of themselves struggling to breathe while asleep used CPAP three more hours per night than those who did not view such videos.

Food Allergies Affect Adults, Too

Ruchi Gupta, MD, MPH, associate professor of pediatrics and medicine at Northwestern University Feinberg School of Medicine, Chicago, and clinical attending physician at Ann & Robert H. Lurie Children's Hospital of Chicago. She is also director of Science and Outcomes of Allergy and Asthma Research (SOAAR) at Northwestern. Dr. Gupta is author of *The Food Allergy Experience.*

Shrimp may have always been your favorite indulgence. But one night, after a luscious dinner at a seafood restaurant, you break out in itchy hives or, even worse, find yourself struggling to breathe. What's the problem?

It could be a food allergy…completely out of the blue. Because food allergies are so commonly associated with children, many adults are shocked to learn that a food that they have enjoyed for decades can suddenly trigger alarming—or even life-threatening—symptoms.

Surprising statistic: In a recent national survey that included more than 40,000 American adults, an astounding 45% of those with a food allergy developed the condition after age 18.

Even though the research showed that more adults are developing new food allergies, science hasn't yet pinpointed *why.* Researchers theorize that the uptick could be due to a number of different factors, including changes in our environment…increased hygienic practices…increased exposure to antibiotics or antibacterials…changes to our *microbiome* (microorganisms, such as bacteria and fungi, in an environment)…and/or overall changes in dietary habits.

CULPRIT FOODS

What food allergies are most common in adulthood? Shellfish tops the list, with just under 4% of study participants reporting that they developed this allergy after age 18. In addition to shellfish, seven other foods (milk, peanuts, tree nuts, fish, eggs, wheat and soy) are responsible for 90% of food allergies in adults and children.

But this list is by no means complete. You can develop a food allergy to many other foods.

SYMPTOMS TO WATCH OUT FOR

How do you know that a food allergy is making you feel lousy—or even putting your life at risk by making it difficult to breathe?

Unlike a food intolerance or sensitivity, which tends to cause milder symptoms, such as abdominal discomfort (stomach pain and bloating, for example), that can occur even a day later, a food allergy triggers symptoms that are acute, more immediate and tough to ignore.

Within a few hours or even minutes of eating the questionable food, you might experience itching, swelling, rash or hives…wheezing, difficulty breathing and/or a feeling that your throat is closing…vomiting (combined with hives or rash)…and even a precipitous drop in blood pressure that can lead to fainting.

Important: If someone is experiencing any of these symptoms due to a known or possible food allergy, it's imperative for the person to be given *epinephrine* as soon as possible to reverse an allergic reaction. Call 911 to get medical help. Whether epinephrine is self-administered or given by another person, the treated individual should receive medical care immediately following its use.

GUESSWORK ISN'T ENOUGH

Why are food allergies in adulthood so frequently missed?

The symptoms, of course, aren't easily overlooked. But what often happens is that the sufferer simply stops eating the problematic food. If shrimp makes you break out in hives, you can just stop eating it, right? (This tactic is why the incidence of food allergies in adults is likely underdiagnosed.) Or you simply may not recognize what is behind some annoying symptom, such as a chronic cough.

But food avoidance—without knowing for sure why the reaction occurred—isn't always the answer. Getting a proper diagnosis is crucial, because completely dodging a food isn't always realistic (hidden ingredients, anyone?) and you need to know how to manage the problem in any circumstance.

IDENTIFYING A FOOD ALLERGY

The first step to unearthing a food allergy is to keep a food diary that documents the food(s) you're eating that cause symptoms. This will give you an accurate history to discuss with your physician—ideally an allergist,* who has special training in diagnosing and treating allergies. You also can record the information with an app on your phone.

To make an actual diagnosis, your physician may draw from an array of clinical tests. However, it is important that this testing be based on a supportive clinical history after ingestion of an allergen. *The different types of testing that are useful in confirming a clinical food allergy are…*

•**Skin prick tests** involve placing a drop of allergen onto the surface of the skin, then pricking it through to introduce the allergen into the top layer of the skin on the forearm or back. If specific immunoglobulin E (IgE) antibody toward the allergen is present and attached to the allergy cells, then redness and an itchy bump should develop within about 15 minutes. Some doctors prefer this type of testing over blood tests (see next column) because they consider skin prick tests to be more accurate.

*To find an allergist near you, consult the American Academy of Allergy, Asthma & Immunology at Allergist. AAAAI.org or the American College of Allergy, Asthma & Immunology at ACAAI.org/locate-an-allergist.

•**Blood tests** that measure the presence of IgE antibodies to questionable food(s) in the blood.

•**Oral food challenge,** considered the gold standard to identify food allergies. Increasing amounts of the problematic food are consumed in the doctor's office, where you're observed for a reaction in a controlled environment.

Note: You do not need the oral food challenge if you get a positive test result from a skin prick or blood test *and* you've had a past reaction to the offending food. Because the blood test and skin prick test have a high false-positive rate, you need both the positive test result and a past food reaction to be considered to have that allergy.

If you're diagnosed with a food allergy, your allergist will advise you on the foods to avoid and give you coping strategies in case of an allergic reaction. For example, you'll get a prescription for an epinephrine auto-injector, along with specific instructions on how and when to use it. If you have a known food allergy, you also may want to wear a medical ID bracelet, available online.

On the horizon: Several exciting treatment advances soon may offer other options. These include oral or skin patch–based immunotherapies that slowly release an allergen into the body in small quantities, desensitizing the immune system to its effects…and vaccines to prevent a food allergy from taking hold among those considered at risk.

Why Some Fruits Make Your Mouth Itch

Beth Corn, MD, associate professor of medicine at Icahn School of Medicine at Mount Sinai, New York City. She also is a spokesperson for the American College of Allergy, Asthma and Immunology and past president of the New York Allergy and Asthma Society. ACAAI.org

Some people who suffer from pollen allergies also suffer from an underreported condition called "oral allergy syndrome"—their mouths, lips, tongues and/or throats feel tingly or itchy and sometimes swollen after they eat certain fruits or vegetables. Symptoms can be so severe that they feel like their throats are closing. On very rare occasions, oral allergy syndrome can cause a potentially fatal allergic reaction.

The first thing to know is that these people typically are not allergic to the fruits and vegetables they react to. They have this reaction because of their pollen allergies—the proteins in the fruits or vegetables are so similar to the proteins in pollens that their immune systems mount an allergic response to them.

Apples, pears, peaches, nectarines, plums, cherries, apricots, carrots, celery, cantaloupe and honeydew are among the most common triggers, but this can vary by person and depends in part on which pollen someone is allergic to. People who are allergic to ragweed pollen might experience oral allergy syndrome when they consume bananas, cucumbers, melons, sunflower seeds and/or zucchini. People allergic to grass pollen are more likely to cite celery, melons, oranges, peaches and/or tomatoes. And people allergic to birch pollen can experience this with apples, almonds, cherries, hazelnuts, peaches, pears and/or plums.

What to do: Stop eating the food, and take an antihistamine such as Benadryl immediately.

Important: If your symptoms include difficulty breathing or dizziness, call 911.

If you wish to continue consuming a fruit or vegetable that causes you mild symptoms, talk to your health-care provider. He/she may suggest cooking it first. The heat will break down the proteins that are confusing your immune system.

Example: Eat a baked apple rather than a raw apple.

Smelling Smells That Aren't There...

Ronald Devere, MD, FAAN, director, Taste and Smell Disorder Clinic, Austin, Texas.

Smelling something (generally unpleasant, such as smoke or garbage) that simply isn't there is known as *dysosmia*. Such episodes typically last 10 minutes to an hour.

This condition is commonly caused by medications (such as diuretics, cardiovascular drugs or neurology medications such as the Parkinson's drug levodopa), pregnancy, a zinc deficiency, diabetes or even severe colds or recurrent sinus infections. Dysosmia also has been linked to migraines—in these cases, the smell disappears when the headache resolves.

For most people, dysosmia is not a serious issue and will generally go away after several months. If it doesn't, consult an ear, nose and throat specialist, who may suggest a nasal endoscopy to rule out abnormalities such as a polyp in your nasal passageways (often the result of chronic inflammation due to asthma or allergies). Corticosteroid medications can shrink polyps, but if that doesn't work, they can be removed surgically. In rare cases, an MRI may be required to determine if the cause is a brain tumor, stroke or head trauma (following an injury such as a concussion)—in some cases, all of these conditions can trigger abnormal electrical discharges in the brain that result in dysosmia.

Many people find relief by "cleaning out" the nasal passageways with saline drops or the regular use of a neti pot (a teapot-like device used to irrigate your nasal passages with a saline solution). Medications such as *gabapentin* (Neurontin), generally prescribed for seizure disorders, may be prescribed to block abnormal electrical discharges in patients whose quality of life is affected by these smells.

CHAPTER 2

Brain Health and Memory

You Can Lower Your Risk for Alzheimer's

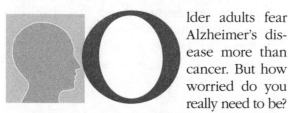

Older adults fear Alzheimer's disease more than cancer. But how worried do you really need to be?

Let's start with the good news…if you have a first-degree relative with the disease (a parent or sibling), you're only at a slightly greater risk than someone who does not have a first-degree relative with Alzheimer's. That's because there are many factors that affect your risk for Alzheimer's…not just your genes (more on this later).

Poor lifestyle choices (such as an unhealthy diet and/or not exercising regularly) also increase your risk—much more so than genetics. That's why one twin in a set of identical twins can get Alzheimer's while the other twin stays healthy.

There's even more good news—a diagnosis of Alzheimer's is not necessarily the disaster you probably imagine it to be. Alzheimer's is now viewed by most medical professionals as a so-called "spectrum disorder," rather than a single disease, because different people have different symptoms and different rates of progression.

Most people diagnosed with Alzheimer's are not on the catastrophic end of that spectrum—they are not going to forget who they are or the names of their loved ones. Most will live at home and die at home, particularly if the disease is detected early and symptoms are well-managed with treatments such as medication, a healthy diet and regular exercise.

Bottom line: Even if you are at genetic risk, you can use lifestyle modifications to reduce

Gayatri Devi, MD, director of New York Memory and Healthy Aging Services and an attending physician at Lenox Hill Hospital, both in New York City, and clinical professor of neurology at SUNY Downstate Medical Center in Brooklyn. A board-certified neurologist, Dr. Devi is author of *The Spectrum of Hope: An Optimistic and New Approach to Alzheimer's Disease.* NYBrain.org your risk to below that of someone who has no family history of Alzheimer's.

HOW TO TWEAK YOUR LIFESTYLE

Most cases of late-onset Alzheimer's disease are preventable—with simple lifestyle changes that reduce one's risk for the disease.

The brain changes of Alzheimer's (the so-called plaques and tangles, which are accumulations of toxic proteins) can start 20 to 30 years before the onset of symptoms. But research shows that preventive measures can stop plaques and tangles as well as symptoms from ever developing...and even prevent symptoms if your brain is riddled with plaques and tangles.

Factors that increase Alzheimer's risk for everyone—regardless of one's genetic predisposition—and how to counteract them...

•**Sedentary lifestyle.** Exercising for 45 minutes, at least three days a week (at an intensity that is 50% higher than your resting heart rate) is a must for reducing your risk for Alzheimer's. It stimulates blood flow to the brain, allowing new neurons to grow. Research shows that it decreases your risk for Alzheimer's by 40%.

Surprising fact: Cognitive abilities such as memory improve by 10% immediately after exercise.

•**Poor diet.** A diet loaded with saturated fats, refined sugar and processed foods increases the risk for Alzheimer's. A Mediterranean-style diet—rich in whole foods such as vegetables, fruits, beans, whole grains and fish—is proven to reduce the risk for Alzheimer's by 50%.

Also helpful: A healthy breakfast, which consists of protein, fiber and fruit. Research shows that if you take in less than 7% of your daily calories at breakfast, your risk for heart disease and Alzheimer's more than doubles.

•**Limited mental stimulation.** Regular mental stimulation reduces Alzheimer's risk—in fact, research shows that even reading a newspaper every day can help prevent the disease.

Best: Engage in a type of mental stimulation that is different from what you do at work, thereby stimulating a different part of your brain.

Example: If you are a computer programmer, learn how to play golf.

•**Social isolation.** Healthy social relationships—with family, friends and in the community—decrease the risk for Alzheimer's disease. Feeling lonely doubles the risk...living alone raises it fivefold.

•**Heart disease.** Circulatory problems cause heart disease and Alzheimer's disease. Medical and lifestyle treatments for cardiovascular issues, including high blood pressure, reduce Alzheimer's risk.

Bottom line: What's good for your heart is good for your brain.

•**Diabetes.** Some experts label Alzheimer's "type 3 diabetes" because of the established link between chronically high blood sugar and the risk for Alzheimer's disease—a person with diabetes has a 57% higher risk of developing the disease. Controlling high blood sugar with medical and lifestyle treatments is crucial for reducing Alzheimer's risk.

Helpful: Keep your glucose level below 100 mg/dL.

•**Insomnia.** Poor sleep increases risk for Alzheimer's, probably because brain plaque is cleared most effectively during sleep. But sleep medications aren't the answer—they also interfere with the clearance of brain plaque.

What works better: Good sleep hygiene, such as going to bed and waking up at the same time every day.

Also helpful: Don't work on your computer in bed or keep your cell phone on your bedside table.

WHAT'S YOUR GENETIC RISK?

Genetics is a strong factor when Alzheimer's begins at a young age. The early-onset form is an aggressive familial illness that can occur, in extremely rare cases, as early as in one's 20s, with most people developing the disease in their 50s or 60s. The child of a parent with early-onset Alzheimer's has a 50% chance of developing the disease. Fortunately, early-onset constitutes only 5% of all cases of Alzheimer's disease.

On the other hand, most cases of late-onset Alzheimer's (beginning after age 65) are not inherited. Instead, many medical and lifestyle factors contribute to the development of the illness.

Compelling scientific research: In one of the largest scientific studies that I have ever completed, published in *Archives of Neurology*, I looked at more than 5,500 siblings and parents of patients with Alzheimer's—alongside age-matched adults who did not have the disease.

Presuming (for uniform statistical analysis) that everyone in the study lived to age 90, I found that those with a first-degree relative with Alzheimer's had about a one-in-four chance of developing late-onset Alzheimer's—whereas those without an afflicted relative had a one-in-five chance of doing so.

In other words, if neither your parents nor siblings have (or had) Alzheimer's (and you live to age 90), you still have a 20% chance of getting the disease—while a person whose parent or sibling had Alzheimer's has a 26% chance.

Takeaway: Having a parent or sibling with Alzheimer's puts you at a relatively small increased risk for the disease.

Exception: A person with late-onset Alzheimer's who also has a variant of the apolipoprotein E gene—APOE e4 (the most damaging of the so-called "Alzheimer's genes")—is more likely to have rapid progression of the disease.

GENETIC TESTING

My take on genetic testing for Alzheimer's: It may be appropriate only for people with a family history of early-onset Alzheimer's disease (before age 65). If a parent has early-onset Alzheimer's, as mentioned earlier, the child has a 50% chance of developing the disease. An estimated 200,000 Americans have the early-onset form of the disease.

If you have this type of family history, consult your doctor and a genetic counselor about genetic testing. Not all the genes that trigger early-onset Alzheimer's are known, but some are. If you decide to have a genetic test—and the test finds that you have one of the genetic mutations for Alzheimer's—you and your family can take that fact into account in various ways.

For example, you would want to create a step-by-step action plan for dealing with the disease, even before symptoms develop, by preparing for the future with advanced directives and financial planning…and perhaps consider entering one of the clinical trials that are testing new drugs to slow Alzheimer's development. (To find such a trial, consult ClinicalTrials.gov and search "early-onset Alzheimer's.")

Important: If you don't have a family history of early-onset Alzheimer's, I typically do not recommend genetic testing. The results would not accurately quantify your risk, and it's crucial that you implement key medical treatments (such as those for high blood pressure or diabetes) and lifestyle changes to reduce your risk for Alzheimer's whether or not you have a genetic variant for late-onset Alzheimer's.

Is It Normal…Alzheimer's …or Something Else?

Jason Brandt, PhD, professor of psychiatry and behavioral sciences, professor of neurology and director of the division of medical psychology, all at Johns Hopkins University School of Medicine, Baltimore. He also directs the Cortical Function Laboratory at Johns Hopkins Hospital and has developed several widely used neuropsychological tests.

The pot you forgot boiling on the stove. The longtime neighbor whose name you suddenly can't recall. The car keys you think you've lost, only to discover they're…in your pocket.

Chances are you have had a momentary memory lapse like these, often called a "senior moment." Though they happen to everyone on occasion, there's a reason for the moniker—these slipups may reflect the gradual loss of one's mental sharpness with aging.

It's no wonder, then, that repeated lapses can be alarming, especially for those with a family history of Alzheimer's disease or some other form of dementia. The good news is that the minor memory misfires that tend to affect people over age 50 often are caused by normal age-related changes in the brain and nervous system.

But still, memory lapses can be an early marker of Alzheimer's or another type of dementia. So if you have been noticing more of those senior moments, it is perfectly reasonable to see your doctor about it and ask about undergoing a cognitive assessment. These tests can put your mind at ease…or help diagnose a potential problem at the earliest possible stage.

TESTING 1, 2, 3

To gauge cognitive function, your physician likely will observe your responses to standardized memory and thinking exercises. Many physicians give patients the Mini-Mental State Examination (MMSE). This exam starts with a set of simple questions that measure orientation—*What year is it? What season? What is today's date? What town are we in?* Next, the doctor will read a short list of words and ask the patient to repeat them back immediately and then five minutes later.

The doctor also will ask the patient to write a sentence and copy a geometric design. Finally, the doctor will ask the patient to perform a series of actions (such as "touch your left shoulder and then tap your head twice"), which gauges the ability to understand language and follow commands.

Helpful: A perfect MMSE score is 30, and a healthy adult should approach that number (anything above 27 is usually fine).

If your physician is concerned, he/she may refer you to a neuropsychologist for further diagnostic testing. Just as a neurologist and radiologist can decipher the images of a brain MRI scan, this kind of doctor examines patterns of scores on a variety of brain-function tests to try to identify specific disorders.

Among the more commonly used tests for assessing a patient with possible Alzheimer's is the Boston Naming Test. Here, the patient looks at drawings of objects and names them. It begins with common nouns (a dog, a tree) and advances to increasingly obscure ones (a padlock, a zebra) that require the test taker to retrieve rarely used words from memory. This is valuable information, as Alzheimer's patients tend to have trouble recalling the names of objects.

Alzheimer's also diminishes the ability to learn and remember new things. Doctors measure this by reading a brief story and asking the patient to repeat it right away, then 20 minutes later.

Finally, since people in the early stages of Alzheimer's tend to develop spatial confusion, we see whether they have difficulty copying, say, a geometric design or drawing common objects (for example, a daisy) upon request.

Important: Don't look up these tests or "prepare" for them in advance. They are useful only if you don't know exactly what to expect and haven't "practiced."

WHAT A DECLINE MEANS

Many patients who visit my clinic have parents or other relatives with Alzheimer's. They're acutely aware of their own periodic memory failures and are understandably worried about how well their minds are working.

Good news: As often as not, after running these tests, I end up telling them, "You're functioning like an average person your age. What you're experiencing looks like typical age-related decline."

That may not sound comforting, but face the facts. Your brain is affected by "wear and tear" as you age. You probably can't run as fast at age 55 as you could at age 35, and your mind isn't quite as efficient as it was two decades ago, either. But if you perform within the average range for your age, there's no cause for concern.

If your results fall below that level, you might be diagnosed with mild cognitive impairment (MCI). If so, your brain function is below the norm for your age even though you don't have dementia.

Keep in mind: MCI is a broad category and encompasses a variety of different things. A patient with MCI who finds it difficult to recall events or the right word to describe an object or who displays spatial confusion, may be in the very earliest stage of Alzheimer's.

In contrast, someone who possesses a solid memory but struggles with executive function (for example, he can't plan well or solve problems effectively) may be at greater risk of developing a frontotemporal dementia—a type of dementia in which personality and language changes are common.

Important: While 10% to 15% of people over age 65 who have MCI will progress to Alzheimer's each year, the diagnosis is not necessarily dire. Many published studies show that patients with cognitive impairment in only one area—just memory or just language or just spatial cognition—have a very strong chance (perhaps as high as 50%) of returning to normal within one year.

How? It could be that the patient who fell into the MCI category was feeling ill the day of assessment…or was sleep-deprived…or drank too much (or not enough) coffee…or even was just in a very bad mood.

Although many factors affect an individual's cognitive performance, these tests are extremely useful when interpreted by an expert neuropsychologist. Recent studies indicate that the brains of patients with Alzheimer's disease undergo changes (observable with special brain-imaging methods) many years before a diagnosis is typically made. So getting a baseline neuropsychological assessment in middle age or a little older may help identify people who should be targeted for more active Alzheimer's prevention.

YOUR NEXT STEPS

If you do well on the cognitive tests but remain worried about memory decline, work hard to keep what you have.

To achieve this (as well as maintain good overall health), follow these lifestyle choices: Eat a healthful diet…get regular exercise…participate in brain-stimulating activities you enjoy…keep your blood pressure under control…and moderate your alcohol intake.

For a patient who is newly diagnosed with early-stage Alzheimer's, I often recommend that he stop driving as a safety measure, advise him to keep written notes and calendars to aid recall and suggest that he talk with his doctor about whether a prescription Alzheimer's drug might help improve mental function. I also recommend beginning a discussion of future care needs and end-of-life plans with family.

As for people who fall in the middle and display some signs of MCI, I often explain that the "senior moments" they're experiencing might be the beginning of something more serious… or they might mean nothing at all.

Best way forward: Follow the blueprint for patients who tested well cognitively—live

a healthful lifestyle, and try to avoid "stressing out." (I frequently recommend mindfulness-based stress reduction programs.) Then I'll re-evaluate them in a year and take other measures if needed.

Your Brain Is Hungry!

Drew Ramsey, MD, an assistant clinical professor of psychiatry at Columbia University College of Physicians and Surgeons in New York City, and a leading expert in the use of nutrition for improving mood, brain function and mental health. He produced the *Eat to Beat Depression* e-course and is the author of *Eat Complete: The 21 Nutrients That Fuel Brainpower, Boost Weight Loss, and Transform Your Health, 50 Shades of Kale* and *The Happiness Diet*. DrewRamseyMD.com

---

I f you had a doughnut and coffee for breakfast, you probably wouldn't be that surprised if you felt sluggish and even a little blue afterward. Had you started your day with, say, eggs and whole-grain toast or a veggie-and-fruit-packed smoothie, you'd expect to feel much better.

While most of us know from our own experience how our diet affects our moods and energy levels, scientific evidence now shows just how crucial food is as "brain fuel."

Latest development: For the first time, high-quality scientific research has confirmed that dietary changes can dramatically improve depression. In fact, diet plays such a fundamental role in mental health that nutritional psychiatry is increasingly being incorporated into evidence-based mental-health practices to help prevent and treat depression and anxiety and even guard against dementia.

To learn more about this important new approach, we spoke with Drew Ramsey, MD, a psychiatrist and leading proponent of the use of dietary changes to improve brain health.

How do the foods we eat affect our brains?

Let's begin with the idea that all the molecules in your brain start at the end of your fork. For example, for your brain to produce serotonin, a brain chemical that regulates moods (and sex drive) along with weight, you must consume tryptophan, an amino acid found in higher amounts in some foods such as pumpkin seeds, asparagus, fish and meats.

Other nutrients, such as zinc and omega-3 fatty acids, are key building blocks of the brain and affect neurogenesis (the creation of new brain cells)...levels of brain-derived neurotrophic factor (a hormone that you need to stave off depression)...and chronic inflammation, which is also linked to depression.

Do foods make a big difference or just a little?

There isn't a single "superfood" for treating depression or other mood disorders. But dietary changes—eating more plant foods and seafood and cutting out fast food and simple sugars—clearly help, whether they're used alone or in combination with antidepressants or talk therapy.

Haven't we known for a while that nutrition plays a role in brain health?

Many studies have suggested that nutritional changes can help patients with mood problems, but there's never been conclusive proof. That changed with the SMILES (Supporting the Modification of Lifestyle Intervention in Lowered Emotional States) trial, which was published in early 2017 in the journal *BMC Medicine*.

It was the first-ever randomized, controlled clinical study to investigate dietary interventions for treating clinical depression. The study looked at 67 men and women with moderate-to-severe depression, most of whom were taking an antidepressant or receiving regular psychotherapy. Half were put on a Mediterranean-style diet for 12 weeks...the other half continued to follow their usual (and largely unhealthy) diets.

After three months, nearly one-third of those who made dietary changes had improved so much that they no longer met the clinical criteria for clinical depression. In other words, they had full remissions. Those who hadn't improved their diets had only an 8% remission rate.

Can nutrition help with dementia?

A healthy diet can help prevent vascular causes of dementia, such as stroke. There's also good evidence that many of the plant-based molecules such as lycopene (found in tomatoes and other red fruits and vegetables) and

flavonols (found in onions, wine, chocolate and many other healthy foods) can produce brain changes that reduce the risk for different forms of dementia, including Alzheimer's disease.

What foods do you usually recommend?

I focus on overall dietary patterns and categories of brain healthy foods (such as seafood, leafy greens and colorful "rainbow" vegetables)...complex carbohydrates (such as whole grains)...grass-fed meat and dairy...and free-range poultry and eggs.

Important: Seafood is a crucial food category that's missing from most Americans' diets. I advise everyone to eat more salmon, bivalves (such as oysters and mussels), anchovies and other types of seafood.

What about supplements?

Several clinical trials have shown that specific supplements—fish oil, zinc, B vitamins, etc.—might be helpful for alleviating depression and other mood problems. Supplements are convenient if you don't eat seafood (a main source of omega-3s), follow a restrictive diet (vegans need to take vitamin B-12) or have a deficiency in need of rapid correction. I tend to emphasize food because no one sits down to a fine meal of vitamins and supplement shakes!

WHAT ARE YOUR NUTRIENTS LEVELS

To rule out medical causes of depression, including thyroid disorders, and to check levels of certain nutrients (such as vitamin D and vitamin B-12), psychiatrists routinely order blood tests. A nutritional psychiatry assessment can also be conducted to understand what patients are eating...when they eat...what their favorite snacks are...and so on.

While physicians typically haven't learned much about nutrition in medical school beyond basic biochemistry, this is changing! A culinary medicine curriculum developed by Tulane Medical School is being adopted by 28 medical schools around the country. And the American Psychiatric Association has recently offered the Brain Food Workshop, developed by researchers at Columbia University, at its professional meetings.

Foods That Trash Your Brain

Joel Fuhrman, MD, a board-certified family physician, nutritional researcher and president of Nutritional Research Foundation in Flemington, New Jersey. Dr. Fuhrman has coauthored numerous studies in peer-reviewed medical journals and is author of six books. His most recent book is *Fast Food Genocide: How Processed Food Is Killing Us and What We Can Do About It.* DrFuhrman.com

Most of us know that fast food is bad for us—contributing to obesity, heart disease, stroke and diabetes.

But did you know that fast food can also affect your brain, quickly turning you into a fast-food addict—someone helplessly compelled to overeat this unhealthy fare? Plus, eating fast food can lead to mental issues such as depression, chronic anger, lack of focus and much more due to the toxicity and nutritional deficiencies it causes.

WHAT EXACTLY IS FAST FOOD?

"Fast food" doesn't just mean the food you buy at a fast-food restaurant chain. It can be any commercially made, highly processed food that you can get fast, eat fast and digest fast.

Fast food is typically highly flavored and delivers lots of calories but offers few vitamins, minerals and phytochemicals (the active compounds found in plants). It's high in harmful ingredients such as sugar and white flour (which is quickly converted to sugar)…salt…unhealthy oils…artificial ingredients, including artificial color and flavor…preservatives…and thickeners. Plus, it's low in fiber.

Examples of fast food other than a burger and fries: Most deli sandwiches, frozen pizza, many breakfast cereals, a bag of chips, cookies, candy and soda. You might be surprised to know that plenty of organic packaged foods also fall under the fast-food category.

Startling: The majority of Americans get more than half of their calories from fast food.

FAST-FOOD ADDICTION

Fast foods can be as addictive as cocaine and other drugs. Food manufacturers design them that way so you'll buy more of their products. *How they hook you…*

The low-fiber calories from fast food quickly flood the bloodstream—a typical fast-food meal is absorbed far faster than a serving of beans. That rush of calories produces a surge of dopamine, the neurotransmitter (brain chemical) that gives us feelings of pleasure. In fact, the amount of pleasure we derive from eating a food directly correlates with the amount of dopamine released in the brain. To repeat and sustain these pleasurable feelings, you desire and eat more fast food.

Additionally, dopamine levels that skyrocket daily quickly lead to dopamine insensitivity—the same amount of dopamine no longer creates the same amount of pleasure.

Upshot: A person who eats a lot of fast food, will crave fast food…overeat fast food…and become literally addicted to fast food. Trying to break the cycle of overeating fast food is like trying to stop taking drugs. When you stop eating fast foods, you'll experience withdrawal symptoms as your body starts to detoxify—you may feel shaky, weak, fatigued, headachy, anxious, irritable—and crave more fast food to end those symptoms.

THE MALNOURISHED BRAIN

Modern medical science regularly warns that eating fast food can cause heart disease, fatty liver and kidney failure but ignores the fact that fast food also affects the brain—our most vulnerable organ.

Multiple studies have found a link between an unhealthy diet and impaired brain function and emotional problems. Depression and other mood disorders don't have one specific cause, but research shows that a bad diet can be a major risk factor.

Recent research: A meta-analysis including studies from 10 countries published in 2017 in *Psychiatry Research* found that a diet high in refined grains, sweets and red and/or processed meat is associated with an increased risk for depression.

Additionally, anger, irritability and aggression …mood swings…poor concentration…brain fog (mental confusion that can include lack of focus, poor memory and reduced mental acuity)

and other mental problems can be caused by the toxins in fast food, and/or by the nutritional deficiencies that arise from consuming fast food regularly. Fast food is also linked to Alzheimer's and other forms of dementia.

New research: A study published in *American Journal of Clinical Nutrition* shows that the brains of people who eat a sugary diet that floods the brain with glucose—in other words, a fast-food diet—have much higher levels of *beta-amyloid*, the toxic protein that accumulates in the brain and is linked to Alzheimer's disease.

That's the bad news. The good news is that there is an easy way out of fast-food addiction and the emotional and intellectual symptoms caused by eating fast food…

RESTORING BRAIN HEALTH

The first step in ending fast-food addiction is to start eating more high-nutrient foods—foods that contain all the vitamins and minerals we require, as well as the phytochemicals and antioxidants that allow brain cells and other cells damaged by fast food to repair themselves. Just cutting back on the fast food you've been eating is not sufficient—people who try to do this almost always fail.

My advice: Eat plenty of Greens, Beans, Onions, Mushrooms, Berries and Seeds, or "G-BOMBS," the superstars of the whole foods menu. To get more of these foods, include them in a big salad every day and add them to whatever you are cooking.

Also: Make a big batch of vegetable-bean soup on Sunday, freeze several servings in pint-size containers, and eat it all week long.

By eating more high-nutrient, high-fiber foods, you'll gradually develop less desire for fast foods.

Try to crowd out all the fast food you've been eating within one week. With this approach, withdrawal symptoms should last no more than three days. After four to six months, the taste buds—dulled by too much sugar and salt—will typically recuperate, allowing you to once again enjoy subtle natural flavors…and you will have lost your emotional attachment to fast foods.

Also: Whenever possible, don't eat alone! Research shows that when people are isolated and lonely, they tend to make bad food choices. When you're experiencing love and connection—and the positive reinforcement and encouragement that go with it—it's much easier to choose healthy food.

Helpful: Join a group (in-person or online) of others interested in eating healthfully so that you can encourage one another. Check with your local health-food store or cooperative, or look online for a Meetup group.

When Dementia Doesn't Start with Memory Loss

James M. Ellison, MD, MPH, the Swank Foundation Endowed Chair in Memory Care and Geriatrics at Christiana Care Health System in Wilmington, Delaware, and a professor of psychiatry and human behavior at the Sidney Kimmel Medical College of Thomas Jefferson University in Philadelphia.

Jane thinks she needs new eyeglasses because she's having trouble reading and seeing objects right in front of her. Joe's personality has dramatically changed, with the formerly genteel man making impulsive purchases and saying rude things. And Jack has begun to make things up, telling his family members grandiose stories they know aren't true.

What do all three have in common? You might never guess that each is suffering from dementia—a devastating condition that most people associate with memory loss.

It's true that declining thinking and reasoning skills, including memory loss, are signature characteristics of the "Big 3"—Alzheimer's disease, vascular dementia and Lewy body disease—which account for about 90% of all dementia cases.

However, the red flags suffered by the other 10% of dementia patients are surprising to many people because they deviate from "typical" symptoms, especially when the disease first develops. *Dementias that don't fit the norm…*

•**Posterior cortical atrophy (PCA).** Visual problems—such as blurry vision, difficulty reading and/or problems with depth perception and identifying objects—can signal PCA, which often strikes in one's mid-50s to early-60s. But these vision issues aren't caused by an eye condition. Instead, they stem from shrinkage in the back of the brain, where the occipital lobes, which control vision, are located.

PCA is actually a visual variant of Alzheimer's or frontotemporal dementia (see below), with the brain no longer properly interpreting what the eyes are seeing. Other symptoms, including diminished memory, reasoning and other cognitive skills, can occur at the same time as the visual disturbances or can come on after a year or two.

How it's diagnosed: If a person is having vision issues, a visit to the eye doctor (an ophthalmologist or optometrist) can determine if he/she needs glasses or contacts or a new prescription. An eye doctor will also test for macular degeneration (for more on this, see page 272), cataracts and other eye problems.

If there are no issues with vision, the patient should see a neurologist, who can perform an exam and order imaging tests. When PCA is present, structural brain scans such as a CT or an MRI will likely show shrinkage in the brain's occipital lobes. These scans can also rule out other potential causes of symptoms, such as a stroke or tumor.

Treatment approaches: The same medications that may temporarily boost brain cell function in people with Alzheimer's can also help some people with PCA. These drugs include cholinesterase inhibitors, such as *donepezil* (Aricept), *rivastigmine* (Exelon) or *galantamine* (Razadyne), as well as *memantine* (Namenda), which blocks a particular brain receptor to enhance the effectiveness of synapses.

To make daily life easier and safer, PCA patients can ask a certified geriatric care manager (usually a social worker or nurse) to assess their homes. To find one in your area, contact the Aging Life Care Association at AgingLifeCare.org.

Examples of what helps: Removing clutter…labeling drawers and items…installing better lighting…and making glass doors and windows more visible with stickers.

•**Frontotemporal dementia (FTD).** Changes in personality, behavior, language or movement may point to FTD, which accounts for about 5% of all dementia cases. Often diagnosed between one's mid-40s and early-60s, FTD is caused by progressive nerve cell loss in the frontal lobes, an area in the front of the brain responsible for cognitive functions including problem solving, memory and judgment, and the temporal lobes, which are involved in short-term memory and emotion.

Uncharacteristic and even disruptive behavior changes are often the first noticeable symptoms of FTD, with patients becoming more irritable, impulsive, euphoric or compulsive. As the disease progresses, people with a language variant of FTD will eventually become mute or have more trouble speaking or understanding others. Memory loss is also a later feature of FTD.

How it's diagnosed: In addition to assessing clinical symptoms, a neurologist will use imaging tests such as CT or MRI scans, which may show wasting in the brain's frontal and temporal lobes, to help diagnose FTD. Additionally, about one-third of FTD cases are inherited, so genetic testing can be performed in those with a family history.

Treatment approaches: The medications most often used by Alzheimer's patients don't always ease FTD symptoms—and may actually worsen them. But other medications, including antipsychotics and antidepressants, can target specific symptoms as they arise. For example, some of the selective serotonin reuptake inhibitor (SSRI) antidepressants, such as *citalopram* (Celexa), may help behavioral symptoms, such as irritability.

Behavioral programs run by hospitals, dementia centers or psychologists can also help FTD patients and give their families the information they need to support their loved ones. Consult The Association for Frontotemporal Degeneration (TheAFTD.org) for information.

•**Korsakoff syndrome.** This disorder is triggered by a severe thiamine (vitamin B-1) deficiency, typically stemming from alcohol abuse or bariatric surgery. Because thiamine is needed to help brain cells convert glucose to energy, its absence causes brain damage that can lead to bizarre symptoms (see next page).

Those with Korsakoff syndrome have a type of short-term memory loss (anterograde amnesia) that prevents them from learning new information and remembering recent events. Also, they may speak coherently and appear normal but "confabulate"—that is, they make up things they can't recall and may even believe their made-up stories.

How it's diagnosed: Since Korsakoff syndrome is typically preceded by a condition known as Wernicke encephalopathy—an acute, life-threatening brain reaction to lack of thiamine—it's easier to diagnose. Wernicke encephalopathy is characterized by impaired walking, confusion and abnormal eye movements. With the presence of these symptoms, a thiamine blood test can be used to support diagnosis.

Treatment approaches: Oral thiamine supplements will help about one-quarter of those with Korsakoff syndrome to recover (although it may take weeks or months). For others, thiamine deficiency causes permanent brain damage. These patients may need institutional care if their impairment is severe.

Power Up Your Brain!

W. Jack Rejeski, PhD, director, Behavioral Medicine Laboratory, Wake Forest University, Winston-Salem, North Carolina.

Concentrated beetroot juice before a workout may boost brainpower.

Recent study: An hour before a 50-minute workout, 26 sedentary adults consumed beetroot juice or a placebo. Over six weeks, beetroot drinkers showed increased brain plasticity, which aids in learning. Beets are rich in nitrates, which help the blood carry oxygen—including to the brain.

Caution: If you are at risk for kidney stones or take medications for heart conditions or erectile dysfunction, consult your doctor before trying the juice.

The 4 Best Supplements to Prevent Alzheimer's

James M. Greenblatt, MD, psychiatrist and chief medical officer and vice president of medical services at Walden Behavioral Care in Waltham, Massachusetts. He has 30 years of experience treating adults of all ages for cognitive decline and mental health challenges. His most recent book is *Finally Focused*, which covers the integrative treatment of ADHD.

Many biochemistry factors contribute to the "neurodegeneration" that leads to Alzheimer's disease. These include brain inflammation...high levels of insulin in the brain, triggered by high blood sugar...nutritional deficiencies...and poor breakdown and elimination of the waste products generated by normal brain activity.

The four supplements I recommend work together to balance brain biochemistry, thereby preventing, stopping or even reversing neurodegeneration. They are safe for anyone to take, but always check with your doctor first. The best time to start supplementation is today even if you have no symptoms. It takes decades of neurodegeneration to develop Alzheimer's disease.

LOW-DOSE LITHIUM

Low doses of nutritional lithium (lithium orotate...not lithium carbonate, which is best-known as a pharmaceutical treatment for bipolar disorder) can shield you against neurodegeneration.

Animal research shows that lithium can stop the development of beta-amyloid and tau, the abnormal proteins in the brain that are the hallmarks of Alzheimer's disease...double the activity of an enzyme that protects the membranes of brain cells—an enzyme that is low in people with Alzheimer's...and prevent the onset of Alzheimer's in mice that have been genetically programmed to develop the disease.

More remarkably, several studies on people show that low-dose lithium can help prevent and even treat Alzheimer's.

Standout research: In a study published in *The British Journal of Psychiatry*, Brazilian researchers studied 45 seniors with mild cognitive impairment, the stage of memory loss and mental decline that precedes Alzheimer's. The researchers divided the seniors into two groups, giving one group low-dose lithium and the other a placebo. After one year, more of the people taking lithium had "stable cognitive performance"—meaning no mental decline. And fewer of those taking lithium developed Alzheimer's disease.

Another important new finding: In a small study recently published in *Alzheimer Disease & Associated Disorders*, doctors from Columbia University Medical Center gave 150 milligrams (mg) to 300 mg of lithium daily to people with typical Alzheimer's symptoms, such as agitation, psychosis (hallucinations, delusions) and sleeping problems. After two weeks, the researchers noted improvements including a "normal sleep cycle, with a marked decrease in paranoia, auditory hallucinations, agitation and aggression." If low-dose lithium can treat mild cognitive impairment and Alzheimer's, it's likely that it can prevent it.

If low-dose lithium can treat mild cognitive impairment and Alzheimer's, it's likely that it can prevent it.

My advice: If you are over age 50, talk to your doctor about taking 10 mg of lithium orotate daily. If you are under age 50, ask about taking 5 mg. Brands of lithium orotate include Pure Encapsulations, Swanson, KAL and many others.

VITAMIN D

Vitamin D influences more than 200 genes including many that play a role in maintaining a healthy brain. It also reduces neuroinflammation—a chronic inflammation of the central nervous system and a key driver of Alzheimer's disease. And vitamin D is a must for the manufacture of serotonin, the neurotransmitter that regulates memory and mood. Not surprisingly, vitamin D plays a key role in preventing Alzheimer's.

New scientific evidence: A 12-year study of 916 seniors, published in *Alzheimer's & Dementia: The Journal of the Alzheimer's Association*, found a link between low vitamin D levels and cognitive decline. Seniors with low blood levels of vitamin D had faster cognitive decline and were nearly three times more likely to develop Alzheimer's, compared with people with normal blood levels of vitamin D. The only way to determine if your blood levels of vitamin D are normal is a vitamin D blood test. You can have your physician order the test.

My advice: Maintaining a blood level of 50 nanograms per milliliter (ng/ml) is best for preventing Alzheimer's. If your blood level is lower, talk to your doctor about taking 5,000 IU of vitamin D-3 daily for three months. If levels still are lower than 50 ng/ml, continue this dose and check again in three months. Once you have achieved 50 ng/ml, take a maintenance dose of 2,000 IU daily. Have blood levels checked yearly.

VITAMIN B-12

Vitamin B-12 plays a key role in the synthesis of every neurotransmitter—the chemicals that relay messages from neuron to neuron. It also is a must for the health of the myelin sheath, which protects neurons. B-12 also helps lower levels of homocysteine, an amino acid that is toxic to brain cells. But as you age, your ability to absorb vitamin B-12 decreases—and if blood levels are low, you're more likely to get Alzheimer's.

Standout scientific research: A study published in *Current Alzheimer Research* found a link between B-12 and Alzheimer's—people with low blood levels of B-12 were about four times more likely to have Alzheimer's disease. (People with low levels of B-12 and high levels of homocysteine were about 30 times more likely to have Alzheimer's.)

And in an eight-year study of 501 people age 60 and older, published in *JAMA Psychiatry*, those with the highest blood levels of vitamin B-12 had the slowest rate of brain atrophy—that is, the higher the B-12 level, the less the brain shrank with age. That's an important finding because brain atrophy is another hallmark of Alzheimer's disease.

My advice: Anyone who wants to prevent Alzheimer's should take at least 1,000 micrograms (mcg) of vitamin B-12 daily—for maximum absorption, take a sublingual form. (A sublingual capsule or liquid supplement is put under the tongue.) Brands include Pure Encapsulations, Nature Made and more.

Superfood for Your Brain

Blueberries can improve brain function in people diagnosed with mild cognitive impairment (MCI).

Recent finding: After 16 weeks of consuming the equivalent of one cup of blueberries a day, people with mild MCI had better cognitive performance than people given a placebo. Other studies have shown that antioxidants in blueberries protect against heart disease, cancer and other diseases.

Study by researchers at University of Cincinnati Academic Health Center, presented at a recent meeting of the American Chemical Society in San Diego.

Go "green" for your brain. People who ate the most leafy greens daily (just over one serving, such as one cup of raw spinach or one-half cup cooked) over a 10-year period had brains that were roughly 11 years "younger" in terms of memory and cognition than people who reported rarely or never eating greens, according to a study of 960 adults ages 58 to 99 without dementia. Whether cooked or raw, spinach, kale and other leafy greens are rich in vitamins E and K, lutein and other substances that may slow cognitive decline.

Martha Clare Morris, ScD, director of nutritional epidemiology, Rush University Medical Center, Chicago.

Beware: In the US, B-12 levels are considered "normal" as long as they are above 200 picograms per milliliter (pg/ml). In Europe and Japan, normal levels are at 500 pg/ml and above. I consider the US "normal" range one of the tragedies of American medicine, dooming many people to cognitive decline. If your physician tells you that your B-12 levels are "normal," ask what your levels are.

CURCUMIN

Curcumin is the principal component of turmeric, the spice that flavors curries. Research shows curcumin is neuroprotective in many ways, including stopping the formation of beta-amyloid.

Standout research: People age 40 to 60 who took a daily curcumin supplement had lower blood levels of beta-amyloid, according to a study conducted by researchers at The Ohio State University and published in *Nutrition Journal*.

My advice: Take 500 mg of curcumin twice daily with meals. Good brands include Doctor's Best, Jarrow Formulas, Now, Source Naturals, Thorne Research and many others.

My favorite brain-protecting curcumin supplement is one I formulated myself—Curcumasorb Mind from Pure Encapsulations. It contains Meriva, a highly absorbable form of curcumin, as well as many other plant extracts shown to be neuroprotective.

Dirty Air and Dementia

Jiu-Chiuan Chen, MD, ScD, associate professor, Keck School of Medicine, University of Southern California, Los Angeles.

Older women who live in areas where fine-particulate air pollution (emitted by vehicles and power plants) exceeds EPA standards are 92% more likely to develop dementia than those in EPA-compliant areas.

Implication: Based on estimates that 30% of the population reside in areas exceeding EPA standards, fine-particulate air pollution may be responsible for 21% of dementia cases in the US.

Losing Track of Your Thoughts?

Gurinder Singh Bains, PhD, associate professor, Loma Linda University School of Allied Health Professions, Loma Linda, California. He has researched the effects of laughter on short-term memory.

Sometimes during the day or before you fall asleep at night, you could be be mulling over a problem and then completely forget your last thought. Are you suffering from short-term memory loss?

Alcohol and Your Brain

Even moderate drinking is bad for the brain. Over a 30-year period, people who drank as few as four pints of strong beer or five large glasses of wine a week had hippocampal atrophy, a type of brain damage often found in people with Alzheimer's disease. Light drinkers—up to three small glasses of wine or two pints of beer a week—showed no decrease in brain function.

Anya Topiwala, MD, PhD, is clinical lecturer in old age psychiatry in the department of psychiatry at University of Oxford, UK.

Heavy drinking triples dementia risk. For women, heavy drinking is three or more alcoholic beverages a day…four or more for men. Early-onset dementia (before age 65) appears to be especially alcohol-related. After years of alcohol abuse, dementia-related brain damage may be irreversible, so early intervention to treat alcohol problems is crucial.

Michaël Schwarzinger, MD, PhD, is an epidemiologist based in Paris, France, and lead author of a study of 1,109,343 patients, published in *The Lancet*.

This could be a form of short-term memory loss. But don't be too quick to assume the worst. Memory naturally declines as we get older. It becomes a real problem only when such instances become persistent and begin to interfere with your daily functioning—for example, you have difficulties performing at your job because of such memory lapses. In this case, you should definitely see your doctor for an evaluation.

Certain medications, such as sleeping pills and antidepressants, can lead to memory problems. Other causes could be smoking, alcohol and/or drug abuse, a head injury or a stroke. A vitamin B-12 deficiency, which is most common in older people, who tend to have trouble absorbing this vitamin from their food, could also be playing a role.

Other possible causes include lack of sleep and stress. Chronic lack of sleep impairs the brain's ability to consolidate memories. With chronic stress, levels of the so-called "stress hormone"

cortisol increase throughout our bodies. When cortisol enters the brain, it can damage the neurons that are needed for learning and memory.

If you think stress is to blame, try some laughter. A recent study found that adults who watched a funny video for 20 minutes had significantly lower cortisol levels than those who did not watch it.

Even better: Those in the study who watched the funny video scored 20% higher on memory tests, including short-term memory, than those in the control group. So get a regular dose of humor, and your memory may kick back into gear!

Diabetes Drug for Brain Health

Boston University Medical Center

A new memory booster may be on the horizon. A single injection of the diabetes drug *pramlintide* improves memory in Alzheimer's patients. It reduces brain levels of the amyloid proteins that accompany Alzheimer's disease and may provide a new treatment option.

Dizzy–Dementia Link

Andreea Rawlings, PhD, postdoctoral researcher, Johns Hopkins Bloomberg School of Public Health, Baltimore.

People who feel dizzy upon standing are 40% more likely to develop dementia than those who don't, according to a 20-year study of nearly 12,000 adults.

Theory: That quick drop in blood pressure, which often leads to dizziness (a condition known as orthostatic hypotension), may cause lasting damage by reducing blood flow to the brain.

Temporary dizziness may indicate an underlying condition such as dehydration or anemia or may be caused by prescription medications.

A Sniff Test for Alzheimer's Disease

Study titled, "Odor Identification Screening Improves Diagnostic Classification in Incipient Alzheimer's Disease," by David R. Roalf, PhD, research assistant professor, department of behavioral neuroscience and psychiatry, University of Pennsylvania, Philadelphia, and colleagues, published in *Journal of Alzheimer's Disease.*

A simple sniff test can help in the early diagnosis of Alzheimer's disease. Combined with standard cognitive tests, it enhances the ability to identify the disease before there are any other symptoms. That means better care.

Background: Brain degeneration can begin as early as 10 years before a definitive diagnosis. Many people develop mild cognitive impairment (MCI) first—a condition marked by problems with memory and thinking that are not serious enough to affect daily functioning. Many people with MCI don't know they have it—and while having MCI increases your risk of developing Alzheimer's, it's not a sure thing. Better tests are needed to identify people with MCI in the first place—and to figure out which ones are at highest risk for Alzheimer's.

Smell might be key. A sharp decline in the sense of smell is one of the earliest warning signs—areas in the brain that process odors are often the first to be affected by the disease. Smell affects taste, too—one reason why many Alzheimer's patients often complain that food doesn't taste as good as it once did. So researchers decided to test a commercially available "sniff" test to see if it could improve early diagnosis.

Study: Researchers at University of Pennsylvania studied 262 people with Alzheimer's disease, 198 with mild cognitive impairment and 292 healthy older adults. On average, subjects were in their early-to-mid-70s. Some with MCI were further classified based on the severity of their condition, since people with more severe memory loss and other symptoms are more likely to progress to Alzheimer's.

Each participant had been painstakingly diagnosed by an experienced clinician using a battery of tests including neuroimaging and advanced cognitive testing. Then researchers used the "Sniffin' Sticks Odor Identification Test," which asks participants to identify 16 common odors and takes about eight minutes. Everyone also took a standard cognitive test called the Montreal Cognitive Assessment (MoCA). It's a one page, 30-point test that measures such skills as short-term memory recall. A health professional can give it in about 10 minutes.

Findings: The healthy older adults did best on the smell test, followed by those with MCI, followed by those with Alzheimer's. Within the MCI group, the test also sniffed out those most at risk—patients on the milder side did better identifying odors than those who were more impaired.

Surprising finding: The sniff test was pretty good on its own but it really made a difference when combined with MoCA, the standard cognitive test. By itself, MoCA correctly identified 77% of those with mild cognitive impairment and 93% of those with Alzheimer's. Add the sniff test, and the accuracy rate went up to 92% of those with MCI and 98% of those with Alzheimer's.

Bottom line: This finding may change the landscape of Alzheimer's screening, making it easier to identify people at highest risk of developing the disease quickly and relatively inexpensively.

Here's why that matters: Knowing you're at high risk means you can get targeted medical care if symptoms develop, work with your doctor to stop taking medications that can increase dementia risk, improve lifestyle factors

Your Brain Stays Alert While You Are Sleeping in Strange Surroundings

Part of the left hemisphere remains more active than normal during the first night of sleep in a new place and remains sensitive to sounds. This may be so that we stay alert for possible threats in a new place—and may explain why many people sleep poorly on their first night in a hotel or other unfamiliar location.

Study by researchers at Brown University, Providence, published in *Current Biology.*

linked to improved cognition, make plans for future care and finances—and perhaps sign up for new clinical trials in the future. That's why an annual "cognitive checkup" is now covered by insurance.

Should you try the sniff test yourself? You could buy it—it's commercially available and easy to self-administer—but it's pricey ($325 for a 12-odor version), and best given along with cognitive testing, as this study showed. If your doctor orders it, it's at least possible that insurance might pick up all or part of the tab.

Do see your doctor if you find that your sense of smell or taste seems to be declining. Rest assured—a loss of smell or taste can be caused by many things other than incipient dementia, including medical problems such as a thyroid condition, certain drugs such as nasal steroid sprays, even a zinc deficiency. Best to find out.

Questions to Ask If You Are Diagnosed with Alzheimer's Disease

Alzheimer's Association, American Academy of Neurologists, Harvard Medical School, Mayo Clinic.

A diagnosis of Alzheimer's can be terrifying. But the more you know about what to expect, the better off you'll be. *If your doctor tells you that you have Alzheimer's disease, here are important questions to ask...*

•**Are you sure it's Alzheimer's disease?** Doctors can diagnose "probable Alzheimer's disease" with about 90% accuracy. But there's always room for error because many forms of dementia can mimic Alzheimer's. Ask your doctor how he/she will confirm that you actually have Alzheimer's and not another form of dementia that could possibly be more treatable (such as dementia caused by thyroid problems or a vitamin deficiency).

•**What will happen to me first?** With early Alzheimer's, you might notice occasional (and slight) memory lapses. Your cognitive abilities will continue to worsen over time. Some people misplace things, and some make poor decisions or engage in uncharacteristically aggressive behavior. Your doctor can tell you what's typical for each of the three stages of Alzheimer's, but the specific symptoms will vary from person to person.

•**How will my moods change?** You might become suspicious of close friends or family members. You might get angry more than you used to or become increasingly agitated toward the end of each day. If you do notice mood changes, ask your doctor what you can do to cope. In some Alzheimer's patients, certain behavior changes are due to something else altogether—such as depression.

•**What medications are you going to prescribe for me, and why?** Depending on your symptoms and stage, you might be given *donepezil* (Aricept) or *memantine* (Namenda). A newer drug, Namzaric, combines both of these drugs in a one-a-day capsule. The drugs can help improve memory/confusion and delay the worsening of symptoms, although they cannot cure the disease. You might need other drugs—such as antianxiety medications—as well.

•**Could nondrug treatments make a difference in my case?** Preliminary research finds that omega-3 fatty acids may slow cognitive declines in Alzheimer's patients who are missing a particular gene. (The US Food and Drug Administration recommends no more than three grams daily from food and supplement sources combined.) A supplement called huperzine A (a moss extract) has shown some benefit—it has properties that are similar to some Alzheimer's drugs. Check with your doctor before starting (or continuing to take) any supplement.

•**Should I increase my exercise?** There's some evidence that vigorous exercise can slow or temporarily stop cognitive declines in those with an early stage of Alzheimer's disease. But hard exercise isn't safe for everyone—and it might or might not help. Your doctor can help you design the best exercise program for you.

•**Is it safe for me to drive?** Personal safety is always an issue as Alzheimer's progresses. The American Academy of Neurologists says that no one with Alzheimer's (regardless of the stage) should drive a car, though other experts advise deciding case-by-case. Get your doctor's opinion on your situation.

Zapping the Brain During Sleep May Improve Memory

Study by researchers at Neuroscience Center at University of North Carolina at Chapel Hill, published in *Current Biology.*

A procedure called transcranial alternating current stimulation (tACS) stimulates a targeted area of the brain with small doses of weak electricity. In a recent study, men given a memory test showed substantial improvement when given tACS during sleep, compared with those given a sham stimulation.

When Tinnitus Is More Than a Hearing Problem

Thomas J. Balkany, MD, the Hotchkiss professor and chairman emeritus of the department of otolaryngology at the University of Miami Miller School of Medicine. He is also a coeditor of the book *Clinical Pediatric Otolaryngology* and coauthor of *The Ear Book: A Complete Guide to Ear Disorders and Health.*

Most people with tinnitus commonly refer to it as "ringing in the ears," but the "ghost sounds" can also sound like whooshing, popping, buzzing, humming or clicking…or even musical melodies.

If you are among the estimated 45 million Americans affected by tinnitus (pronounced tin-EYE-tus or TIN-uh-tus), you quickly realize that the sounds you're perceiving are not coming from any actual external source. You may also assume that you're the only one who can hear the odd sounds you're hearing. But that's not always true.

An important distinction: For some tinnitus sufferers, the condition is caused by physical problems that can sometimes be heard by an examining physician. Quick treatment for this type of tinnitus may eliminate the bothersome sounds…and stop a potentially serious medical issue. *What you need to know about the two main types…*

SUBJECTIVE TINNITUS

This form of tinnitus accounts for more than 95% of all tinnitus cases. The ghost sounds, as described above, may come and go, but when present are continuous and audible only to you. Loudness and pitch tend to vary from time to time.

Main cause: Damaged cells in the *cochlea,* the spiral-shaped structure in the inner ear that converts external sound waves into electrochemical signals that you "hear" in the brain. These cells can produce false signals that the brain interprets as sounds.

Cell damage within the inner ear is usually due to long-term noise exposure or age-related hearing loss. Sometimes, the cause is as simple as a buildup of earwax. Tinnitus may also result from long-term use of aspirin or other medications that can damage the ears, such as chemotherapy drugs or diuretics.

Note: In rare cases, subjective tinnitus is associated with a benign tumor pressing on the auditory nerve. Hearing tinnitus sounds in only one ear can be a warning clue.

OBJECTIVE TINNITUS

Objective tinnitus is less ghost-like—it can be heard (and measured) by a doctor. It is much less common, affecting less than 5% of tinnitus sufferers.

The sound is mainly caused by the noisy movement of blood through abnormal veins/arteries in the head or neck. Doctors call these sounds *pulse-synchronous* because there's one sound with each heartbeat.

Important: Pulsatile tinnitus, or vascular tinnitus, as this condition is often called, is worrisome because it typically signals an underlying vascular disease, such as atherosclerosis…brain aneurysm (a bulge in a weakened artery in the brain)…or a vascular tumor.

Much less often, clicking sounds, like those from a typewriter, can occur with objective tinnitus. Involuntary muscle contractions of the palate or middle ear could be the cause. This type of tinnitus is usually temporary and associated with stress or head trauma or, more rarely, with multiple sclerosis or a brain stem tumor.

TINNITUS TREATMENT

If you think you might have either type of tinnitus, see an otolaryngologist (an ear, nose and throat doctor) for an evaluation. The doctor will check your hearing and blood pressure. He/she will also listen for pulsatile tinnitus by pressing a stethoscope over the ear canal or major blood vessels in the head, neck or heart. If sounds are present, you'll probably need an MRI or a CT scan. Just knowing that tinnitus is not caused by anything serious (*as most often is the case*) goes a long way toward relief.

Treatment for subjective tinnitus: This type of tinnitus can rarely be eliminated altogether, but it almost always can be reduced. *Best approaches…*

•**Deal with stress.** Emotional stress is *strongly* linked to tinnitus. The fight-or-flight stress hormones enhance the transmission of nerve impulses, making the ghost sounds louder and more distressing. Patients with tinnitus should manage their stress with the help of a psychotherapist…self-help approaches such as exercise, yoga and/or meditation…and/or complementary therapies such as massage, biofeedback or acupuncture.

•**Consume less caffeine.** Coffee, tea and caffeine-loaded soft drinks can make tinnitus much worse. Caffeine stimulates the nervous system and makes tinnitus louder. Some people notice a difference when they reduce their intake of caffeinated beverages to one or two a day, but avoiding caffeine altogether is usually more effective.

•**Improve sleep.** Good sleep hygiene (going to bed at the same time every night and getting restful sleep) is beneficial for overall health and can help alleviate tinnitus. If you have trouble falling asleep or wake up during the night, try introducing more exercise into your routine so that you are more physically tired at night.

•**Limit the use of aspirin and other over-the-counter (OTC) pain relievers.** Aspirin is known to cause reversible damage to the nerve cells in the cochlea of the inner ear. In addition, a Harvard study found that people who took *ibuprofen* (Motrin) or *acetaminophen* (Tylenol) most days of the week had a 20% increased risk for hearing loss, which increases the risk for tinnitus.

Low-dose aspirin therapy (81 mg daily) for heart health and occasional use of these other medications shouldn't be a problem. Tinnitus usually occurs only with regular high doses. If you're taking higher doses of aspirin or these other medications and develop tinnitus, stop taking them. The sounds will usually disappear within a day or two.

•**Sound therapy.** Sound therapy uses external sources of sound to reduce the severity of tinnitus. By introducing a louder sound, the softer sound of tinnitus can be blocked out. *Various methods…*

•Background sound masking. Tinnitus sounds become less noticeable when you're listening to other sounds. Some people keep a fan running or listen to low-volume background music. You can buy inexpensive sound generators that produce birdsongs, the sounds of running water, white noise and other constant sounds. If you mainly notice tinnitus at night, you can buy inexpensive pillow speakers that will mask the noises without bothering your bed partner.

•Wearable maskers. Many people with tinnitus also have hearing loss. Using hearing aids can help reduce the tinnitus sounds by making surrounding sound louder…and there are some models that also include a masking component—they simultaneously enhance hearing and block tinnitus sounds.

Important: You can buy wearable maskers online, but it's best to get a customized device from an audiologist. The audiologist will test different volumes/frequencies to find one that precisely matches your tinnitus. The device will then be adjusted as low as possible until it just covers up the tinnitus sounds but doesn't interfere with normal hearing.

These combination devices are similar in appearance to hearing aids and cost about $1,000 to $2,500 for a pair. The cost is very rarely covered by insurance.

Some people use these devices indefinitely. Others find that masking gradually results in reduced loudness over time, even when the maskers are not in use. After a few months, some people discover that they no longer need the devices for tinnitus control.

•**Neurophysiology-based treatment.** One of the most recent and effective treatments for tinnitus, neurophysiology-based treatment uses sound therapy along with intensive counseling to dampen the anxiety associated with tinnitus sound. The goal is for the patient to learn to ignore the tinnitus until it fades into the background.

In the past, surgeries were done to cut the hearing nerve with the hope of alleviating subjective tinnitus, but this did not improve the condition and sometimes made it worse. However, surgery may be needed in the rare case when a tumor is causing subjective tinnitus.

Treatment for objective tinnitus: Fewer than 5% of objective tinnitus cases require surgery to manage a serious underlying condition, such as severe narrowing of the carotid artery, an aneurysm or a vascular tumor. Botox is sometimes used to help spasms in the soft palate and one or both tiny muscles in the middle ear can be divided to stop spasms in the middle ear.

Music-Making: The Ultimate Brain Booster

Roy Ernst, PhD, founder and adviser to the board of directors of New Horizons Music, a nonprofit organization dedicated to music education for older adults. He is also professor emeritus at the Eastman School of Music, University of Rochester, New York.

For people who like to do brain "exercise," working crossword puzzles or playing computer games is pretty standard fare. But you'll likely get a better brain workout by picking up a guitar, cello or clarinet instead—and, for good measure, joining a band or orchestra.

CREATE YOUR OWN NEURAL SYMPHONY

Why is music so great for brain health? Scientists know that it's one of the few activities that engages many areas of your brain at the same time.

When you read a musical score, for example, your brain processes several notes per second, taking in each note's pitch, duration, intensity, volume, articulation and tone quality. Then the brain sends out signals to your nerves and muscles so you can physically turn those notes into a melody.

If you're playing in a band or orchestra, you must listen even more carefully, blending your sounds with those of your fellow players. This involves constantly making small adjustments to stay in time and in tune—a process that requires total focus and engages even more areas of your brain.

Scans show that parts of the brain that govern auditory, visual, sensory and motor and emotional function are all engaged when musicians practice and perform. It's not surprising that scans have also revealed that musicians have superior memories and executive function—brain processes tied to planning, solving problems and focusing.

The perks are more than cognitive. Playing an instrument requires your undivided attention, giving you the same stress-reducing advantages as meditating does.

There are also health benefits—music-making can lower your heart rate and blood pressure, according to a study from the Netherlands. Plus, your body pumps out extra *oxytocin*, a hormone that can make you feel less anxious and more connected to your fellow players.

AGE IS AN ADVANTAGE

Many people assume that they're past the age when they can learn how to make music. But that's not true. Adult learners actually have an edge over children in several ways. *For example, adults tend to…*

•**Practice more effectively.** Adult learners take their goals seriously and often have more discipline, thanks to years in the workforce.

•**Draw on experiences.** A lifetime of ups and downs lets you create music in a richer, more emotional way than younger folks.

•**Have been lifelong listeners.** Years spent hearing different genres of music make it easier to grasp music's basic structures, such as chords, phrases and form.

HOW TO START AND KEEP PLAYING

To succeed when learning a new musical instrument, follow these steps…

•**Choose your instrument.** Don't base your decision on instruments you may have stored in your attic (for example, an instrument your child used to play). If you just love the sound of a particular instrument, that should be your first choice. However, it's best to rent initially instead of buying in case you change your mind.

Note: Medical issues or physical limitations can impact your instrument choice. For example, if you have arthritis or dental work, certain instruments may not be advisable. Check with your doctor if you have any questions.

•**Practice, practice, practice.** Once you have some basics down, pick a few songs that you love and play them repeatedly. When doing so, focus on making your music more creative and expressive.

•**Expect plateaus.** You may well reach a point when you feel you are no longer improving. Don't get frustrated. Instead, go back and review the basics that got you this far. Keep polishing those skills, and you may find that you break through to the next level.

For example, maybe you are discouraged because you can't play high notes on your instrument. If you are patient and keep playing the notes you can play comfortably, the higher notes will probably eventually come.

•**Don't let an ailment set you back.** Poor vision, hearing or mobility isn't an obstacle to playing music. You can get your eyeglass prescription tweaked or read your music from an iPad so you can enlarge the notes. A hearing aid might help.

Find out from fellow players what they've done to overcome physical challenges. They may have ingenious solutions. And with practice, your fingers are sure to get nimbler and those music-centric regions of your brain will wake up.

•**Look for inspiration.** Listen to music you love…as often as you can. There's nothing like a rousing rendition of your favorite melodies to keep you motivated.

Helpful: Go to YouTube.com and search your favorite songs and/or performers. Whether you want to play sax like Charlie Parker or violin like Hilary Hahn, you'll find hours of enjoyment—and inspiration!

JOIN A MUSIC GROUP!

New Horizons Music, a nonprofit organization that encourages adults to get together to make music, sponsors more than 200 ongoing music groups in all regions of the US. Most of these musicians are beginners, though others are returning to skills learned in childhood.

To find a group in your area, go to NewHorizonsMusic.org. If you don't find one in your specific location, New Horizons can help you start one. The cost to join a group ranges from zero to several hundred dollars, depending on the particular group. Music camps are also available for a fee that covers the cost of instruction, room and food.

Another option: Check out community and church choirs and orchestras. You can also search online with your hometown and the word "band" or "orchestra." You can check local music stores or community centers for leads on an individual teacher.

Helpful: Look for someone with a pleasant personality, patience and a good sense of humor.

Strokes Can Cause Memory Loss, Too

Majid Fotuhi, MD, PhD, a neurologist and medical director at NeuroGrow Brain Fitness Center in McLean, Virginia. He is author of *The Memory Cure* and *Boost Your Brain*.

Alzheimer's disease is the most widely recognized form of dementia. But there's another cause of memory loss that people should know about—but usually don't.

Vascular cognitive impairment (VCI), which is typically caused by multiple small strokes, has been estimated to affect 1% to 4% of adults over age 65. However, because there is no agreement on the exact definition of this condition, the actual number of affected individuals is not known. Most older adults with vascular risk factors—such as high blood pressure (hypertension) and diabetes—may have varying levels of VCI.

BLOOD VESSELS AND YOUR BRAIN

The brain requires a hefty amount of blood—about 20% of the heart's output—to function normally. Even a slight reduction in circulation—such as that caused by small strokes—can result in symptoms, including slowed thinking, that can mimic Alzheimer's disease.

While genetics can play a role in Alzheimer's disease, VCI is widely recognized as the most preventable form of dementia. Even if you've begun to suffer early signs of this form of cognitive impairment (see symptoms below), you may be able to avoid the devastating effects of full-blown dementia.

HIDDEN BLOCKAGES

Most people imagine stroke as a life-threatening event that causes dramatic symptoms. This is true of major strokes. It is not the case with mini-strokes, also known as transient ischemic attacks (TIAs).

When Johns Hopkins researchers looked for evidence of microscopic strokes—areas of brain damage that are too small to be visible on a magnetic resonance imaging (MRI) scan—they found that such strokes are extremely common. Millions of Americans with normal cognition, including healthy adults, have probably experienced one or more of these minor mini-strokes.

What happens: Small, transitory blood clots can momentarily prevent circulation to small areas of the brain. Or vascular hypertrophy, an abnormal growth of cells inside blood vessels, may impede normal circulation. In either case, certain parts of the brain receive insufficient blood and oxygen. The damaged areas can be much smaller than a grain of rice.

Symptoms—assuming that there are noticeable symptoms—tend to be minor. People who have experienced multiple mini-strokes that affect larger or more diverse areas of the brain are those most likely to develop dementia, but it might take years or even decades before the problem is severe enough to be diagnosed. Symptoms to watch for…

Specific symptoms of VCI depend on the part of the brain affected. Patients who have suffered multiple mini-strokes may walk or think more slowly than they did before. Some have trouble following directions. Others may feel apathetic or confused.

Some mini-strokes, however, affect only the part of the brain involved in decision-making and judgment. The changes might be so subtle that a patient isn't aware of them—at least, until subsequent mini-strokes affect larger or different areas of the brain.

GETTING THE RIGHT DIAGNOSIS

People who exhibit marked cognitive changes usually will be given an MRI or computed tomography (CT) scan. These tests sometimes reveal white, cloudy areas in the brain (infarcts) that have suffered damage from impaired circulation due to mini-strokes.

Often, however, the mini-strokes are too small to be detected. In these cases, patients may be incorrectly diagnosed with Alzheimer's disease. (The abnormal proteins that are characteristic of Alzheimer's cannot be detected by standard imaging tests.)

The distinction is important. There is no cure for Alzheimer's disease. In patients with VCI, there are a number of ways to stop the disease's progression and maintain long-term cognitive health.

BETTER VASCULAR HEALTH

Brain damage that's caused by mini-strokes can't be reversed. Medication—including cholinesterase inhibitors, such as *donepezil* (Aricept)—may modestly reduce some symptoms in patients with dementia but cannot cure it.

Preventive strategies, however, can be very effective in people with VCI alone. *Most important…*

•**Don't let high blood pressure shrink your brain.** Chronic hypertension is one of the main causes of dementia because the vascular trauma is constant. People with uncontrolled hypertension actually have smaller brains because of impaired circulation. Their risk of developing dementia is two to three times higher than that of people with normal blood pressure.

My advice: Blood pressure should be no higher than 120/80 mm Hg—and 115/75 mm Hg is better. Most people can achieve good blood pressure control with regular exercise and weight loss, and by limiting sodium and, when necessary, taking one or more blood pressure–lowering drugs, such as diuretics, beta-blockers or ACE inhibitors.

•**Avoid the other "D" word.** By itself, diabetes can double the risk for dementia. The actual risk tends to be higher because many people with diabetes are obese, which is also a dementia risk factor.

Important research: One study found that patients with multiple risk factors, including diabetes and obesity, were up to 16 times more likely to develop dementia than those without these risk factors.

My advice: By adopting strategies that prevent hypertension, including weight loss and regular exercise, you'll also help stabilize your blood sugar—important for preventing or controlling the health complications associated with diabetes.

•**Keep an eye on your waist.** Obesity increases the risk for hypertension and diabetes and has been associated with damage to the hippocampus (the brain's main memory center). Obese patients also have a much higher risk for obstructive sleep apnea, interruptions in breathing during sleep that can increase brain shrinkage (atrophy) by up to 18%.

My advice: Measure your waist. For optimal health, the size of your waist should be no more than half of your height. Someone who's 68 inches tall, for example, should have a waist measurement of 34 inches or less.

•**If you drink, keep it light.** People who drink in moderation (no more than two drinks daily for men or one for women) tend to have higher HDL, so-called "good," cholesterol…less risk for blood clots…and a lower risk for stroke and dementia.

My advice: If you already drink alcohol, be sure that you don't exceed the amounts described above. Drinking too much alcohol increases brain atrophy.

•**Get the right cholesterol-lowering drug.** People with high cholesterol are more likely to develop atherosclerosis (fatty buildup in the arteries) and suffer a mini-stroke or stroke than those with normal cholesterol levels.

My advice: Talk to your doctor about statins, such as *atorvastatin* (Lipitor) and *simvastatin* (Zocor). These drugs not only reduce cholesterol but also may fight blood-vessel inflammation. Other cholesterol-lowering drugs—such as resins, which bind in the intestines with bile acids that contain cholesterol and are then eliminated in the stool—don't provide this dual benefit.

•**Ask your doctor for a vitamin B-12 test.** If your blood level is low, you may benefit from B-12 supplements or injections.

NFL Brain Disease Starts Early

JAMA.

Professional football players have a high risk of developing a degenerative brain disease called chronic traumatic encephalopathy.

A worrisome discovery: Signs of disease were present in the autopsied brains of 21% of high school players, 91% of college players and 99% of NFL players.

Want to Boost Your Brain Power? Have More Sex

Hayley Wright, PhD, research associate, Coventry University, Centre for Research in Psychology, Behaviour and Achievement, in Coventry, UK. She was the lead author of "Frequent Sexual Activity Predicts Specific Cognitive Abilities in Older Adults," published in *The Journals of Gerontology.*

Finally, there's a way to improve your brain function that doesn't involve Sudoku, crossword puzzles or an hour on the treadmill. According to researchers in the United Kingdom, you can give your brain a boost by having sex more often!

Recent finding: A study of 28 men and 45 women—all ages 50 to 83—found that those who engaged in more frequent sexual activity scored higher on verbal fluency (this can be tested for by asking a person to name all the animals he/she can think of, for example, followed by as many words beginning with "F" as possible in 60 seconds) and visuospatial ability (this is often measured by asking a person to draw a clock face from memory). These tasks may seem abstract, but they give important clues about how the brain coordinates more complex behaviors in everyday life—for example, how people organize and prioritize information and tasks (such as remembering and ticking off items from a shopping list in your head as you navigate around the store). The participants who reported weekly sexual activity scored highest, with the verbal fluency tests showing the strongest effect.

Background: Previous research conducted in 2016 found that older adults who were sexually active scored higher on cognitive tests than those who were not sexually active. For the new study, the researchers specifically examined the impact of the frequency of sexual activity and used a broader range of tests to investigate different areas of cognitive function.

Participants divulged—via questionnaire—whether they engaged in sexual activity never, monthly or weekly, on average, over the past 12 months, and answered questions about their general health and lifestyle. They also took tests of attention, memory, verbal fluency, language and visuospatial ability. Language was assessed with basic tests of spelling and sentence construction—in the more traditional sense of reading, writing, speaking and listening. While the verbal fluency tests did require language, they relied much more on executive control to shift to new information (for example, from zoo animals to pets), update their memory and inhibit responses that had already been given.

Results: The study findings suggest that frequency of sexual activity is not linked to attention, memory or language. In these tests, the participants performed just as well regardless of how often they reported having sex, if at all. But weekly sexual activity was linked to better verbal fluency and visuospatial ability.

Implications: Lead researcher Hayley Wright, PhD, a research associate at Coventry University's Centre for Research in Psychology, Behaviour and Achievement, said, "We can only speculate whether this [result] is driven by social or physical elements—but an area we would like

You're Not Wasting Time with Video Games

Video games may help protect the brain. Older adults who played Super Mario 64, a 3-D logic-and-puzzle game, for 30 minutes a day, five days a week, for six months, had increased volume of gray matter in the brain's hippocampus and cerebellum regions—and their short-term memory improved. The effects were not seen in people who took piano lessons for six months or in a control group that did neither activity. Gray matter normally atrophies as people age. Learning new things may help slow the atrophy—but the reason for the specific effectiveness of the video game in this study remains unknown.

Gregory West, PhD, associate professor of psychology, Université de Montréal, Canada, and coauthor of a study published in *PLOS ONE*.

Computer games protect against delirium. Playing computer games, using e-mail, reading and singing do more than just help reduce dementia risk. These activities also reduced delirium (a state of sudden confusion) in older adults after orthopedic surgery, according to a new study.

Why: Older adults who regularly engage in these pastimes strengthen cognitive reserve, the mind's resistance to age-related brain changes.

Joe Verghese, MD, professor of neurology and medicine, Albert Einstein College of Medicine, New York City.

to research further is the biological mechanisms that may influence this." For example, future research could look at how the neurotransmitters that are often increased by social interaction, such as dopamine, might influence the relationship between sexual activity and brain function. Dr. Wright adds, "We need to…look at what impact sexual activity can have on those aged 50 and over, beyond the known effects on sexual health and general well-being."

Volunteering Can Stop Your Brain from Shrinking

Brain shrinkage is a normal part of aging and causes a decrease in memory and mental sharpness. When retired people served as mentors to young children in public schools in a two-year program—helping students learn to read—the gray matter and a key memory region in their brains stayed the same size and, in some cases, grew slightly. This may be associated with a reduced risk for Alzheimer's disease. Any type of sustained purposeful activity that involves leaving your house and interacting socially with others may have similar benefits.

Michelle C. Carlson, PhD, professor, department of mental health, Johns Hopkins Bloomberg School of Public Health, Baltimore.

Bottom line: Even though the causal link between frequent sex and better brain power is still not established, do you really need more research in order to try it? Give it a go…it's surely more fun than doing another crossword puzzle.

Bonus: This welcome news comes on the heels of earlier research that links sexual activity to overall happiness!

Could a Memory-Boosting Brain Implant Help Those With Dementia?

Study titled "Closed-loop Stimulation of Temporal Cortex Rescues Functional Networks and Improves Memory," led by researchers at University of Pennsylvania, published in *Nature Communications*.

You know what it's like. There's a word that's on the tip of your tongue…but you can't quite access it. Wouldn't it be nice if you could get a little brain boost in those moments? A whiz-bang brain implant may be the first step.

Recent finding: Neuroscientists at the University of Pennsylvania have made a remarkable discovery—a surgically implanted brain device that stimulates specific areas of the brain with electrical pulses at just the right moment can improve memory performance by up to 15%.

Study details: The research, published in the journal *Nature Communications*, focused on 25 patients who were being treated for epilepsy. As part of that treatment, the patients already had electrodes implanted in their brains. An earlier study involving these patients had shown that delivering electrical stimulation to their brains boosted memory when it was predicted to fail.

As part of the new investigation, the electrodes determined and recorded the exact patterns that indicated when each patient's brain memory functions were working well and when that brain needed a little nudge. This information was used to create a computer algorithm that could identify those patterns in the brain and predict when a memory lapse was likely to happen.

To test the effectiveness of the new brain-stimulation system, the patients were asked to memorize a list of words…and recall as many as they could after a short distraction. They performed this test and other similar tests repeatedly—some with the implant that delivered the electrical pulses turned on and some with it turned off. The patients weren't told by the researchers whether the device was on or off—and they couldn't feel any difference. When the device was turned on, the study participants performed 15% percent better, on average, on the word-recall test.

What this means: This level of memory improvement may not sound earth-shattering, but it's about the same amount of memory that patients with Alzheimer's disease lose over about two-and-a-half years. The development of this technology is in its early experimental stage, but scientists believe that it may suggest a new type of treatment to help people who have serious memory problems, such as those with dementia (including Alzheimer's disease) or traumatic brain injuries.

Bottom line: Even though the test on patients with epilepsy was a success, the researchers don't know yet whether the results will be similar in a broader population. It's also worth noting that the memory boost provided by the brain implant does not offer the kind of help you need to remember, say, where you left your keys. The implant tested here also requires an extremely delicate surgical procedure to the brain, which would make it a choice for only the most severe cases of memory impairment. Even so, it's an exciting development—and one that could well play an important role in future treatments.

―――――――――――――――――――――――

CHAPTER 3

Cancer Breakthroughs and Care

Get an Extra Edge Against Cancer

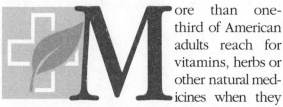**M**ore than one-third of American adults reach for vitamins, herbs or other natural medicines when they have colds or other routine (and hopefully mild) health problems. Similar remedies can help when you have cancer.

To learn more about the best and safest ways to use natural therapies—also known as complementary and alternative medicine (CAM)—to fight cancer and its complications, we spoke with Mark A. Stengler, NMD, a naturopathic physician who treats cancer patients.

HOW CAM CAN WORK

Research has shown that many so-called "alternative" treatments can enhance the effects of conventional cancer care such as surgery, radiation or chemotherapy...reduce treatment side effects...and possibly improve survival.

This type of integrative care doesn't replace conventional cancer treatments. Rather, with the guidance of a doctor, complementary therapies are added to a patient's treatment plan.

Important: To ensure that the following therapies would be appropriate for you, consult the Society for Integrative Oncology (Integrative Onc.org) to find an integrative oncologist near you...or check with The American Association of Naturopathic Physicians (Naturopathic.org) to locate a naturopathic doctor who also treats cancer patients.

Mark A. Stengler, NMD, a naturopathic physician and founder of The Stengler Center for Integrative Medicine in Encinitas, California (MarkStengler.com). He has served on a medical advisory committee for the Yale University Complementary Medicine Outcomes Research Project and is author of *Outside the Box Cancer Therapies: Alternative Therapies That Treat and Prevent Cancer* and coauthor of *Prescription for Natural Cures* and *Prescription for Drug Alternatives* (both from Bottom Line Books, BottomLineStore.com).

37

Also: Be sure to ask the doctor you choose to be in touch with your oncologist. *Here's how CAM can help with problems that plague most cancer patients...*

•**Get relief from "chemo brain."** It's estimated that three-quarters of cancer patients will experience some degree of mental cloudiness. Known as "chemo brain," it can include mood swings, memory loss and mental fatigue. It eventually improves, but some patients will feel like they're in a mental fog years after their treatments have ended.

What helps: The omega-3 fatty acids in fish oil supplements—a typical daily dose is 1,000 mg total of *eicosapentaenoic acid* (EPA) and *docosahexaenoic acid* (DHA) combined—help regulate acetylcholine, a neurotransmitter that increases nerve growth factor and improves memory as well as energy levels.

The omega-3s also increase the effectiveness of 5-fluorouracil and other chemotherapy drugs, according to a study published in *Clinical Nutrition Research*. In research published in *Cancer*, lung cancer patients who took fish oil along with chemotherapy had a greater one-year survival rate than those who didn't take the supplements.

Note: Fish oil may cause stomach upset in some patients, along with bleeding in those who are taking anticoagulant medications such as *warfarin* (Coumadin), *apixaban* (Eliquis) and *rivaroxaban* (Xarelto).

•**Boost energy levels.** Ginseng is one of the more effective supplements for cancer patients. A number of studies have shown that it reduces treatment-related side effects, including weakness and fatigue. A double-blind study in *Journal of the National Cancer Institute* found that patients who took ginseng had less fatigue than those given placebos.

My advice: The American form of ginseng (*Panax quinquefolius*) is more effective than the Asian form.

Typical dose: 1,300 mg to 2,000 mg daily. It rarely causes side effects, although it may lower blood sugar in those with diabetes.

Also helpful: Glutathione, a "super antioxidant" that can be combined with chemotherapy to reduce toxin-related fatigue and other side effects. It's usually given in an IV solution. Side effects are unlikely, but it may interfere with some chemotherapy drugs. Be sure to consult an integrative oncologist to see whether you will/won't benefit from glutathione.

•**Improve immune response.** Turkey tail is one of the best-studied medicinal mushrooms. Available in capsule form, the supplement has chemical compounds (beta-glucans) that stimulate many aspects of the immune response, including antibody activity—important for inducing the death of cancer cells.

Impressive research: A study published in *Cancer Immunology and Immunotherapy* found that postsurgical remissions in colorectal cancer patients were twice as common in those who were given turkey tail.

Typical dose: 3,000 mg daily. Side effects are unlikely.

A NUTRITIONAL BOOST

Conventional oncologists receive little training in nutrition, but it's a critical issue for cancer patients. One study found that 91% of cancer patients had nutritional impairments, and 9% were seriously malnourished. Research shows that malnutrition contributes directly or indirectly to a significant number of cancer deaths due to poor appetite and the disease process of advanced cancer.

Loss of appetite is a major cause of malnutrition and muscle loss (cachexia). I advise patients who are losing weight to address these problems by getting more calories.

With every meal, include high-fat foods such as olive oil, coconut oil, avocado, nuts and seeds. A 10-year study, published in *Archives of Internal Medicine*, looked at more than 380,000 adults and found that a Mediterranean-style diet, which is high in olive oil and other healthy fats, reduced cancer deaths in men by 17% and 12% in women.

Also helpful: Protein shakes. They can provide the extra protein that's critical for cancer patients. Up to 80% of those with advanced cancer experience muscle loss. Protein shakes can help reverse it.

Best option: Ready-made whey protein or pea protein shakes—both are nutritious, have

5 g of sugar or less per serving and are readily available in health-food stores.

My advice: Get 1 g to 1.2 g of protein per kilogram (2.2 pounds) of body weight daily. This means that someone who weighs 150 pounds will need about 68 g to 82 g of protein daily. You can get that much from two or three servings of a typical whey protein beverage, which comes ready-mixed or in powdered form.

Caution: If you have moderate or severe kidney disease, check with your doctor for advice on your protein intake.

Breakthrough Cancer Therapy: Blood Cancers Have Up to an 80% Response Rate

Caron A. Jacobson, MD, medical oncologist and assistant professor of medicine at Dana-Farber Cancer Institute and Harvard Medical School, both in Boston. She is the medical director of the Immune Effector Cell Therapy Program at Dana-Farber, which houses its CAR T-cell program. Dr. Jacobson, who specializes in lymphoma treatment and is affiliated with Brigham and Women's Hospital in Boston, is the principal investigator of CAR T-cell trials in lymphoma there and at Dana-Farber.

When it comes to the development of cancer treatments, the decades-long arc of progress is slow and incremental. Then something truly significant happens to change the course of the disease. What's happening now appears to be one of those moments.

Latest development: A type of blood-cancer treatment that has already shown remarkable success in clinical trials is beginning to receive FDA approvals. Two of these treatments, for example, have recently been approved (see page 40).

With the new treatment, known as CAR T-cell therapy, blood is drawn from a patient to isolate his/her T-cells, the powerhouses of the body's immune system. The T-cells are genetically altered and reprogrammed to recognize and kill tumor cells and then infused back into the patient.

The treatment has been called a "living drug" because it's hoped that the enhanced T-cells will continue to multiply and remain active in the body, possibly providing lifelong protection against the cancer.

A GAME CHANGER

Researchers at universities and pharmaceutical companies have now developed CAR T-cell therapy for leukemia, multiple myeloma and lymphoma—blood cancers that account for about 10% of all cancer cases diagnosed in the US each year.

The hope is that similar treatments eventually will be used for tumors affecting the breast, lung, prostate and other parts of the body.

Important: The treatment of "solid" tumors with this type of gene therapy still presents formidable obstacles that will have to be overcome.

CAR T-cell therapies have mainly been studied in patients with lymphoma or other blood cancers that didn't respond well to standard treatments or that later recurred.

Example: Lymphoma patients are typically given several types and/or protocols of standard chemotherapy without a sure result. These patients are thought to be good candidates for CAR T-cell therapy—and the early results are promising. Studies show that up to 80% of such patients respond to CAR T-cell therapy, and about 30% to 40% of patients were still in remission after six months. In earlier studies, some patients have remained in remission for more than five years.

Important caveat: So far, hundreds of patients have been treated with CAR T-cell therapy. We're seeing remarkable response rates, with many patients achieving a "complete" response—meaning that no cancer is detectable in the body with current methods. But the treatments are too new—and patients haven't been followed for a long enough time—to say for sure that the treatments promise a cure.

HOW IT WORKS

Except for cases for which FDA-approved CAR T-cell therapy now is available (see page 40), adult patients who are eligible for this treatment receive it by participating in a clinical trial. They report to a laboratory or clinic, where they undergo a four-to-six-hour process to collect blood cells, which are then sent to a company that reengineers the patient's T-cells, giving them the ability to recognize a protein (for example, CD19) on the surface of blood-cancer cells. The engineering process takes two to four weeks.

The patients are given several days of routine chemotherapy. After that, the engineered T-cells are given back to the patient via infusion. This treatment, which takes about 15 minutes, usually is administered just once, though some studies allow a second infusion if there is a partial response or relapse. The cell infusion and period of observation thereafter are typically done on an inpatient basis.

The reengineered cells circulate throughout the body and quickly begin to multiply and attack the tumor cells. Even though it's hoped that the reengineered cells will stay active in the body indefinitely, it's too early to know if this will happen. The cells might last for six months, 12 months…or forever.

NOT RISK-FREE

With the treatment beginning to get FDA approval, it is expected to be very expensive—possibly costing hundreds of thousands of dollars. At this point, it's unclear the extent to which insurance will cover the cost.

For now, the CAR T-cell treatments are somewhat risky. The genetically altered T-cells, when activated by cancer cells, can trigger a condition known as cytokine release syndrome. Many patients experience intense flulike symptoms, including a high fever, aches and fatigue. About 10% to 15% will get sick enough that they require ICU-level care, but these side effects can be treated with steroids and other drugs. Mild-to-severe confusion may develop in up to 30% of patients. While this too is reversible, there have been cases of fatal brain swelling.

The cardiac stress and respiratory distress due to the "inflammatory cascade" that is triggered by the treatment also can be life-threatening. The risks will undoubtedly decline as doctors gain more experience with the therapy.

How to access this therapy…

Recent approvals: Based on the results of trials of CAR T-cells in children and young adults with acute lymphoblastic leukemia, in August 2017, the FDA approved a CD19-targeted CAR T-cell therapy called *tisagenlecleucel* (Kymriah). In October 2017, a second CAR T-cell therapy, *axicabtagene* (Yescarta), was approved for patients with large B-cell lymphomas who have not responded to other treatments.

For patients with lymphoma, leukemia or multiple myeloma for whom an FDA-approved CAR T-cell therapy is not available, a clinical trial may be an option. If your doctor believes that you're a candidate for CAR T-cell therapy, discuss whether it makes sense for you to participate in an ongoing study. Your oncologist can advise you about clinical trials in your area. If accepted into the trial, the CAR T-cell therapy is covered but supportive care is billed to insurance.

Fat and Cancer Risks

Watch where you store fat. A 12-year meta-analysis of 43,000 people concluded that excess fat around the waist and hips—even for someone of normal weight—may present a cancer risk similar to that of overall obesity.

Details: About four excess inches around the waist caused risk for obesity-related cancers, such as pancreatic and breast, to jump by 13%. About three extra inches at the hips increased risk for bowel cancer by 15%.

Theory: Excess fat alters hormone levels and can lead to inflammation—both linked to cancer risk.

Heinz Freisling, PhD, section of nutrition and metabolism, International Agency for Research on Cancer, Lyon, France.

Overweight cancer risk. Risk for cancer rises by 7% for every decade a woman is overweight. Breast, endometrial, colon and kidney cancers showed the clearest connection. While the study results do not prove that being overweight causes these cancers, it suggests that excess weight can influence cancer development, possibly because weight affects estrogen levels and feeds chronic inflammation.

Study of nearly 74,000 US women from the Women's Health Initiative, led by researchers at International Agency for Research on Cancer, Lyon, France, published in *PLOS Medicine*.

Unusual Signs of Brain Cancer...and New Hope

Keith Black, MD, chair and professor of the department of neurosurgery at Cedars-Sinai Medical Center and director of the Maxine Dunitz Neurosurgical Institute and the Johnnie L. Cochran, Jr. Brain Tumor Center. Dr. Black has operated on more than 6,000 patients with brain tumors. He is author of *Brain Surgeon: A Doctor's Inspiring Encounters with Mortality and Miracles.*

The late senator John McCain made headlines after being diagnosed with a glioblastoma, the deadliest of all brain tumors. That description and his eventual death may seem as if it's over for anyone afflicted by this aggressive cancer.

But survival rates vary widely. Some of these tumors respond better than others to treatment, so it's important to recognize easy-to-miss symptoms of this disease. Early diagnosis means treatment can start sooner. And while it can't be cured, there are advances that may improve the odds of living longer.

WHAT IS A GLIOBLASTOMA?

This cancer is a primary brain tumor—it originates in the brain in contrast to cancers such as lung cancer, skin cancer or breast cancer that start somewhere else and may spread to the brain.

About half of primary brain tumors are benign (not cancerous)—and these have a high cure rate. The rest are malignant and tend to be aggressive and life-threatening. A glioblastoma is both the most common and the most aggressive kind of malignant primary brain tumor. It is a tumor that grows from cells that make up the gluelike supportive tissue of the brain, and tumor cells migrate throughout the brain, so it's hard for a surgeon to remove it entirely. Average survival after diagnosis is only 18 to 24 months, with 25% of patients alive after two years and 10% alive after five years.

Glioblastomas strike both men and women, often in their 40s, 50s or 60s. Few causes are known—exposure to high levels of radiation to treat a childhood cancer is one, and cell-phone use is a suspected cause (see page 42). There is rarely an identifiable genetic predisposition. The frustrating reality is that most cases, like Senator McCain's, are seemingly spontaneous—no one knows what brings them on.

SIGNS AND SYMPTOMS

With a glioblastoma, as the malignant cells spread, they increase pressure in the cranium, which leads to headaches in about half of patients. Blurry vision and/or seeing double can also occur. So can mood changes such as sudden-onset depression or anger. Muscle weakness or numbness in the arms and/or legs, which can lead to trouble walking, is another possible symptom. *More symptoms...*

• **Seizures.** Brain tumors can interfere with communication between nerve cells, causing abnormal electrical activity that manifests as seizures. Nearly one-third of brain tumor patients will experience at least one seizure. A seizure can range in intensity from a subtle twitching on one side of the body to a loss of consciousness. It may be preceded by an aura, an abnormal change in sensation such as tingling, sensing flickering lights or smelling an unpleasant odor.

• **Trouble reading.** While memory loss and confusion can be glioblastoma symptoms, some are more specific. Other commonly affected areas of the brain are the frontal, temporal or parietal lobes, which are responsible for language comprehension, math or spatial orientation. If a tumor grows in the left frontal or temporal lobes, a person may have difficulty speaking or understanding others or comprehending sentences containing cross-references or comparisons. With tumors in the parietal lobe, math may become unusually challenging and so may interpreting material shown in formats such as columns or charts—the parietal lobe also governs recognition of left-right or up-down positioning.

Just having one of these symptoms, or even more than one, does not mean that you have brain cancer, of course. One clue is how quickly symptoms come on. With a glioblastoma, several serious symptoms often arise in a matter of weeks or at most a few months.

NEW TREATMENTS

The first option after discovery of a glioblastoma is often surgery, followed by radiation and chemotherapy. A glioblastoma can't be cured, but it can be managed to extend life. *Some promising newer treatment options now being studied in humans…*

•**Immunotherapy.** A cutting-edge class of drugs known as checkpoint inhibitors ignite the immune system by blocking certain signals released by tumors. That allows tumors to be "seen" and attacked by the immune system. Several clinical trials are now under way to test immunotherapies for glioblastomas.

•**Drugs that cross the blood-brain barrier.** There is a dense lining of cells that surrounds and protects the brain. Most drugs can't cross it, including many chemotherapy drugs. But the budding field of nanomedicine—including the use of drugs as tiny as molecules—is leading to investigational agents that breach the barrier, enter tumor cells and block key proteins.

•**Brain tumor vaccine.** Vaccines containing a patient's own immune cells—specifically, dendritic cells (cells that identify foreign invaders in the body)—may be able to activate a patient's immune system to attack the tumor. In a small 2017 study of 16 glioblastoma patients who received such a vaccine plus chemotherapy, published in *Clinical Cancer Research*, four were still alive after five years. More trials are under way.

On the horizon…

•**Blood test before symptoms arise.** Changes in tumor protein activity indicative of a future brain tumor may one day be detectable via a blood test.

•**Could Zika help?** Scientists are exploring whether the Zika virus, which can cross the blood-brain barrier, might in a deactivated form destroy brain tumor cells.

THE CELL-PHONE/BRAIN CANCER CONNECTION

Wireless devices including cell phones emit radiation, which we know can penetrate into the brain and, over time, may cause normal cells to become cancerous. Some studies have found a link between cell-phone use and brain cancer, including glioblastomas. But others have failed to do so. *It makes sense to err on the side of caution…*

•**When speaking on a cell phone,** minimize radiation exposure by using wired earphones (not a wireless version) or use the speakerphone function.

•**Limit use to areas with good reception,** which enables your phone to function at reduced power and therefore with reduced radiation.

Melanoma: The Major Good News

Marianne Berwick, PhD, distinguished professor, department of internal medicine, University of New Mexico School of Medicine, and former chief, Division of Epidemiology, Biostatistics and Preventive Medicine, University of New Mexico Comprehensive Cancer Center, both in Albuquerque.

Many adults grew up during the sun-loving era of the 1950s, '60s and '70s. *Now:* It's believed to be partially responsible for the quadrupling of melanoma cases over the past several decades. More than 9,000 Americans die from the disease each year.

Patients and doctors also are paying more attention to skin changes that might be cancer—and spotting melanoma earlier.

Major good news: Early-stage melanoma is usually cured by lesion-removing surgery. The five-year survival rate for early-stage melanoma

Melanoma Alert

Waiting to remove melanoma can be deadly.

New study: Data from 153,000 adults diagnosed with this cancer revealed that patients with stage 1 melanoma were 5% more likely to die over an eight-year period if they were operated on 30 to 59 days after their biopsies than those treated sooner. Risk for death rose to 41% for those who waited longer than 120 days.

Brian Gastman, MD, plastic surgeon and director of melanoma surgery, Cleveland Clinic, Ohio.

is 99%. But even stage III melanoma, cancer that has spread to nearby skin or lymph nodes, has a five-year survival rate of 63%. Stage IV melanoma, in which cancer has metastasized or spread to other sites in the body, has a five-year survival rate of 20%—but even for these advanced cases, new therapies designed to contain or reverse the disease are extending lives. *Here's what's new…*

ABCDE Warning Signs of Melanoma

- Asymmetry
- Irregular Borders
- More than one or uneven
- Distribution of Color
- Diameter larger than one-quarter inch
- Evolution, such as changes in color and/or size.

DIAGNOSIS

Examination of all the skin on your body by a savvy dermatologist at least once a year—and a biopsy of any suspicious moles—is still the best first-line of defense against melanoma. Be alert to the "ABCDE" warning signs for melanoma (see box above). Bring any skin changes to your doctor's attention immediately (even if it isn't time for your yearly skin check).

Diagnostic danger: Melanoma is tough to diagnose, particularly in its early, or "thin," stage, when the mole is less than one-millimeter thick.

My advice: If your doctor tells you that you have melanoma, ask to have your biopsy slide sent to another pathologist for a second opinion. Check first with your insurance provider to see if that's covered and if you need preauthorization.

Also important: Most people think of melanoma as a brown or black spot that is changing. But amelanotic melanoma is pale and reddish and has a poor prognosis because it's usually detected after it has spread.

What to do: Alert your doctor to both dark and light unusual skin changes.

New option: If you have a suspicious lesion, you may be able to avoid surgical biopsy. Ask your doctor about having genetic testing instead, such as the Dermtech Pigmented Lesion Assay (PLA). It is highly accurate in distinguishing malignant melanoma from benign nevi, and may be covered by your insurer.

NEW THERAPIES

New therapies are brightening the previous grim outlook for advanced melanoma.

For example, several recently approved oral drugs inhibit a genetic mutation called BRAF that drives approximately 40% to 60% of melanomas. These drugs, which slow the growth of tumors and extend life, include *vemurafenib* (Zelboraf) and *dabrafenib* (Tafinlar).

A new class of drugs called MEK inhibitors—*trametinib* (Mekinist), *cobimetinib* (Cotellic) and others—inhibit the MEK protein, which helps speed the growth and spread of melanoma tumors.

New development: Combining dabrafenib and trametinib more than doubles average survival for advanced melanoma from five months to 11 months. Unfortunately, these drugs do have side effects, ranging from headaches and fatigue to kidney and heart problems—and even, ironically, basal cell carcinoma, another type of skin cancer. Also, although they can slow and shrink tumors and extend life for months, even years, the cancer eventually returns.

What to do: Make sure your oncologist tests your tumor for genetic mutations.

Immunotherapy—drugs such as *pembrolizumab* (Keytruda), *nivolumab* (Opdivo) and *ipilimumab* (Yervoy) that stimulate the immune system to fight cancer—is another new way to treat advanced melanoma. But the drugs work only in a small percentage of patients, control cancer for a limited time, are very expensive and have a range of debilitating and even deadly side effects.

New development: Combination immunotherapy—such as the immunotherapeutic drug Keytruda with cellular therapy, which uses immune cells such as interleukin or interferon—is showing better results in clinical trials. FDA-approved interferon and interleukin-based treatments for melanoma include *aldesleukin* (Proleukin), interferon alfa-2b (Intron A) and peginterferon alfa-2b (Sylatron).

FEWER SURGICAL COMPLICATIONS

Once melanoma is diagnosed, a sentinel-lymph-node biopsy can determine whether it has spread to nearby lymph nodes. Often, all lymph nodes in an area are removed if cancer is found in the sentinel lymph node. However, removing all the lymph nodes in an arm or a leg can cause lymphedema—permanent, painful swelling of the limb that limits activity and can lead to frequent infections.

New scientific finding: Less extreme surgery is just as effective, according to a study conducted at 63 medical centers and reported in *The New England Journal of Medicine*.

Details: 1,900 patients with melanoma that had spread to at least one lymph node either had all their lymph nodes in the area of the affected node immediately removed…or had only the affected lymph node or nodes removed, while the other nodes in the area were tracked with ultrasound. If melanoma occurred in a new node, the other lymph nodes were removed. After three years, the two groups had the same survival times. But patients who had all their lymph nodes removed had four times the risk for severe swelling in the affected arm or leg.

New Clue for Melanoma

Rebecca Shannonhouse, editor, *Bottom Line Health*, BottomLineInc.com.

You probably know the ABCDEs of detecting skin cancer. The early letters of the alphabet—Asymmetrical…irregular Borders…dark or multiple Colors…a Diameter of more than 6 mm (about the size of a pencil eraser)…and Evolving in size, shape or color—signal that a mole may no longer be just a harmless skin spot.

What's new: Researchers have now discovered that melanoma, the deadliest form of skin cancer, is more likely to be found in new spots on the skin instead of existing moles.

After reviewing 38 previous studies that looked at a total of more than 20,000 melanomas, researchers found that 29% arose from

Protect Your Face from Skin Cancer

Outside this winter? Don't forget sunscreen, especially on your eyelids and the area surrounding your eye sockets. These spots are prone to skin cancer, yet people often miss them when applying sunscreen.

Tip: Sunscreens labeled "for sensitive skin" are less likely to sting if they get in your eyes.

Study by researchers at University of Liverpool, UK, published in *PLOS ONE*.

existing moles. However, a whopping 71% occurred as new skin spots, according to the research, which was published in the *Journal of the American Academy of Dermatology*.

Takeaway: People who are conscientious about performing regular skin checks should pay close attention to spots and growths that weren't there before. These growths—as well as any spots that fit the ABCDEs described above—should be examined by a dermatologist.

Very helpful: Go to the website of the American Academy of Dermatology (AAD.org) and search for "Body Mole Map." You can download a printable chart that allows you to note the location of new skin spots and growths and track any changes in old ones. If you notice a mole that's markedly different from the others—or one that changes, itches or bleeds—be sure to see a dermatologist right away.

Does a Birthmark Pose a Health Risk?

Andrew Bronin, MD, associate clinical professor of dermatology, Yale School of Medicine, New Haven, Connecticut. He is an editor for *Journal of the American Academy of Dermatology*.

Most birthmarks are harmless. That said, you should keep an eye out for any signs of change. And, although it's rare, some kinds of birthmarks can indicate a serious medical problem.

Birthmarks, as the name indicates, are skin abnormalities that you're born with. There are two main categories—vascular, caused by blood vessels (these include purplish marks referred to as port-wine stains and bright-red hemangiomas)…and pigmented, caused by cells called melanocytes, which are pigmentated differently than the rest of the skin and include moles.

Although not all moles are present from birth, most people are born with a few. It's also common to acquire moles as we age. They're usually not a health problem. But if a pigmented lesion (a mole) starts to change—such as if it grows, changes color, becomes irregular in shape, crusts or bleeds—bring it to your doctor's attention. It could be a sign of malignant melanoma, a cancer of pigment cells that is potentially fatal. Malignant melanoma can develop within a pre-existing mole or birthmark, and it can also develop on normal skin where there wasn't a mole previously.

Vascular birthmarks come in a variety of forms. Port-wine stains are flat red blotches on the skin and usually represent only a cosmetic problem, treatable if desired by laser. But some port-wine stains can indicate underlying bone and nerve development abnormalities. Babies with port-wine stains should be evaluated by their physicians to rule out such problems.

Hemangiomas are rubbery, bright red nodules of skin and often disappear spontaneously over time. But sometimes hemangiomas break down, ulcerate and bleed—in which case they require treatment. Also, depending on their location, hemangiomas can grow and interfere with vision, breathing, hearing or elimination. Any hemangioma present at birth should be evaluated by a physician to assess its potential risk and to develop a management plan even if that plan is just watchful waiting.

Bottom line: All birthmarks should be evaluated by a physician just to make sure there isn't an underlying health problem—or a risk for one. Fortunately, though, most are only cosmetic—beauty marks, in fact!

Skin Cancer…Parkinson's Link

Study of nearly 4,000 people by researchers at Mayo Clinic, Rochester, Minnesota, published in *Mayo Clinic Proceedings.*

A recent study backs up past speculation that there is a link between the risk for Parkinson's disease and the risk of developing the skin cancer melanoma. The research found that people who have melanoma are about four times more likely to develop Parkinson's disease and vice versa. Study authors suggest that those who develop melanoma might benefit from counseling about their likely higher risk of developing Parkinson's. In addition, those with Parkinson's, or a family history of the disease, may benefit from more proactive melanoma screening.

Liver Cancer Has the Fastest-Rising Death Rate…but It's Very Preventable

Pankaj Vashi, MD, AGAF, FASPEN, chair of the department of medicine and chief of the department of gastroenterology/nutrition at Cancer Treatment Centers of America at Midwestern Regional Medical Center, Zion, Illinois.

In June 2017, a team of scientific experts from the American Cancer Society issued a special report about liver cancer.

Sobering statistics: Death rates from liver cancer (hepatocellular carcinoma) are rising faster than those of any other cancer—with rates doubling since the mid-1980s, said the report, published in *CA: A Cancer Journal for Clinicians.* This year, about 41,000 Americans will be diagnosed with the disease. The report also grimly notes that only one in five people with liver cancer is alive five years after diagnosis.

That is the bad news. Here's the good…

"A substantial proportion of liver cancer deaths could be averted" by prevention and early detection and treatment of the leading causes of liver cancer, the experts wrote.

More good news: The main risk factors behind the rise in deadly liver cancer have been identified, and medical care and lifestyle changes usually can keep them under control.

Here's how to protect yourself from this deadly disease…

CRITICAL RISK FACTORS

The three-pound liver is the largest internal organ and for good reason—it performs a wide array of indispensable functions.

It filters and detoxifies your blood and makes proteins that help the blood clot. Food would be unusable without the liver—it's a must for the digestion of carbohydrates, protein and fat. The liver also stores glycogen, a type of carbohydrate called a polysaccharide that is used for fuel when blood sugar (glucose) is low. And the liver helps produce several crucial hormones such as angiotensin, which regulates blood pressure.

Because the liver is involved in such a broad range of metabolic activities, it is exposed to many factors that can weaken and damage it, increasing the likelihood of liver cancer. The two main factors are blood-borne viruses such as hepatitis C…and excess dietary fat.

●**Hepatitis C virus.** Half of all cases of liver cancer are caused by hepatitis C, which infects liver cells. Over the decades, a chronic case of hepatitis C can first cause liver inflammation and damage and then lead to cirrhosis (liver scarring, or fibrosis) and liver cancer. About 3.5 million Americans are infected with hepatitis C, and 81% of them are baby boomers, people born from 1945 to 1965. Not surprisingly, baby boomers have the highest death rates from liver cancer, but older and younger people get it, too.

In the case of baby boomers, most with hepatitis C were probably infected in the 1960s, '70s and '80s by blood transfusions and organ transplants…contaminated medical equipment or procedures that exposed them to other people's blood…sharing needles in recreational drug use…or having sex with someone who was infected. This virus was discovered in 1989 and eliminated from America's medical blood supply in 1992.

Hidden time bomb: Most people (of any age) who have chronic hepatitis C infection don't know that they're infected—because the infection rarely creates symptoms until the disease has reached an advanced state.

What to do: If you're a baby boomer, you must be tested for hepatitis C—it's that simple. (It also is the recommendation of the Centers for Disease Control and Prevention.)

If you're not a baby boomer, you still should be tested for the hepatitis C virus if you had a blood transfusion before 1989 or if you have a history of intravenous drug use.

The test detects antibodies to the virus. Some people infected with hepatitis C "clear" the virus and are no longer infected—but they still will test positive for antibodies that were formed at the time of the infection. That's why positive antibody tests are followed up with liver scans that can detect cirrhosis, and if you have cirrhosis, you definitely have an active infection. A liver biopsy is the medical "gold standard" for confirming hepatitis C.

If you find out that you're infected, be happy you found out—and don't despair. A few years ago, it was next to impossible to stop chronic hepatitis C from damaging the liver. But in the past few years, the FDA has approved daily drug regimens that can cure hepatitis C, eradicating the virus from the body in more than 90% of cases. The risk of developing liver cancer depends on the damage already done by the virus. But after successful treatment of hepatitis C, the risk decreases with time. If you're diagnosed with hepatitis C, talk to your doctor about the drug regimen that is best for you.

●**Hepatitis B virus.** Infection with hepatitis B is the main cause of liver cancer worldwide, but it is less common in the US, where it causes about 15% of cases.

What to do: As with hepatitis C, most people who are infected with hepatitis B don't know it. You should be tested for hepatitis B if you were born in Asia or Africa, where it is more common…you were never vaccinated for hepatitis B (a standard vaccination in the US)…you had sex with a person known to be infected with hepatitis B…you have an HIV infection…you're on hemodialysis for kidney failure…you are on chemotherapy or another immunosuppressive treatment…or you have ever used recreational drugs intravenously.

If you are infected with hepatitis B, treatment will depend on whether the infection is acute or chronic and the degree of liver damage. Talk to your doctor about the liver-protecting regimen that's right for you.

•**Obesity and diabetes.** The twin US epidemics of obesity and diabetes have led to a third epidemic—nonalcoholic fatty liver disease (NAFLD)—and NAFLD can lead to liver cancer. Obesity, of course, includes excess fat…and in diabetes, excess blood sugar eventually gets stored as excess fat. Fatty liver afflicts an estimated 20% to 30% of American adults, including more than 60% of those who are obese.

What happens: Between 10% and 20% of people with NAFLD develop an even more serious form of fatty liver disease called nonalcoholic *steatohepatitis* (NASH). In NASH, liver cells are inflamed and swollen, and there often is cirrhosis.

Warning: NASH puts you at the same risk for liver cancer as someone with hepatitis C.

What to do: There are no long-term medical therapies that successfully control NASH. But lifestyle changes have proved to both prevent and reverse the condition.

HEALTHY LIVER LIFESTYLE

If you're obese or have diabetes, you probably have NAFLD, and it's possible that you have NASH. Either way, your risk for liver cancer is elevated. Make the following lifestyle changes—starting today.

Note: The same lifestyle changes also are effective for strengthening the liver in people diagnosed with hepatitis C or hepatitis B.

•**Eat a Mediterranean diet.** It's the best dietary approach for managing NAFLD and NASH.

Latest development: A scientific paper in the July 2017 issue of the medical journal *Liver International* declared the Mediterranean diet "the diet of choice" for NAFLD. The paper's authors point out that the diet can reduce fat in the liver even without weight loss…reduces liver inflammation and liver scarring (cirrhosis)…can

prevent or treat diabetes…and is better than a low-fat diet for weight loss. (Losing as little as 7% to 10% of your total body weight can reverse NASH.)

Bottom line: Eat more fruits, vegetables, beans, whole grains, olive oil, nuts and seeds, and fish. Eat less saturated fat from red meat and dairy products, less sugar and less processed food, and drink fewer or no sodas, including diet sodas (which, research shows, increases the craving for sugar).

•**Don't fail to exercise.** The more physically active you are, the less likely it is that you will develop NAFLD.

My recommendation: Go for a brisk walk of 30 minutes at least five days a week—a study shows that this regimen reduces liver fat by up to 43%.

•**If you're drinking coffee, don't stop.** Many studies link coffee intake to a healthier liver.

Standout scientific research: Coffee drinkers have a 40% lower risk for liver cancer than people who don't drink coffee, according to a study published in *Clinical Gastroenterology and Hepatology*. Those who drank the most coffee—three or more cups a day—had a 56% lower risk. The beverage is proved to reduce liver enzymes (a sign of inflammation) and to slow the progression of fibrosis.

•**Consider taking liver-supporting nutritional and herbal supplements.** Scientific studies show that certain nutritional and herbal supplements can decrease liver fat and fibrosis and improve liver function. *Check with your doctor about taking these top three supplements…*

•Omega-3 fatty acids. *Typical dose:* 500 milligrams (mg) to 2,000 mg daily.

•Vitamin E. *Typical dose:* 400 IU, twice daily.

•Silymarin (active ingredient in milk thistle). *Typical dose:* 250 mg, three times daily.

Biopsy Breakthrough—A Simple Blood Draw May Be All That's Needed

Stanley R. Hamilton, MD, head of the division of pathology and laboratory medicine and the Frederick F. Becker Distinguished University Chair in Cancer Research at The University of Texas MD Anderson Cancer Center in Houston.

I n the near future, a vial of blood may be all that's needed to track cancers and make important decisions about chemotherapy and other treatments—without the need for risky and potentially uncomfortable biopsies.

Latest development: Blood tests known as "liquid biopsies" are already used routinely for certain lung cancer patients. The genetic information of other cancers, including melanoma and malignancies of the breast and pancreas, can also be found in a vial of blood.

What you need to know about this new type of biopsy…

AN EASIER TEST

Traditional biopsies, known as tissue biopsies, are a standard part of cancer care. They are done to confirm or rule out a cancer diagnosis…to identify and characterize different types of cancer…and to track cancer changes over time.

With tissue biopsies, small portions of tissue are surgically removed or extracted with a needle and sent to a laboratory for analysis. The procedure comes with the risk for tissue damage, infection or other complications. It's also highly stressful for patients who are already dealing with the challenges of having cancer.

Another drawback: Up to 20% of tumors can't be biopsied at all. They may be located in an inaccessible part of the body or too close to a vital structure (such as an important blood vessel). Or the procedure might be too risky for a patient who's already seriously ill.

With liquid biopsies, all the doctor needs is a blood sample. What information can be gleaned from a vial of blood? When tumor cells die, they cast off small amounts of DNA into the bloodstream. A blood test can analyze the DNA

and map genetic abnormalities that may affect subsequent treatments. The tests can also detect whole tumor cells that malignancies sometimes shed. The cancer cells themselves can be analyzed for important abnormalities that may guide treatment decisions.

WEALTH OF INFORMATION

The genetic information provided by image-guided tissue biopsies and liquid biopsies can be used to tailor treatments for specific cancer patients. Genetic alterations that drive certain cancers can be detected before cancer treatment begins, or they can emerge during therapy or at some time in the future. *Examples of genes that could be detected with either a liquid or tis-*

Nuts to Cancer!

Nuts fight stomach cancer. A study involving 566,000 older adults found that regularly eating nuts and peanut butter was associated with a 27% lower risk for gastric noncardia adenocarcinoma (cancer of the lower stomach), compared with people who reported consuming these foods infrequently.

Possible reason: The beneficial polyphenols, fiber, vitamins and minerals in nuts and peanuts (which are technically legumes).

Christian C. Abnet, PhD, MPH, senior investigator, division of cancer epidemiology and genetics, National Cancer Institute, Bethesda, Maryland.

Tree Nuts Linked to Colon Cancer Survival

Stage-3 colon cancer patients who ate at least one ounce of tree nuts (such as walnuts and almonds) twice a week had a 42% lower chance of cancer returning and a 57% reduced chance for death from the disease, compared with patients who did not eat nuts. No benefit was found from peanuts, which are legumes. All patients studied already had surgery and chemotherapy—diet, including nuts, is not a substitute for standard therapy.

Temidayo Fadelu, MD, a postdoctoral fellow at Dana-Farber Cancer Institute, Boston.

sue biopsy and potentially affect cancer care for certain malignancies...

•**Breast cancer.** About 20% of breast cancer patients have genetic factors that cause them to produce high levels of the HER2 protein. Standard chemotherapy drugs don't work well for these patients, but they often respond to targeted therapy drugs such as *trastuzumab* (Herceptin).

•**Melanoma.** For the 40% to 60% of melanoma patients with a specific mutation of the BRAF gene, targeted therapy drugs such as *vemurafenib* (Zelboraf) are a good choice.

•**Lung cancer.** About 5% of lung cancer patients have a mutation in the ALK gene and may not respond (or may stop responding) to standard chemotherapy. However, these patients often do respond when they are given targeted drugs such as *ceritinib* (Zykadia).

Promising research: Scientists recently used liquid biopsies to identify genetic mutations in patients with colorectal, biliary (related to the bile duct) and other gastrointestinal cancers. They found that nearly 80% of patients who had become resistant to drug therapy had a specific genetic alteration...and about half had multiple genetic mutations. With this information, oncologists will know what treatments to start—or when it's time to switch treatment strategies.

THE RESEARCH

Liquid biopsies are still so new that there's no definitive research on their reliability.

The largest study done so far: Research presented at the 2016 annual meeting of the American Society of Clinical Oncology looked at 15,000 blood samples taken from patients with a variety of cancers. For several hundred of the patients, tissue biopsies were also available. In a head-to-head comparison, the same genetic mutations that appeared in tissue biopsies were also found to be present in the liquid biopsies between 94% and 100% of the time.

More good news: In the same study, the genetic changes were detected in nearly two-thirds of patients and provided critical information for oncologists—when to choose certain drugs, for example, or when to encourage patients to enroll in a genetic abnormalitydirected clinical trial.

WHAT COMES NEXT?

It is too soon to conclude that liquid biopsies will become the new gold standard for identifying and tracking cancer-related gene abnormalities.

The current tests have inherent limitations. Some cancers, particularly those that are small and early stage, don't shed detectable levels of DNA into the blood. A blood test would miss these cancers, but an image-guided tissue biopsy may not.

Expense is another factor. A liquid biopsy can cost more than $5,000. It's covered by some, but not all, insurers. While the test isn't cheap, it might be a bargain compared with some traditional biopsies. A lung cancer tissue biopsy usually costs about $14,000 and has a known rate of complications, including pneumothorax (air in the chest cavity), bleeding and infection. A blood "stick" is much easier—and safer.

GETTING TESTED

The Guardant360, one of the most widely used "liquid biopsies," looks at 73 different genes that could be tied to melanoma as well as lung, breast, colorectal and pancreatic cancers. Since the testing can be done with a routine blood sample, there are no additional risks—and you will be spared the discomfort of a traditional biopsy.

The Right Team to Treat Your Cancer

Richard A. Ehlers II, MD, associate professor, department of breast surgical oncology and associate vice president in the Division of Houston Area Locations at The University of Texas MD Anderson Cancer Center. He is also adjunct assistant professor in the department of surgery at The University of Texas Medical Branch at Galveston.

If you or a loved one is being treated for cancer, you may not be aware of so-called "tumor boards." But if you're getting care at a major academic or cancer-specific medical center, these regular face-to-face gatherings of cancer specialists—oncologists, radiologists, surgeons, pathologists, psychologists and others—play a key role in assessing individual cases. This may involve reviewing the pathology report...tracking disease progression...and discussing the treatment options for different types of cancer.

What gets reviewed: If your case comes before a tumor board, the doctors likely will address a variety of issues. Is surgery an option or will radiation and/or chemotherapy be more appropriate? If surgery can be done, should it or chemotherapy be used first, followed by other treatments? Is this patient battling mental health issues…or getting the runaround from insurance to get coverage for certain drugs?

HOW TUMOR BOARDS HELP

Cancer care is rarely a straightforward process. From the time you are diagnosed until your treatments end, your care will depend on the opinions of a surprising number of specialists—and good communication among those experts can strongly affect how well you do.

Important recent finding: Among nearly 5,000 patients with colorectal and lung cancers, those whose doctors participated in weekly tumor boards lived longer, according to a study presented at a symposium of the American Society of Clinical Oncology.

To ensure that the medical center where you're being treated relies on a tumor board's guidance, you should seek out a cancer center designated by the National Cancer Institute or accredited by the Commission on Cancer.

Large cancer centers usually have separate tumor boards for different types of cancer. At smaller programs, a single board will review all or most cancer cases.

Tumor boards provide important oversight because what seems like a perfect treatment plan can fall short in real-world circumstances. For example, chemotherapy might be the recommended treatment for a specific cancer, but a tumor-board oncologist might argue that a particular patient isn't healthy enough to withstand the treatment. A psychologist or social worker at a meeting might point out that the patient will need transportation to and from the chemotherapy clinic.

WHO GETS REVIEWED?

At MD Anderson Cancer Center and other large cancer centers, virtually all cases are discussed at a tumor board, although doctors give most of their attention to rare/complicated cases. There's no separate charge to patients for the review.

My advice: If you're not sure that your case has been discussed at your treatment center's tumor board, ask your doctor whether it has been (or will be). Your doctor should not be offended by this question—especially if he/she will be presenting the case. If your case hasn't been reviewed, ask why not. You have the right to request a tumor board review, but it might not be available at a smaller medical center.

Most tumor boards meet weekly or twice a month and are comprised of a dozen or more specialists, including surgeons, medical oncologists, radiation oncologists and pathologists. Depending on the cancer, other doctors—gynecologists, urologists, etc.—may participate. Meetings often include a nutritionist, nurses, mental health experts and a social worker.

THE BENEFITS

Your case might go before a tumor board prior to treatment…after a preliminary treatment plan has been initiated…or during treatment when there is an important change in clinical circumstances.

Important finding: When the records of more than 200 pancreatic cancer patients collected from various institutions without tumor boards were later evaluated by a panel at Johns Hopkins University School of Medicine that included medical and radiation oncologists, surgical oncologists, pathologists and other experts, treatment changes were recommended in nearly 25% of these cases.

Research also shows that patients tend to have better outcomes in terms of treatment responsiveness, recovery times and survival, among other factors, when their cases are discussed at a tumor board.

Also: Patients whose cases are reviewed are more likely to be guided to a clinical trial—one that their primary oncologist might not be aware of. Many cancer patients are eligible for these trials, which provide excellent care…yet only about 3% of patients ever participate. The more patients there are enrolled, the more quickly important clinical questions can be answered.

The National Cancer Institute website lists thousands of clinical trials that are looking for participants—to compare drug treatments, study new surgical techniques or radiation treatments, etc. Most tumor boards have a "checklist," which includes the question of whether there is a trial for which the patient might be eligible.

THE PERSONAL TOUCH

The services provided by tumor boards go beyond the nuts and bolts of treatment. For example, many cancer patients lose weight during chemotherapy or radiation treatments. If poor nutrition is threatening your recovery—or even your ability to continue treatments, a nutritionist might recommend nutritional counseling, or even help you find a free meal service in your area.

Many cancer patients suffer from mental health issues—depression, bipolar disorder, etc. The best cancer plan won't help if you're unable (or unwilling) to continue treatments. A tumor board will attempt to address—or correct—all the issues that can affect how well or poorly you respond to treatments.

Patients don't typically attend tumor boards. Many different cases are reviewed at any one meeting. The presence of a patient would affect the confidentiality of others' personal health information.

Got Cancer? Protect Your Heart from Harmful Therapies

Anju Nohria, MD, director of the Cardio-Oncology Program at Dana-Farber/Brigham and Women's Cancer Center in Boston. Dr. Nohria is also a cardiovascular medicine specialist at Brigham and Women's Hospital, an assistant professor of medicine at Harvard Medical School and the author of more than 60 peer-reviewed articles. BrighamAndWomens.org

First, the good news: Thanks to advancements in prevention, detection and treatment, the overall number of cancer deaths has been significantly reduced.

Now, some bad news: For some patients, this success comes at a high cost—many cancer treatments are considered cardiotoxic, meaning they can damage the heart.

In fact, 99% of 303 oncologists included in a 2017 study published in the *International Journal of Cardiology* said that they prescribe cardiotoxic therapies.

While these are among the most effective treatments for cancer, they can cause dangerous heart conditions such as high blood pressure (hypertension), heart failure, arrhythmia and more…or make preexisting conditions worse—either during treatment or years later.

PROTECTING YOUR HEART

The risk for heart damage from these treatments depends on such factors as the type of treatment and dose…the location of the cancer…and the patient's age, preexisting cardiac risk and overall health status.

When developing a treatment plan for cancer, an oncologist should carefully weigh the risks and rewards of treatments that are considered to be cardiotoxic and discuss this in detail with his/her patient.

Cancer therapies that have been shown to have negative effects on the heart—and how to protect yourself…

•**Anthracyclines,** such as *doxorubicin* (Adriamycin) and *epirubicin* (Ellence). This class of chemotherapeutic drugs, commonly used to treat lymphoma, ovarian cancer and breast cancer, kills cancer cells by damaging their DNA. However, in the process of attacking the cancer, these drugs can weaken the heart, increasing the risk for heart failure. About 9% of patients taking an anthracycline medication will experience a weakening of the heart muscle known as cardiomyopathy. Cardiomyopathy tends to occur within the first year after treatment but may not manifest for 10 to 20 years.

To protect your heart: Your oncologist should check for cardiomyopathy with a baseline echocardiogram (ultrasound of the heart) prior to anthracycline chemotherapy, and again within one year of completing treatment. If cardiomyopathy is caught early, heart medication, such as a beta-blocker combined with an ACE inhibitor, can be started. New research suggests that this drug combination may have a protective effect on a patient's heart during cancer treatment. Ask your doctor if this strategy is right for you.

•**Radiation.** Radiation to the chest—especially the left side, where the heart is—can damage the blood vessels that bring blood to the heart, the heart valves and the heart muscle, contributing to coronary artery disease, heart failure and arrhythmia. Thanks to advancements in targeted radiation (radiating only the tumor, not the entire chest), the risk of having a heart issue after radiation is lower than ever. Still, many patients who have had radiation will experience cardiac issues sometime in the 40 years following treatment. For this reason, the effect is more concerning for younger cancer patients than older patients.

To protect your heart: If you have had radiation treatment to the chest, see your cardiologist or internist annually for a thorough physical aand make sure that any cardiovascular risk factors you might have—such as hypertension, diabetes and/or excess weight—are addressed.

My advice: Ten years after radiation treatment, have an echocardiogram and stress test, repeating these tests every five to 10 years, or sooner if you're experiencing any of the cardiac symptoms mentioned on page 53.

•*Trastuzumab* **(Herceptin).** This cancer medication, used to treat more aggressive breast cancers (HER2-positive, specifically), causes weakening of the heart muscle, typically during treatment. Thirteen percent of patients taking trastuzumab plus an anthracycline drug experience heart issues. Most at risk are those who have a prior history of cardiac risk factors such as hypertension and diabetes and those who are over age 65.

To protect your heart: You'll need an echocardiogram before and after treatment, and possibly during treatment as well, to check for warning signs. Fortunately, cardiomyopathy caused by this drug tends to be reversible—if your oncologist notices any problems, he/she can halt treatment, begin medication such as a beta-blocker and ACE inhibitor to help heal the heart, then restart trastuzumab.

Important: Recent research suggests that taking a combination of trastuzumab and an anthracycline along with a blood pressure drug

called *candesartan* (Atacand) successfully treats early breast cancer while protecting the patient's heart. And a new study indicates that women with early, localized breast cancer can now take trastuzumab for just nine weeks instead of the customary year with the same anticancer effect but much less cardiotoxicity.

•**Tyrosine kinase inhibitors,** such as *bevacizumab* (Avastin) and *sunitinib* (Sutent). These newer cancer medications, used to treat kidney, esophageal, stomach and colon cancers, block a receptor required for new blood vessel formation, starving tumors of blood needed for growth. That's bad news for tumors and for the heart, which needs a steady blood supply to thrive. Because of this, 20% to 60% of patients taking a tyrosine kinase inhibitor will experience hypertension during treatment and, in some cases, cardiomyopathy and heart failure.

To protect your heart: Your oncologist will monitor your blood pressure throughout treatment with this drug, adding blood pressure medication if necessary. No echocardiogram is needed. Once treatment is complete, your blood pressure usually returns to normal.

Note: Patients who have a preexisting heart condition or cardiac issues while receiving these therapies should get treated at a cardio-oncology program or see a cardio-oncology specialist. To find one near you, check with your oncologist.

Better Colon Cancer Testing

One in six colorectal cancer patients diagnosed before age 50 has a mutation in one or more of 25 cancer-susceptibility genes that may be helpful in determining optimal treatment and possible risk for other malignancies, such as breast cancer, according to a new study of 450 patients.

New recommendation: Use of multigene testing in all early-onset colon cancer patients—even if they have no family history of the disease. The testing may also signal whether other family members could be at risk.

Heather Hampel, MS, LGS, The Ohio State University Wexner Medical Center, Columbus.

Watch out for: Anyone receiving cardiotoxic cancer therapy who has symptoms such as shortness of breath, chest pain, difficulty breathing when walking or lying down or changes in heart rhythm should alert his/her doctor.

Note: Many cardiotoxic effects cannot be felt by the patient, so vigilant monitoring of cardiac function during (and sometimes after) treatment is also vital.

Common Heart Drug Can Treat a Rare Cancer

Brad Bryan, PhD, biomedical scientist, Texas Tech University Health Sciences Center, El Paso, and leader of a study of propranolol, published in *JAMA Dermatology*.

Propranolol, available in generic form for about $4 a month, has been shown effective in treating soft tissue sarcoma, a rare cancer with only a 40% survival rate. Prescription drugs for sarcoma can cost more than $10,000 a month. The European Commission has granted propranolol orphan drug designation, recognizing its treatment value even though it is not officially labeled for sarcoma treatment.

Nail Salon Caution

Elizabeth K. Hale, MD, senior vice president, The Skin Cancer Foundation, New York City.

Lamps used in nail salons to dry nails—both the ultraviolet (UV) lamps and the LED—emit UV radiation. These lamps predominately produce UVA rays, which have been linked to both premature skin aging (such as age spots and wrinkling) as well as skin cancer. Still, they present only a moderate UV risk—far lower than using a tanning bed, for example.

While using nail lamps occasionally is not a cause for alarm, you should minimize UV exposure whenever you can. It's best to let nails air-dry. However, if you're getting a gel manicure, the nail lamp is necessary. Protect your hands by applying sunscreen 20 minutes before using the lamp, but keep sunscreen off your nails, as it could interfere with polish application. Keep in mind that nails will still be unprotected (squamous cell carcinoma is often found underneath the nail plate). For that reason, keep gel manicures to a minimum.

For the Very Best Cancer Care

Charles B. Inlander is a consumer advocate and health-care consultant based in Fogelsville, Pennsylvania. He was the founding president of the nonprofit People's Medical Society, a consumer advocacy organization credited with key improvements in the quality of US health care, and is the author or coauthor of more than 20 consumer-health books.

Hospitals—especially the bigger regional medical centers—are in an all-out war for your business. Whether it's in a TV ad or on a billboard, there are images of white-coated doctors with headlines suggesting that you can get world-class medical care right near your home. It's a powerful claim and, in many instances, may be true. But for certain conditions—particularly cancer—you should do a lot of homework before you commit to your local medical center for care.

Diagnosing and treating cancer is complicated and often requires the expertise of several specialists, such as a surgeon, radiologist, oncologist, pathologist and others, who are highly trained in cancer care. These specialists need to work as a team to make sure that your care is coordinated from the minute you enter the system throughout the ongoing follow-ups that all cancer patients need. Spending on cancer care will reach up to $207 billion by 2020—far more than what it was in 2010. As a result, hospitals all around the country see this as a massive revenue stream and are erecting new buildings that they're calling "cancer centers." But there are no established guidelines for these cancer centers. *To get the best possible cancer care for yourself or a family member...*

•**Seek out an NCI-Designated Cancer Center.** The National Cancer Institute, the federal government's world-renowned agency overseeing research and care strictly related to cancer, has chosen 69 programs in 35 states and the District of Columbia as NCI-Designated Cancer Centers. Most of these programs are affiliated with major teaching hospitals and medical schools, although some are freestanding cancer centers. Hospitals and medical centers must apply for the designation and demonstrate that they meet a set of standards established by the NCI and must undergo regular reviews. NCI-Designated Cancer Centers not only have the resources needed to provide the highest quality in diagnosis and treatment but also are the sites where most clinical trials originate and are coordinated. This is especially important for people with advanced cancers or otherwise hard-to-treat malignancies.

To find an NCI-Designated Cancer Center: Go to Cancer.gov and search for "NCI-Designated Cancer Centers." Or call the NCI at 800-4-Cancer.

•**Look for an affiliated hospital.** If you can't travel to an NCI-Designated Cancer Center or your insurance plan will not pay for it, seek out the nearest local facility that has an affiliation with one of these cancer centers. Highly regarded facilities, such as New York's Memorial Sloan Kettering, have made affiliations with top-notch regional medical centers, allowing certain local medical facilities to communicate with some of the most renowned specialists and access to many clinical trials not normally made available to local hospitals. To find out if your local medical center has such an affiliation, call and speak to someone in the oncology department.

•**Look for experience.** Not all cancer care needs to be provided at an NCI-Designated Cancer Center or even an affiliated program. Many early-stage or slow-growing cancers, such as most prostate and even some breast cancers, can be treated by local physicians who have a history of successful care handling your specific type of cancer over a period of several years. Ask your family doctor for a referral based on his/her experience with similar cases.

Cancer Links

B-vitamins linked to lung cancer in men. The lung cancer risk for male smokers taking the highest daily doses of B-6 (20 milligrams a day for years) was three times that of men who did not take the vitamin. The lung cancer risk for those taking high doses of B-12 (more than 55 micrograms a day) almost quadrupled.

Possible reason: The vitamins may hasten the development of lung cancer in male smokers who already have the disease at a subclinical level. There was no sign of increased risk in women taking high doses of the vitamins.

Theodore M. Brasky, PhD, research assistant professor in the department of internal medicine at The Ohio State University Comprehensive Cancer Center, Columbus.

Gum disease linked to cancer. Postmenopausal women with a history of periodontal disease have a 14% higher risk for any cancer—and a risk for esophageal cancer three times higher than that in women without gum disease. Periodontal disease also is associated with a higher risk for lung, breast and gallbladder cancers and melanoma. The study did not prove cause and effect, but it is known that periodontal disease can cause general inflammation, which increases risk for cancer.

Jean Wactawski-Wende, PhD, is dean of the School of Public Health and Health Professions, department of epidemiology and environmental health, University at Buffalo, New York.

Many Expensive Cancer Drugs Are Useless (or Worse)

Diana Zuckerman, PhD, president, National Center for Health Research and the Cancer Prevention and Treatment Fund, Washington, DC

First comes the shock of a cancer diagnosis. *Then comes the flurry of questions:* Is there a cure? Is there a treatment? What drug do I take? Will it work?

Sometimes the answers are easy to find. People with chronic myeloid leukemia, for example, can take *imatinib* (Gleevec) and have an 80% chance of surviving for 10 years.

But other cancer patients aren't so lucky. They may be given an option of taking a chemotherapy medication that won't help them live longer—and that will make their lives more miserable in the bargain.

This is especially true of the spate of cancer therapies that have come on the market in the last 10 years, according to recent studies. Despite these new drugs, cancer deaths for men and women decreased by just approximately 1% from 2004 to 2013, according to the National Cancer Institute.

We asked Diana Zuckerman, PhD, president of the National Center for Health Research, a nonprofit organization in Washington, DC, to explain why many new cancer medications have so few benefits…and what you or your loved ones can do to get the treatment you need and deserve—at a reasonable cost.

RUSHING CANCER DRUGS TO MARKET

One big reason these drugs aren't very effective is a sped-up approval schedule that puts many new cancer drugs in the hands of patients before they've been thoroughly vetted.

Consider this: From 2002 to 2014, the Food and Drug Administration (FDA) approved 71 drugs for a variety of types of cancer—but fewer than half of these drugs have been shown to extend patients' lives by at least two-and-a-half months, the minimum standard. Many of them came with hefty price tags of more than $10,000 a month. For some of these chemo drugs, the story is even worse—they didn't improve survival at all. As if that weren't bad enough, some of these new drugs have side effects that are as dangerous as the cancer they are supposed to treat.

How did this happen? In the quest to get potentially lifesaving medications to people who desperately need them, the FDA approves drugs before the information about their real benefits has been determined. Two-thirds of these drugs were approved because they showed some evidence that they might work, such as shrinking the tumor in the first few months, but without any evidence that they helped patients live longer.

While stopping tumor growth or reversing it is a promising sign, physicians know that it can be temporary and sometimes followed by rapid tumor growth. In some cases, the treatment is so toxic that it kills healthy cells in addition to cancer cells and the patient may die sooner or with terrible side effects. Nevertheless, pharmaceutical companies prefer to measure the effect on tumor growth because the results can be measured months or even years sooner than overall survival.

But that's a mistake. If you have cancer, you're probably more interested in living longer than in simply avoiding death from cancer. For example, if the drug you take causes liver toxicity or a stroke that can kill you before the cancer would, it's not doing you any good.

NOT ALL DRUGS GET FOLLOW-UP STUDIES

When drugs are approved only on the basis of the way cancerous tumors respond, the FDA usually requires follow-up studies to prove that the drugs are truly beneficial, such as helping patients live longer or improving their quality of life for the weeks, months or years that they have left.

That process makes sense—as long as the FDA enforces it.

Example: In 2008, *bevacizumab* (Avastin) was approved to treat metastatic breast cancer because studies showed that it improved progression-free survival (how much time the patient lives with breast cancer without the disease getting worse). Later research showed that the drug offered no survival benefit and it came with an increased risk for heart attacks and strokes, among other harmful and debilitating side effects. In 2011, the FDA revoked the drug's approval for breast cancer. That follow-up decision has helped breast cancer patients avoid an expensive, ineffective drug, although thousands of breast cancer patients took the drug between 2008 and 2011.

Unfortunately, that's a rare example. Between 2008 and 2012, 36 out of 54 cancer drugs were approved on the basis of tumor shrinkage and similar preliminary measures. Later studies showed that only five of those 36 drugs improved overall survival. Eighteen of the drugs proved unable to improve survival, and there's no information about the final 13 because they either haven't been tested or the results haven't been reported.

Yet all these drugs are still on the market. One reason is that postapproval studies that could result in removing a drug from the marketplace are very difficult to conduct.

Example: It is difficult to conclusively prove whether these cancer drugs are effective because patients are less willing to participate in further clinical trials on a drug that's already been approved.

The problem may get worse. The FDA is currently evaluating ways to overhaul its processes and speed up approval of all types of drugs, including cancer treatments, in its effort to get life-saving drugs on the market faster.

LITTLE CONSIDERATION FOR QUALITY OF LIFE

A drug that increases a cancer patient's well-being and comfort is also considered worthy of FDA approval even in cases where living longer is not likely. But a recent study published in JAMA Internal Medicine looked closely at 18 drugs that had no survival benefit to see what effect they had on patients' quality of life. The majority of the drugs either contributed to a worse quality of life—for example, patients suffered from diarrhea, fatigue, sleep disturbances or memory loss—or the evidence was mixed (which means the research was inconclusive, with some studies suggesting that treatment was helpful and other studies suggesting it was harmful).

Some of the worst offenders included…

•*Bendamustine* (**Treanda**). The drug is approved for non-Hodgkin lymphoma and chronic lymphocytic leukemia.

Cost: $53,000 to $85,000 a year, depending on diagnosis.

Results: Research shows that patients taking this drug for either condition do not live longer, even though it is FDA approved for these patients. The drug does not improve quality of life for leukemia and no studies were done to show whether it improves quality of life for patients with lymphoma.

•*Cabozantinib* (**Cometriq**). The drug is approved for thyroid cancer.

Cost: Nearly $170,000 a year.

Results: Even though it is FDA approved for these patients, research shows those who take this drug do not live longer. It makes patients' quality of life worse, usually due to diarrhea, fatigue, nausea and other unpleasant side effects.

•*Everolimus* (**Afinitor**). The drug is approved for kidney, breast and pancreatic cancer.

Cost: Nearly $145,000 a year.

Results: Research shows that this drug does not help patients with kidney, breast or pancreatic cancer live longer, although it is FDA approved for them. There is no clear evidence that it improves quality of life for these patients, either.

•*Peginterferon* (**PEG-Intron**). The drug is approved for melanoma.

Cost: $26,000 a year.

Results: Research shows that this drug does not help patients with melanoma live longer. It makes their quality of life worse. Some of its scarier and more common side effects include anxiety, depression, bloody diarrhea, difficulty breathing, vision loss, stroke and life-threatening infections.

MAKING THE RIGHT TREATMENT CHOICES

A cancer diagnosis is stressful under any circumstances, but if your cancer doesn't respond to standard treatments, the choices get tougher. The choice is always the patient's—for some people, living another two months is worth possible side effects. But there is no excuse for chemotherapy that won't help extend life and makes you more miserable in the final days.

Unfortunately, you can't always count on your doctor to help you sort through the options. Many doctors will list all the drugs out there because they want you to have a say in your own care. They also assume that FDA approval means that the advantages outweigh the dangers and may not realize that the studies are inconclusive.

To make an informed decision, though, you need to know the benefits and risks of the medications that are being offered. *Here's how…*

•**Ask your doctor specific questions.** Will this drug help me live longer, or will it just cause the tumor to shrink? What are the side effects and how dangerous or unpleasant are they? If you don't get answers, ask your health-care provider to do some research and give you a summary of the results. Then do some digging on your own.

• **Use reputable sources for your research.** Google searches can send you straight to a misleading advertisement for a drug as well as other misinformation from a variety of sources. Go to Drugs.com instead, where you'll find the proven risks and benefits of each medication. Look for the sections on risks, side effects, adverse events and contraindications to find out what the problems might be. Check what the drug has been approved to treat. For example, some treatments used for prostate cancer are FDA approved to treat prostate "problems" or "health" but are not proven to treat prostate cancer.

You might also search on Google Scholar or PubMed to find journal articles written by scientists and medical experts who have studied the treatment you are considering. Again, read carefully to see whether there is any evidence that the drug improves "overall survival." If the drug improves "progression-free survival," that doesn't mean patients live longer.

• **Get impartial help.** The Cancer Prevention and Treatment Fund, the primary project of the National Center for Health Research, offers a no-cost cancer help hotline to help patients sift through their choices. This organization doesn't accept any funds from companies that make any medical treatments. Send an email to info@stopcancerfund.org with the type of cancer treatment you're considering, and someone will reply with relevant and meaningful information that can help you make a smart decision.

Radiation Alternative for Lung Cancer

Paula Mulvenna, MBBS, consultant clinical oncologist, The Newcastle upon Tyne Hospitals, UK.

Patients with non-small cell lung cancer that metastasized to the brain who had traditional treatment—whole-brain radiation—had similar survival rates as those who had steroids to reduce swelling but no radiation.

If lung cancer has spread to your brain: Ask your physician if other therapies, such as stereotactic radiation and/or a targeted drug regimen, would be better than whole-brain radiation.

Cancer "Restaging"

Sunil M. Patel, MD, oncologist/hematologist and associate professor, University of Texas MD Anderson Cancer Center, Houston.

According to most textbooks, a tumor is staged only once, at the time of diagnosis. A patient who's initially found to have a stage II tumor, for example, will always be a stage II patient, even if the cancer progresses over time.

But in real life, oncologists often restage tumors based on a patient's response to treatment. This is a bit of a misnomer, as this reevaluation typically does not result in a new stage assignment but simply identifies whether the treatment is working. "Restaging" is typically accomplished through physical exam and imaging, and the oncologist uses these results to guide treatment.

Fighting Cancer Fatigue? Timing Is Everything

Study titled, "Comparison of Pharmaceutical, Psychological, and Exercise Treatments for Cancer-related Fatigue," by researchers at University of Rochester Medical Center, Rochester, New York, published in *JAMA Oncology*.

If you suffer from cancer-related fatigue, an oh-so-common experience, your doctor might prescribe medications to help you… such as the antidepressant *paroxetine*…the narcolepsy drug *modafinil*…the steroid *methylprednisolone*…the ADHD drugs *methylphenidate hydrochloride* or *dextroamphetamine*. Yes, that last one is an amphetamine, which you might expect would give you a burst of energy short-term but wouldn't help with long-term cancer-related fatigue (CRF). Right you are!

In fact, prescription drugs in general are the least effective treatments for this debilitating condition, finds the largest meta-analysis of studies ever conducted on the topic.

Good news: The new analysis found that exercise, along with specific kinds of psychological therapy, work to treat cancer-related fatigue much better than any medication. But timing is key. One approach works better during treatment…another once the surgery, radiation and/or chemotherapy are done.

Background: More than half of cancer patients experience some degree of fatigue—which can be severe. That terrible tiredness can exacerbate depression, sleep problems and pain. At its worst, cancer fatigue is a crushing sensation that's often not relieved by rest and can persist for months or even years.

It is believed that cancer fatigue could be the result of a chronic state of inflammation induced by the disease or its treatment. This fatigue may decrease a person's chances of survival because it lessens the likelihood that he/she will have the energy or the desire to complete medical treatments. That's why the National Cancer Institute clinical oncology research program has named cancer fatigue a top research priority.

Study: Researchers at the Wilmot Cancer Institute at University of Rochester analyzed the outcomes of 113 studies that tested various treatments for cancer fatigue—exercise, psychological therapy, exercise-plus-psychological therapy and pharmaceutical medications. All the studies were randomized clinical trials, the gold standard for evaluating treatments. More than 11,000 patients were involved across these studies. Nearly half were women with breast cancer, and 10 studies focused only on men.

Finding: While there's no miracle cure, exercise alone—either aerobic or strength or a combination—was the most effective at relieving cancer fatigue. Psychological counseling, especially cognitive behavioral therapy (CBT)—already established as an effective way to improve sleep—came in a close second. What was definitive was that drugs for treating cancer fatigue don't work very well.

Surprising finding: Studies that delivered a combination of exercise and psychological therapy had mixed results—some of these combination approaches were more effective than either exercise or therapy alone, but some were less effective. When the researchers took a deeper

Healing Garden

A gardening program helps cancer survivors adopt healthier lifestyles. In a study, Master Gardeners mentored cancer survivors to set up vegetable gardens. Compared with non-gardening people, participants ate more vegetables, gained fewer inches and had improved self-worth. Search online for "cooperative extension" plus your zip code to see if there are gardening classes for cancer survivors nearby.

Wendy Demark-Wahnefried, PhD, RD, is professor of nutrition sciences at University of Alabama at Birmingham.

dive, they discovered that timing plays a role—exercise and counseling each seemed to be more effective at a different stage of treatment…

Exercise by itself was most effective during primary treatment, when a patient is undergoing surgery followed by radiation or chemotherapy or both. (Exercise can also make certain cancer treatments more effective, according to other research.)

Psychological intervention such as CBT, either by itself or in combination with exercise, conferred the most advantage once primary treatment had ended. While the researchers offered no definitive explanations, they did note that it can be overwhelming to commit the time to regular therapy sessions plus exercise when you're already going through treatment. Once it's over, a problem-solving approach such as CBT can help you take the steps that help you deal with emotions, fit in exercise, get better sleep and overcome obstacles to taking better care of yourself.

Bottom line: Medications shouldn't be the first thing your doctor recommends for cancer fatigue—far from it. Cancer patients already take a lot of medications that all come with risks and side effects, and any time you can eliminate a drug from the list it's a good thing.

Instead, talk to your doctor about getting help with an exercise counselor trained in working with cancer patients. Ask about CBT as well.

CHAPTER 4

Cardiovascular Disease

5 Surprising Ways to Prevent a Heart Attack

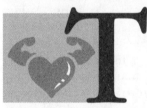There are hopeful signs that Americans are increasingly embracing a heart-healthy lifestyle. The percentage of smokers has plunged to approximately 15% over the last decade. Many people are eating better and doing a better job of controlling high blood pressure and elevated cholesterol.

But despite these gains, cardiovascular disease still accounts for one out of three deaths in the US. Much of the blame goes to the obvious culprits that fuel heart disease—cigarette smoking, elevated blood cholesterol, high blood pressure, obesity, diabetes and a lack of exercise, to name a few. But others might surprise you.

SMALL CHANGES COUNT

Research shows that our daily habits account for 40% to 50% of all deaths caused by cardio-vascular disease. The good news is that even small lifestyle choices may offer big benefits. Five little things you can do to reduce heart attack risk…

SECRET #1: **Avoid secondhand smoke.** Most people associate secondhand smoke with lung disease—but the danger to the heart is worse than you may realize.

Here's why: Exposure to cigarette smoke—from smoking yourself or from secondhand smoke—increases arterial inflammation and impairs the ability of arteries to dilate and constrict normally. It also makes blood more likely to coagulate, the major cause of heart attacks.

If you live with an indoor smoker or spend time in other smoke-filled environments, your risk for a heart attack is 30% higher than in someone without this exposure. Cities (and

Barry A. Franklin, PhD, director of preventive cardiology and cardiac rehabilitation at William Beaumont Hospital, Royal Oak, Michigan. Dr. Franklin has served as president of the American Association of Cardiovascular and Pulmonary Rehabilitation and the American College of Sports Medicine. He is also coeditor of *The Heart-Healthy Handbook*, available at HealthyLearning.com.

countries) that have adopted public-smoking bans have reported reductions in heart attacks of 20% to 40%—with most of the reductions occurring in nonsmokers.

SECRET #2: **Know your family genes.** If you have inherited gene variants known to increase the risk for heart disease, your risk of developing coronary disease and having a cardiac event is higher than you probably think. In an important new study, researchers from Massachusetts General Hospital followed more than 55,000 participants for up to 20 years, analyzing genetic variants and lifestyle data.

Conclusion: People with a genetic predisposition for heart disease had nearly double the risk of developing it themselves.

But bad genes don't have to be destiny. The same study found that people who made positive changes in two or three out of four common areas known to negatively impact heart health—smoking, obesity, lack of regular exercise and an unhealthful diet—were able to reduce their cardiovascular risks by nearly 50%.

SECRET #3: **Get a flu shot.** The flu can be deadly, yet fewer than half of at-risk Americans (including those with chronic health conditions, such as cardiovascular and/or lung disease) get an annual vaccination.

Why it matters: The fever, dehydration and pneumonia that often accompany the flu can be devastating for people who have cardiovascular disease. The flu can worsen preexisting conditions such as heart failure or diabetes or trigger an asthma attack or heart attack in some people.

A 2013 *JAMA* study that looked at more than 6,700 patients (mean age, 67 years) found that those who got a flu vaccination were 36% less likely to suffer cardiovascular events (such as heart attacks) during the following year than those who weren't vaccinated. When researchers looked only at patients who had recent cardiac events, they found that vaccination cut the risk by 55%.

Recommended: An annual flu shot for everyone age 50 or older…and for anyone who has been diagnosed with cardiovascular disease. Adults age 65 and older should discuss the pros and cons of the high-dose flu vaccine with their physicians—it's reported to be about

24% more effective than standard vaccines but may have greater side effects.

SECRET #4: **Don't stop taking a beta-blocker drug abruptly.** Used for treating high blood pressure, irregular heartbeats, rapid heart rates and many other conditions, beta-blockers are among the most commonly prescribed drugs in the US.

Drugs in this class—*propranolol* (such as Inderal), *atenolol* (Tenormin) and many others—are generally safe but may cause side effects including fatigue, light-headedness and even impotence. As a result, patients sometimes decide on their own to stop taking these drugs.

The danger: If these drugs are suddenly stopped, the patient can have a dangerous upsurge in adrenaline activity, which can cause a faster heart rate, heavy sweating, spikes in blood pressure and an increased risk for heart attack and stroke. People who want to stop taking a beta-blocker are advised to slowly decrease the dose over 10 to 14 days.

Important: If you believe that you need to stop taking any prescribed medication, be sure to first check with your doctor. If side effects are a problem, you can probably switch to another drug or a dose that's easier to tolerate.

Secret #5: **Lower your resting pulse.** When you increase your heart rate during aerobic exercise, you're helping to prevent a heart attack or stroke—this signifies that you're getting the cardiovascular benefits of moderate-to-vigorous exercise. Paradoxically, a slower resting heart rate is also protective.

Here's why: In general, a slower resting rate means a longer life—probably because a slower heart rate exerts less stress on blood vessel walls. Studies have shown that healthy men and women with lower resting heart rates (less than 60 beats per minute) have fewer cardiac events and a lower risk of dying from cardiovascular disease than those with faster rates (greater than 80 beats per minute).

A study of heart patients taking beta-blockers found that each 10-beat reduction in resting heart rate reduced the risk for cardiac death by 30%. For example, if someone with a resting heart rate of 80 beats per minute is given a beta-blocker to slow the rate to 60, the risk for cardiac death will drop by 60%.

Recommended: A resting heart rate of 50 to 70, depending on your cardiac history and typical physical activity level. Regular exercise…quitting smoking…maintaining a healthy weight…and avoiding high doses of caffeine can slow the resting heart rate.

Also important: Your recovery heart rate, the time that it takes your pulse to approach its resting rate after exercise. The fitter you get, the more quickly your heartbeat will return to a resting rate.

Being a Sports Fan Can Kill You…and Other Surprising Heart Attack Triggers

Gregory S. Thomas, MD, MPH, medical director for the MemorialCare Heart & Vascular Institute at MemorialCare Long Beach Medical Center in California and clinical professor at University of California, Irvine.

When health experts calculate the likelihood of someone having a heart attack, they typically look at well-known risk factors including high blood pressure, smoking, a sedentary lifestyle and a family history of early heart disease.

What most people don't realize: There are "secret" or little-known risk factors for heart attack that most people (including most doctors) ignore. Many of these factors are as risky as the well-known ones above. *Here are the secret risk factors for a heart attack…*

AN INTENSE SPORTS LOSS

Researchers in Los Angeles tracked causes of death in the counties or states of teams playing in the "high drama" 2008 and 2009 Super Bowls—the New York Giants beating the New England Patriots (Massachusetts) in 2008…and the Pittsburgh Steelers beating the Arizona Cardinals in 2009. The researchers found that in the eight days starting on the day of New England's loss, the number of deaths from heart disease in Massachusetts was 24% higher than it had been after previous Super Bowls…and in the eight days starting on the day of Pittsburgh's win, the number of deaths from heart disease in the Pittsburgh area was 31% lower than it had been after previous Super Bowls. Meanwhile, in Arizona, where researchers had established that fan fervor for the home-state team was significantly lower than in Massachusetts and Pittsburgh, there was little difference in the rate of heart disease deaths after the team's loss. (Data could not be obtained from New York City.)

The disappointment of a losing game after fervently rooting for a team is a form of emotional stress, which can trigger heart attacks—possibly because stress hormones increase heart rate and blood pressure and make blood more likely to clot. (The researchers didn't theorize about what caused the decrease in the death rate in Pittsburgh after its win.)

But forlorn fans aren't the only folks whose hearts are harmed by emotional stress. Research shows that other events that cause emotional stress—holidays such as Christmas and New Year's…a nearby natural disaster…daily problems at work…or the recent death of a spouse—increase the risk for heart attacks. So does the emotional stress of acute anger, chronic hostility and pessimism.

Smart strategy: The risk from emotional stress can be dramatically reduced by regular exercise (see next page).

AIR POLLUTION

Tiny particles of air pollution—congealed specks of floating carbon, metals and other "particulate" substances that emanate from exhaust pipes, industrial smokestacks and coal-fired power plants—cause heart attacks. In fact, in a scientific statement released in 2010, the American Heart Association said that just hours of exposure to these particulates can trigger heart attacks and that long-term exposure increases risk even more.

The people most at risk for heart attacks from air pollution have other risk factors for heart disease—they are over age 60, overweight, have diabetes and/or have had a previous heart attack or stroke. But years of exposure to air pollution can increase the risk for heart attack for any senior.

Scientific evidence: A new study published in *Environmental Research* shows that even a few years of low exposure to air pollution in a city increased the risk of developing heart disease in older people by more than 20%.

Bottom line: Make air pollution less risky to your heart by working with your doctor to reduce other risk factors such as being overweight or having high blood pressure, high LDL cholesterol and high blood sugar.

Also, know when the air is unhealthy, and stay indoors at those times.

Resource: AirNow.gov, which displays daily air-quality levels across the US.

Eat fatty fish two to three times a week or take a daily fish oil supplement for the omega-3 fatty acids.

New research: Harvard Medical School scientists found that boosting blood levels of omega-3s can prevent the artery-damaging inflammation caused by air pollution.

MARIJUANA

In a study of nearly 4,000 people published in *Circulation*, researchers found that smoking marijuana caused a five-fold increased risk for heart attack during the first hour after smoking. In a similar study of nearly 2,000 people published in *American Heart Journal*, those who used marijuana weekly or more often had four times the risk for heart attack and nearly double the risk of dying from heart disease, versus people who didn't use marijuana at all.

Reason: The autonomic nervous system controls your heart's activity, and marijuana delivers a one-two punch to both parts of the autonomic nervous system. It stimulates the sympathetic nervous system, speeding up heart rate and raising blood pressure (making a heart attack more likely)…while suppressing the heart- and artery-relaxing parasympathetic nervous system (also putting you at greater risk for a heart attack).

Bottom line: Avoid using recreational marijuana if you have risk factors for heart disease. If you're using it medicinally, discuss the risk with your doctor.

ERECTILE DYSFUNCTION

Heart attacks occur when people develop atherosclerosis—a blockage of one or more coronary arteries by cholesterol-ridden arterial plaque. And one common sign that an older man has such blockage is erectile dysfunction (ED)—a problem often caused by a blockage of blood flow to blood vessels in the penis.

Compelling scientific evidence: Research shows that ED precedes the symptoms of heart disease (such as chest pain) in seven out of 10 men with heart disease—with ED usually showing up about three years earlier. And a study published in *International Journal of Impotence Research* shows that severe ED nearly triples the risk for heart disease.

Bottom line: The scientific consensus is that a diagnosis of ED is a warning of heart disease. If you are diagnosed with ED, you should have a cardiovascular workup—as soon as possible.

THE EXERCISE ELIXIR

The human cardiovascular system is designed for daily physical activity. Physical activity helps keep blood pressure normal…blood sugar stabilized…cholesterol low…the heart muscle strong…and the risk for heart attack minimized—including the risk from little-known risk factors. In my view, exercise is the best habit for your heart.

Compelling scientific research: In an eight-year study of more than 400,000 people published in *The Lancet,* researchers found that even 15 minutes of daily exercise reduced the risk of dying by 14%—and that includes the risk of dying from cardiovascular disease. And those 15 minutes don't even have to be continuous. To get the benefit, you can exercise for five minutes, three times a day.

My advice: Brisk walking is an ideal exercise. You can do it easily with others, which further reduces your risk for a heart attack. (Social isolation and loneliness increase the risk for heart disease by 29%, according to a recent study published in *Heart.*) And you can build walking into your other daily activities—such as parking five to 10 minutes away from your destination and walking the rest of the way.

"Silent" Heart Attack: Are You at Risk?

Gregory Thomas, MD, a cardiologist, medical director for the MemorialCare Heart & Vascular Institute at Long Beach Memorial Medical Center in California, and clinical professor at the University of California, Irvine.

Most of us think we know what a heart attack looks and feels like. Pain or discomfort in the chest…shortness of breath…a cold sweat…and perhaps even a sense of impending doom. But not so fast. Heart attack symptoms can vary widely from person to person—and may not be noticeable at all.

The reality: Of the 735,000 heart attacks that strike Americans every year, nearly half are silent—that is, there are no obvious symptoms. In fact, people who have had a silent heart attack don't even know they've had one! These heart attacks don't occur only in older adults—they are quite common in middle-aged adults, research shows.

Don't be fooled: Many people assume that a silent heart attack is less harmful than a "real" heart attack, but that's not true. In fact, some studies indicate that a person who has had a silent heart attack has a higher risk of dying from heart disease than a person who has had a recognized heart attack—perhaps because he/she doesn't receive appropriate medical care.

ARE YOU AT RISK?

Some risk factors for a silent heart attack are obvious, such as high blood pressure, smoking and being overweight. But many other risks are hidden and largely unrecognized by doctors and patients alike.

If you have one or more of the risk factors below, make an appointment with an internist or a cardiologist and discuss getting an electrocardiogram (see next page for details) to determine whether you have damage to the heart due to a silent heart attack you may have unknowingly suffered.

If your doctor discovers that you have had a silent heart attack, your treatment—such as medications, a heart-healthy diet and regular exercise—should be the same as that received by a person who has had a recognized heart attack. Your primary care physician can provide much of the care, but if you have had a heart attack, you should be seeing a cardiologist at least yearly. *Important risks for silent heart attack…*

•**Low sensitivity to pain.** Because pain is a major symptom of most heart attacks, it stands to reason that silent heart attacks are more likely in people who are less sensitive to pain—and recent research confirms this theory.

Recent finding: In a study of nearly 5,000 people, published in the *Journal of the American Heart Association*, researchers found that women with lower pain sensitivity were more likely to have had a silent heart attack than those who were more sensitive to pain. According to this study, people who can keep a hand in icy water for up to two minutes have a lower sensitivity to pain.

•**Peripheral neuropathy.** About 20 million Americans—many of them with type 2 diabetes—have peripheral neuropathy, nerve damage that causes symptoms such as numbness, tingling and burning pain, usually in the feet or hands. Having diabetes and peripheral neuropathy more than doubles the likelihood of having a silent heart attack—probably because sensitivity to sensation has been reduced.

•**Elevated blood sugar.** A fasting blood sugar (glucose) test is typically ordered to detect elevated glucose levels and diabetes. You fast overnight for at least eight hours, and your blood is drawn in the morning and sent to a laboratory, where your glucose level is measured. If it's 126 mg/dL or higher, you have diabetes. But if your glucose level is 100 mg/dL or higher, you're 60% more likely to have had a silent heart attack than someone whose glucose level was normal (less than 100 mg/dL). Chronically high levels of glucose (even if they haven't yet reached the point of diabetes) damage arteries, increasing risk for heart attack and stroke. Elevated glucose is common. The average adult in the US has a blood sugar level of 106 mg/dL.

•**Sluggish kidneys.** Two findings on routine laboratory tests that measure kidney function have been linked to a higher risk of having had a silent heart attack…

•Albuminuria. This indicates that there are elevated levels of a protein in your urine that can signal kidney disease. Albuminuria is detected by a combination of two tests—a microalbuminuria test and a creatinine test.

●**Low glomerular filtration rate (GFR).** This shows your kidneys are struggling to do their main job—filtering impurities out of your blood.

Scientific evidence: A study of nearly 19,000 people by researchers from the University of Alabama at Birmingham found that people with the highest levels of albuminuria (greater than 300 mg/g) were 2.5 times more likely to have had a silent heart attack than those with the lowest levels.

They also found that those with the lowest estimated GFR levels (less than 30) were three times more likely to have had a silent heart attack than those with the highest levels. (Normal GFR varies by age but ranges from 60 to 120.)

●**Fatigue, swollen legs and/or breathing problems.** All three can be symptoms of a weakened heart muscle—including one damaged by a heart attack. If you experience these symptoms but you haven't had a detectable heart attack, you may have had a silent heart attack. Especially if one or more of these symptoms come on suddenly or unexpectedly, see a doctor promptly for an evaluation.

SMART STRATEGY

Detecting a silent heart attack is easy to do with an electrocardiogram (EKG or ECG). This five- to 10-minute test measures the electrical activity of your heart. If the EKG detects abnormal "Q-waves"—a lack of electrical activity in areas of the heart—your heart muscle has been damaged by a heart attack.

If you've had a silent heart attack, you should promptly treat your heart disease. In my decades as a cardiologist, I've seen over and over again that treating cardiovascular disease with cholesterol-lowering medications, increasing daily exercise and improving diet dramatically decreases the risk for a second heart attack and premature death.

If you have had a silent heart attack, a second one is also more likely to be silent or have atypical symptoms, such as neck, jaw or back pain, nausea, dizziness and/or fatigue. Be on guard for unusual symptoms and a sense that you're

feeling "not quite right." Also, be sure to see your physician for regular checkups.

Thyroid Hormone Linked to Artery Disease

Arjola Bano, MD, MSc, DSc, is a researcher in the departments of internal medicine and epidemiology at Erasmus Medical Center, Rotterdam, the Netherlands, and leader of a study of more than 9,400 people, published in *Circulation Research.*

Middle-aged and older adults with higher levels of free thyroxine (FT4) had twice the rate of calcified coronary arteries as those with normal levels—and an 87% higher risk for heart attack or stroke. Generally, elevated FT4 levels indicate hyperthyroidism. Symptoms include weight loss, anxiety, weakness, sleep difficulty and increased heart rate.

The Danger of Exercising Angry

Andrew Smyth, MD, PhD, postdoctoral researcher at Population Health Research Institute at McMaster University, Hamilton, Ontario, Canada, and the HRB Clinical Research Facility in Galway, Ireland.

You have a fight with your spouse or someone else, and you're red-hot angry. So you go for an intense run or to the gym. Healthy way to blow off steam, right?

Not so fast. The truth is, you may be putting your heart at risk. Anger spikes adrenaline, constricts blood vessels and increases heart rate and blood pressure—and so does intense exercise. And the combination of exercising while angry is enough to trigger a heart attack in some people.

Surprising recent finding: In a study of 12,461 people in 52 countries who had a first heart attack, what happened in the hour before the attack mattered. Compared with controls who didn't have heart attacks, those who did were three times more likely to have been angry/upset and to have engaged in intense exercise beforehand—specifically, in the 60 minutes preceding the attack.

A new excuse to kick back on the couch? Not at all! Regular physical exercise plays a key role in preventing cardiovascular disease, including heart attacks. Nor should you *avoid* exercise when you're angry. If exercise is your go-to way to relieve stress, go ahead—just stick with your usual workout. That's true even if your regular exercise is intense—the key is not to increase the intensity or duration more than is normal for you.

Save those fitness ambitions for when your emotions are on an even keel. In the meantime, work on ways to have fewer episodes of anger—and better manage those that you do have. You might benefit from yoga, meditation, a walk in the woods, reading—or a combination.

Just remember: When you're feeling stressed, it's not the time to push your physical limits.

Afib Detector

Daniel J. Cantillon, MD, is a cardiologist and electrophysiologist at the Cleveland Clinic.

An Apple Watch device detects atrial fibrillation, we hear from Daniel J. Cantillon, MD. Atrial fibrillation, marked by irregular heart rhythms, increases stroke risk. Kardiaband, the first-ever FDA-approved medical device for an Apple Watch, is a wrist sensor embedded in a watchband. It records an EKG and sends it to a doctor's office. The device detects potentially dangerous heart abnormalities that require evaluation. It costs $199 and requires a $9.99/month or a $99/year subscription.

Medication vs. Stents

Justin E. Davies, MBBS, PhD, is a senior research fellow at Imperial College London, UK, and leader of a clinical trial of 230 coronary patients with severe single-vessel blockages, published in *The Lancet*.

Medication can work as well as stents for certain heart patients. When people in good general health have stable angina caused by a single blocked artery, drug therapy alone may provide relief—adding a stent (a small wire-mesh tube) requires hospitalization and may not bring added relief. But stents may have a place in patients who don't tolerate medications.

Sluggish Circulation? Here's the PAD Exercise RX

Neel P. Chokshi, MD, MBA, assistant professor of clinical medicine at Perelman School of Medicine, University of Pennsylvania in Philadelphia, and medical director of the university's Sports Cardiology and Fitness Program. His research has been published in *American Journal of Cardiology* and other professional journals.

If your calves cramp while walking or climbing stairs—especially if the pain eases when you stop—it's a red flag that you may have peripheral artery disease (PAD). With PAD, your arteries are narrowed due to plaque buildup, which prevents the muscles in your extremities (usually your legs) from getting enough blood flow to keep up with the increased oxygen demand when you are active.

It's no small matter—if PAD goes untreated, the condition can lead to infection, loss of the function of the limb and, in severe cases of blockage, amputation.

Here's the irony of treating PAD: People who have this circulatory problem, with its telltale pain while walking, are often prescribed (you guessed it!) walking to relieve their pain.

Is Heart-Stopping Sex a Myth?

Heart-stopping sex does happen but is very rare. In a study of 4,557 cases of sudden cardiac arrest over a 13-year period, only 34 cases were linked to sex—about one in 100 cardiac arrests in men and about one in 1,000 cases in women.

Sumeet Chugh, MD, associate director, Cedars-Sinai Heart Institute, Los Angeles, and senior author of a study published in *Journal of the American College of Cardiology.*

Even though it hurts, walking—when done according to certain guidelines (see below)—does actually improve the symptoms of PAD and slow its progression. In fact, exercise works as well as any medication or surgery, according to research published in *Circulation.*

WALK THIS WAY

What's so great about walking? When you repeatedly put one foot in front of the other, it brings more oxygen to your muscles, which improves your circulation and eases the pain of PAD. The exact reasons why walking helps aren't known, but it's well-established that the more you walk, the farther you'll be able to walk…and with less pain.

Important: If you suspect that you have PAD but haven't been diagnosed, it's important to see your doctor for an evaluation. This will include an ankle-brachial exam, which compares the blood pressure in your arms to that in your feet, to show how well your blood is flowing, and possibly other tests such as an ultrasound. You may also have other related factors, such as high blood pressure, that need to be addressed.

To get the best results from your walking program…

•**Stretch.** Before getting started, your calf muscles need a good stretch to increase blood flow to the area.

What works best: Stand in front of a low step (a curb works fine, too). Place the toes of one foot on the step and drop your heel just enough to feel a stretch in your calf. Don't overdo it…stop at the point of tightness. Hold it for 10 to 15 seconds, then switch feet.

To warm up your thigh muscles, stand on one leg and raise the other foot behind you by bending the knee. Do not pull up on your foot…just rest that ankle in your hand and hold that position long enough to feel a slight stretch in your thigh (usually 10 to 15 seconds). Switch legs and repeat. (If you can't reach your ankle, try standing with a wall behind you and place that foot against the wall to hold it up.)

•**Walk.** Find a flat, safe surface for your walks (neighborhood streets, a local track, a shopping mall or a treadmill).

What works best: Start by walking for five minutes at a pace that causes some pain. On a pain scale from one to five, where one is mild pain and five is severe pain, aim to walk at a three or four.

•**Rest.** After walking for five minutes with moderate pain, stop and rest until the pain goes away.

Helpful: If you like to walk in an area where there aren't any benches for your rest period, treat yourself to a cane with a folding seat attachment. It's not too heavy to carry and gives you a place to sit during your rest stops.

•**Repeat.** Once the pain has dissipated, try to walk for another five minutes. If you find that it's impossible to do the additional five minutes without severe pain, try slowing down your pace to achieve a few extra minutes.

•**Stay focused on your goal.** Try to walk at least three—ideally, five—times a week. During the first two months, build up slowly to a total of 35 minutes of walking during each session, not counting the rest breaks. After you can manage that, keep adding a few minutes each week until you're at the ultimate goal of walking 50 minutes per session.

•**Cool down.** You should always finish by walking slowly for five minutes. Then stretch your calf and thigh muscles again to help minimize muscle soreness after walking.

SMART STRATEGIES

To give yourself the best possible odds of succeeding at your walking program, you should also…

•**Track your progress.** To stay motivated, jot down the total time and distance of your walks. Or wear a fitness tracker, such as Fitbit, or use a phone app, like MapMyWalk, to help track your time, effort and distance.

•**Avoid boredom!** If you walk outside, vary your route. If you prefer a treadmill, listen to music or a podcast…or watch a 30-minute TV show.

Also helpful: Find a walking buddy—the social aspect can help keep you on target.

FOR AN EXTRA BOOST

Working with a physical therapist to start a walking program is smart, since supervised programs seem to be more effective by helping to ensure that you keep up with your walking program and hit the required pain thresholds.

You're also likely to get help paying for your sessions with a physical therapist.

Recent development: Medicare Part B now covers comprehensive cardiac rehabilitation programs that include exercise, education and counseling for patients with PAD. The specific amount you'll owe may depend on several things, such as the Medigap insurance (if any) you have and the type of facility you choose. Check with your insurer.

AN ALTERNATIVE TO WALKING

If any amount of walking is too painful or too dangerous for you, don't give up. New research shows that you can get comparable results with arm exercises.

Important recent finding: In a study that was conducted at University of Minnesota School of Nursing in Minneapolis, researchers randomly divided 28 people with PAD (average age 65.6) into three different groups—no exercise...treadmill walking...or arm exercise. Participants assigned to arm exercises used an arm ergometer (a device with bicycle-like pedals that are operated by the arms). After three months of training for three hours a week, people in both exercise groups could walk farther without pain.

Other possibilities: It's likely that bike riding, dancing, swimming or pool walking, which haven't yet been tested in people with PAD, may also help relieve symptoms. If you enjoy those activities, talk to your doctor about giving them a try!

Watch Out for This Deadly Family Heart Condition

John A. Elefteriades, MD, chief of cardiothoracic surgery, Yale New Haven Hospital, Connecticut.

Adults whose parents and/or sibling had an aortic dissection (a sudden tear in the main artery from the heart) have a one in eight risk of having it, too, and at roughly the same age, according to a new study.

If a family member has suffered an aortic dissection: Ask your doctor to monitor you with an echocardiogram every five years for an aortic aneurysm.

Blood Thinners Decrease Dementia Risk

Study of 444,106 people by researchers at Karolinska Institute in Stockholm, Sweden, published in *European Heart Journal.*

Recent finding: People with atrial fibrillation who take anticoagulant medications had up to a 48% lower risk of developing dementia, compared with people who don't take the medications.

What's That Mean? Anticoagulants vs. Antiplatelets

American Heart Association/American Stroke Association, Pharmacy Choice, Inc., UC San Diego Health, Circulation, MedicineNet.com, Mayo Clinic, US Food and Drug Administration.

If you or someone you love has some form of heart or blood vessel disease...or if you've had or are at risk of having a stroke...a blood thinner may be living in your medicine cabinet. Put simply, blood thinners keep your blood from forming clots in any part of your body.

But do you really know what they do? Not all blood thinners work the same way. Here's what you need to know.

WHAT'S SO BAD ABOUT CLOTTING ANYWAY?

Clotting is something your blood does naturally—and it's important. Without the ability to clot, a simple cut could cause you to bleed excessively. When you bleed, platelets—small disk-shaped parts of bone marrow cells that circulate in your blood—release a chemical called thromboxane that "calls out" to other platelets to come help. These platelets stick together and stop the bleeding.

But there are times when clotting is not your friend. Some clots are caused by injury, or they can form in arteries where there's no obvious injury. Other clots, such as deep vein thrombosis (DVT) may happen after prolonged sitting. Family history also plays a role in how likely you are to have blood clots. Clots near the heart can cause a heart attack, while those that travel to blood vessels in your brain can cause a stroke. That's where blood thinners come in—they keep platelets from "overdoing it."

There are two main types of blood thinners…

Antiplatelets are what the name implies… they keep platelets from clumping together and forming clots. They also break up existing clots. They are often the first type of blood thinner your doctor may suggest.

Best for: Antiplatelets are a more conservative option than anticoagulants, so they are often the first approach that health-care professionals recommend. They are often recommended for patients who have either had, or are at high risk of having, a myocardial infarction (a heart attack caused by clot) or an ischemic stroke (caused by a clot).

•**OTC prevention.** Over-the-counter aspirin tablets are antiplatelets. Many people at risk for heart attack take low-dose aspirin daily to prevent heart attacks. The benefits need to be balanced against the risks, especially for gastrointestinal bleeding. (Fortunately, there's an app for that.)

•**Omega-3 fatty acids also act as antiplatelets.** While many people take omega-3 capsules as a dietary supplement (a typical daily dose is 1,000 mg), some health-care professionals recommend higher doses to help prevent blood clots for cardiovascular patients—for example, after a heart attack. Because antiplatelets raise bleeding risk in some people, however, anyone taking more than 3,000 mg per day should do so only in consultation with a health-care professional, according to the American Heart Association.

•**Prescription option.** People who have already had a heart attack or stroke, or have another cardiovascular condition such as unstable angina, may be prescribed the medication *clopidogrel* (Plavix) to prevent a future heart attack or stroke. It's also an antiplatelet.

Anticoagulants also work to keep blood clots from forming, in this case by targeting certain proteins that are important to the clotting process.

Best for: These are more effective than antiplatelets but also have more side effects, so doctors prescribe them for specific reasons. People who have had "mini strokes," also called transient ischemic attacks (TIA), or those who have atrial fibrillation (Afib), which is an abnormal heart rhythm, are often prescribed anticoagulants. They can also be helpful if you're at risk for deep vein thrombosis, a clot that forms in a deep vein that may travel to your lungs. (*Warning:* Some people with Afib should not be prescribed an anticoagulant—but often are.)

•**Old standby.** *Warfarin* (Coumadin) is a prescription anticoagulant that's been around a long time. It's proven to reduce stroke risk. But it requires frequent blood tests to finesse the dose, plus you'll need to avoid certain green vegetables.

•**Newer entrants on the anticoagulant** scene are *dabigatran* (Pradaxa), *rivaroxaban* (Xarelto), *apixaban* (Eliquis) and *edoxaban* (Savaysa). They don't require blood tests and there are no food restrictions but they have their own unique risks.

The key one: Only dabigatran has an antidote—the others can put you at risk of uncontrolled bleeding.

Don't Let the New Blood Pressure Guidelines Fool You

H. Gilbert Welch, MD, MPH, professor of medicine at The Dartmouth Institute for Health Policy and Clinical Practice, Lebanon, New Hampshire, and author of three books, including *Less Medicine, More Health: 7 Assumptions That Drive Too Much Health Care* and *Overdiagnosed: Making People Sick in the Pursuit of Health.* TDI.Dartmouth.edu

The definition of high blood pressure has reached a new low—130 is the new 140. According to guidelines set by the American Heart Association and the American College of Cardiology in late 2017, if your systolic (upper) number is 130 mm Hg or higher…and/or your diastolic (lower) number is 80 mm Hg or higher…you have high blood pressure, aka hypertension. The previous threshold was 140 mm Hg. (Diastolic, the lower number, is less important at predicting cardiovascular risk.)

Overnight, more than 30 million Americans "got" high blood pressure. Combined with those who met the earlier threshold, that's a total of about 103 million people. As an advocate for using less medicine whenever possible, I'm worried by these new guidelines. That's why I wrote an article in *The New York Times* titled, "Don't Let New Blood Pressure Guidelines Raise Yours." And it's why I enthusiastically agreed to work on this article. It's not that controlling very high blood pressure isn't important. It's critical. Treating very high blood pressure with medication is one of the most important preventive interventions doctors do.

But doctors also can do too much prescribing. Aggressive medical management to reach the new goals for people at the margin may have only modest benefits that don't outweigh the risks for side effects. In a blow to wide acceptance, the American Academy of Family Physicians (AAFP) declined to endorse the new guidelines because they don't meet that organization's standards for medical evidence. It's sticking with the previous guidelines.

When doctors disagree, it can be confusing for patients. Here are some facts to help you and your physician make the right decision…

MODEST NEW BENEFITS

While the new guidelines emphasize lifestyle changes such as getting more exercise, losing weight if you need to and eating a healthful diet as the first line of defense—good advice for all of us—the likely practical effect will be to push many more people into drug treatment. So let's examine the benefits.

The new guidelines stem from a federally funded study called the Systolic Blood Pressure Intervention Trial (SPRINT). It covered people over age 50 at high risk for cardiovascular disease. Half were treated to bring their systolic blood pressure down to less than 140 and half to bring it down to less than 120.

Result: Compared with those treated to less than 140, those treated to less than 120 had 25% lower risk for heart attack, stroke, heart failure and death from cardiovascular causes. Sounds impressive, right? But in reality, over the course of the three-year study, about 6% of participants who aimed for 120 had cardiovascular "events" such as heart attacks—compared with 8% of those who aimed for 140. That's only a two-percentage-point difference.

The truth is, while reducing very high blood pressure—say, from 160 or 180 to 140—has enormous benefits, going from 140 to 130 doesn't. According to a review that included 74 trials and more than 300,000 patients that was published in *JAMA Internal Medicine*, bringing blood pressure levels below 140 did not help prevent a first heart attack or stroke, reduce the rate of cardiovascular disease or help prevent death overall.

RISKS OF AGGRESSIVE TREATMENT

In the SPRINT trial, getting to a blood pressure goal of less than 120 required an average of three different drugs per patient—compared with two drugs for a 140 goal. While that extra drug didn't substantially increase side effects in that trial, it's still true that 38% of patients in the 120-target group had adverse events, including abnormally low blood pressure, loss of consciousness and acute kidney injury. I'm concerned about adding even one extra prescription medication, especially for many elderly patients who already may take eight or even 10 medications a day.

Blood pressure drugs, like all drugs, have side effects. The type called beta-blockers can cause dizziness, weakness and fatigue, as can ACE inhibitors, angiotensin II receptor blockers and alpha blockers. Dizziness and light-headedness can result in more falls, which is particularly dangerous for older people, making them more prone to fractures—including hip fractures, which can have devastating consequences for health and independence.

These concerns are among the reasons that the AAFP and the American College of Physicians came out with blood pressure treatment

The Right Way to Measure Your Blood Pressure at Home

If you're concerned about your blood pressure, and especially if you've started to take medication to bring it down, consider measuring your blood pressure yourself at home. Many physicians recommend this do-it-yourself approach because it can help you become more aware of the things that move your blood pressure up or down.

Buy a monitor with an inflatable upper-arm cuff—more reliable than those with wrist cuffs or fingertip monitors. *Follow these tips when you measure your pressure…*

•**Relax.** Don't exercise or drink caffeinated drinks or alcohol for at least 30 minutes before measuring. Make sure your bladder is empty…sit quietly for five minutes before you take a measurement…sit still while you measure.

•**Watch your posture.** Sit with your back against a straight-back chair…feet flat on the floor, legs uncrossed. Support your arm on a flat surface with your upper arm at heart level. The middle of the blood pressure cuff should be placed just above where the elbow bends.

•**Place the cuff directly on your bare arm, not over clothing.**

•**Take your pressure at the same time every day.** Either morning or evening is fine. It doesn't matter whether you do it before or after taking medication—just be consistent.

•**Take two or three readings one minute apart.** Print out or write down the results or store them in your device's built-in memory.

Ask your doctor's office if you can do a practice run there. That way you can be sure that you are using the monitor correctly at home.

Caution: Don't rely solely on your at-home readings. Compare them with the readings you get in your doctor's office as a backup.

guidelines specifically for people age 60 and older in 2017.

Recommendations: Doctors should prescribe drugs for healthy patients only when systolic levels are 150 or higher. For patients at high cardiovascular risk, especially stroke patients, doctors are advised to start treatment at 140.

OVERDIAGNOSIS RISK

There's a bigger problem in extrapolating the results of the SPRINT trial to the real world. Blood pressure is an extremely volatile variable, and it can change within minutes in reaction to stress, activity or just the anxiety of sitting in a doctor's waiting room. (For how to get a good blood pressure reading, see the box.) To remove those stressors, the SPRINT researchers had patients measure their own blood pressure (using an automated cuff) after five minutes of quiet rest without staff in the room.

This may be an ideal way to measure blood pressure, but it's not what happens in the real world. You might have had a blood pressure reading of 130 in a situation such as the SPRINT trial, while it might be 140 or even higher when measured in your doctor's office. In practice, that may lead to many people being overmedicated.

WHAT TO DO NOW

Have the new guidelines pushed you into the official "high blood pressure" range? I hope you now realize that it's not a medical emergency if they have. But it's an opportunity to talk to your doctor about what blood pressure goal is right for you, given your age and risk factors.

Even if you wind up needing medication, a lifestyle plan is enormously important. Limit alcoholic drinks to no more than one a day if you're a woman or two a day if you're a man. Revamp your diet to include plenty of fruits and vegetables and whole grains. Reduce your salt intake. Exercise regularly. If you smoke, quit. Lose weight if you need to. Find healthy ways to manage stress.

Ironically, the recent dramatic increase in the number of people with "high" blood pressure can distract patients and doctors from focusing on these important lifestyle changes. Doing those things is good for blood sugar, for better sleep and for overall well-being, regardless of blood pressure.

The Real Secret to Lowering Your Blood Pressure

Janet Bond Brill, PhD, RDN, FAND, a registered dietitian/nutritionist and nationally recognized expert in nutrition and cardiovascular disease prevention. She is a former director of nutrition for Fitness Together, one of the world's largest organizations of personal trainers, and has served as a nutrition consultant for several other large companies. She is author of *Blood Pressure Down: The 10-Step Plan to Lower Your Blood Pressure in Four Weeks—Without Prescription Drugs.* DrJanet.com

Forget everything that you have read about the latest "superfood" for lowering blood pressure. While it's true that certain foods do provide this remarkable benefit, many people mistakenly assume that there must be one nutritional magic bullet that will do the job on its own.

Is it possible to control high blood pressure (hypertension) with diet alone? Yes, many people can—but only when they take advantage of the additive benefits from multiple strategically chosen foods.

Example: Suppose you eat a lot of bananas because you know that this food is high in blood pressure–lowering potassium. That's great, but you'll shave only a point or two off your blood pressure.

To really leverage your diet, you need to also regularly consume other foods that help control blood pressure. When combined, the nutrients in these foods work synergistically to give the greatest blood pressure–lowering effects. Then the benefits accrue quickly—for some people, a five-point drop may occur within a week.

What you may not realize: By eating the right foods, losing weight if you're overweight and cutting sodium if you're salt-sensitive (see page 74), some people can achieve blood pressure drops that equal or exceed the effects of drug therapy—with none of the side effects. And if you must take medication, these foods may allow you to use a lower dose.*

Caution: If you take blood pressure–lowering medication, never change your dose or discontinue it without consulting your doctor.

Some of the best blood pressure–lowering foods are well-known—bananas, leafy green vegetables, etc. *Here are some lesser-known options to add to your hypertension-fighting diet…*

•**Beet juice/beet greens.** As a nutritionist, I usually advise clients to eat whole foods rather than drink juices because of the extra fiber. But beet juice is an exception. It's a concentrated source of nitrates, chemical compounds that quickly lower blood pressure.

When you drink beet juice or eat other high-nitrate foods (such as rhubarb, spinach, beet greens or chard), cells in the linings of blood vessels produce more nitric oxide, a molecule that dilates blood vessels and lowers blood pressure.

Scientific evidence: In a study that was published in *Hypertension* and looked at 64 adults with hypertension (ages 18 to 85), some of the patients drank a daily 8.4-ounce glass of beet juice, while others drank a juice with the active compounds removed (the placebo).

After one month, those given the real juice had average drops in systolic (top number) blood pressure of about eight points, while their diastolic pressure (bottom number) dropped five points. Blood pressure did not drop among those in the placebo group.

You can buy beet juice in health-food stores and juice shops. Or you can make your own by blending/processing cooked beets. To liven up the flavor, add a little lemon juice, ginger or a sweetener such as stevia.

Caution: If you have kidney disease, consult your nephrologist or a registered dietitian/nutritionist who specializes in kidney disease before regularly consuming beet juice—its high potassium level could worsen this condition.

•**Figs.** These delicious jewels are heart-healthy because they are super-high in potassium, with 232 mg in just two fresh figs. They also have a considerable amount of fiber and polyphenols, compounds that when consumed with additional blood pressure–lowering food can reduce systolic blood pressure by up to 12 points, in some cases.

Fresh figs are scrumptious, but dried figs are easier to find in grocery stores—and many people enjoy their intense sweetness.

What to try: Chop dried figs, and use them as a natural sweetener in oatmeal, pancakes, muffins or even soups.

•**Hibiscus tea.** If you enjoy chamomile and other herbal teas, you might like the delicate floral flavor of hibiscus tea, which is high in flavonoids, plant-based antioxidants with anti-inflammatory effects, and other heart-healthy compounds. One study, which compared hibiscus tea to *captopril*, an ACE inhibitor blood pressure drug, found that the tea was just as effective as the medication.

•**Pistachios.** Even though most nuts are good sources of fiber, potassium and magnesium, pistachios are special because they are high in arginine, an amino acid that stimulates the production of nitric oxide (discussed earlier).

Important recent finding: A study at Pennsylvania State University found that people who ate 1.5 ounces of pistachios (about 70 nuts, unshelled) daily had drops in stress-related systolic blood pressure of nearly five points compared with those who ate nuts less than once a week.

Not fattening: Nuts are high in calories, but research has shown that people who eat them regularly actually tend to gain less weight than those who don't eat nuts—probably because the fiber and protein in nuts help dieters feel full longer. At roughly 260 calories per 1.5 ounces, you'll need to cut calories elsewhere to prevent weight gain but can likely do so easily because nuts give such a feeling of satiety.

•**Pomegranate juice.** Pomegranate juice contains many different flavonoids. The juice mimics the effects of ACE inhibitor drugs, such as *lisinopril* (Zestril, Prinivil, etc.), which dilate blood vessels and lower blood pressure.

A recent study found that people who drank a little less than two ounces of pomegranate juice daily for a year had average drops in systolic blood pressure of 12%.

The juice is tart, so some people buy sweetened versions.

My advice: Avoid the added sugar. Instead, add a little stevia or other natural sweetener. One pomegranate yields about half a cup of juice.

•**White beans.** Like many of the other foods described earlier, white beans are chock-full of potassium. One cup contains more than 1,000 mg of potassium. (A cup of black beans has about 800 mg.)

Potassium acts like a natural diuretic and removes sodium from the body. Many people are sensitive to sodium, which means that their blood pressure will rise if they consume too much (the standard recommendation is no more than 2,300 mg daily). Research has shown that one of the best ways to lower blood pressure is to increase your potassium–sodium ratio.

Keep Black Licorice Consumption Moderate

US Food and Drug Administration. FDA.gov

Black licorice contains *glycyrrhizin*, which can cause potassium levels in the body to fall, potentially leading to abnormal heart rhythms. For people age 40 and above, two ounces a day for more than two weeks may trigger arrhythmia—irregular heartbeat—and other cardiovascular effects. A regular black licorice habit also may interact with some medicines, herbs and dietary supplements. Occasional enjoyment is fine.

Is Salt Harmful for Everyone?

James J. DiNicolantonio, PharmD, a cardiovascular research scientist and doctor of pharmacy at Saint Luke's Mid America Heart Institute in Kansas City, Missouri. Dr. DiNicolantonio is also an associate editor of *BMJ Open Heart*, on the editorial advisory board of *Progress in Cardiovascular Diseases* and other journals and author of *The Salt Fix*, TheSaltFix.com.

We've all been told that a high-salt diet is a leading cause of high blood pressure (hypertension), heart attack, stroke and heart failure. What doctors don't tell patients—what many doctors don't know themselves—is that salt doesn't have the same effect on everyone's blood pressure.

A surprising fact: Many people do better when they consume more than the USDA's recommended daily sodium limit of 2,300 mg (roughly the amount in one teaspoon of salt). *Other common misconceptions regarding sodium…*

***MYTH #1:* Salt raises blood pressure in everyone.** It's true that doctors have a right to worry about the salt consumption for some patients. Salt sensitivity—generally defined as an increase of 5% or more in blood pressure when sodium is consumed—is most common in older adults, black people and people of Chinese descent. Important: If you're sensitive to salt, exceeding the recommended daily limit of 2,300 mg of sodium can cause sharp rises in blood pressure.

But what's harmful for this subset of the population is not harmful for everyone. Research shows that salt sensitivity affects about half of people with high blood pressure and about 20% of people who have normal blood pressure.

***MYTH #2:* Salt always increases heart disease.** If a high-salt diet increased blood pressure, it would obviously increase the risk for cardiovascular disease—but, as discussed earlier, this occurs only in some people. When researchers study whether eating highly salted foods increases the rates of high blood pressure and heart disease, the findings are mixed. Meanwhile, the correlation between high-salt diets and improved health is compelling.

BP Monitor Warning

If you are checking your blood pressure at home using an automated blood pressure device, listen up. New research on dozens of such monitors shows that their readings were off by 5 mmHg nearly 70% of the time—an inaccuracy that may influence the decision to start or reduce blood pressure medication.

What to do: Take your device to your next doctor appointment to measure its accuracy against an automated office blood pressure machine. At home, take several readings (to get a range).

Jennifer Ringrose, MD, associate professor of medicine, University of Alberta, Edmonton, Canada.

Example: People consume staggering amounts of sodium in Japan, France and South Korea. The average South Korean, for example, consumes more than 4,000 mg of sodium a day. In France and other Mediterranean countries, very salty foods, such as prepared sardines, anchovies and many aged cheeses, are eaten with most meals. Yet these countries are among those with the lowest death rates from coronary heart disease in the world, and Japan and South Korea boast among the highest longevity.

Most people don't realize that a low-salt diet can sometimes raise blood pressure by stimulating the body's "rescue" system (the renin-angiotensin aldosterone system) that's designed to help the body retain salt and water. When this occurs, low salt intake can increase heart rate, blood clotting and the constriction of blood vessels. It's also been linked to insulin resistance and diabetes.

***MYTH #3:* No one needs more salt.** The ubiquitous advice to reduce sodium intake might be justified if it helped some people and didn't hurt the rest. But this isn't always the case.

To remain in homeostasis, the physiological state that puts the least stress on the body, most people who are not salt sensitive need about 3,000 mg to 5,000 mg of sodium a day.

What's more, many of our food choices (sugar and caffeinated beverages, for example) deplete salt from the body. So do commonly prescribed medications such as some antidepressants, diuretics and diabetes drugs. In addition, the average nonathletic adult sweats out 600 mg of sodium a day.

***MYTH #4:* Healthy diets are naturally low in salt.** The diets that experts recommend for disease prevention, such as the Mediterranean diet, do exclude many of the processed foods that happen to be high in salt (and other unhealthful ingredients)—but they're not low-salt diets overall. If anything, as mentioned above with such countries as Japan and South Korea, they contain more salt than Americans typically eat. Think seafood (clams, lobster, crab), olives, kimchi, etc.

Why do these countries have less cardiovascular disease than the US? While there is no definitive research that a high-salt diet is the reason, it's been my observation that people who indulge their salt cravings tend to eat more heart-healthy vegetables (particularly the bitter ones, such as bitter greens)…nuts…and seeds—most likely because these healthy foods taste better with salt.

What's more, there is often a lot of potassium in naturally salty foods—for example, spinach, Swiss chard and artichokes. When it comes to improving blood pressure and heart health, more potassium is probably more important than less sodium.

MYTH #5: **Everyone should check the sodium content on food labels.** Unless you eat a lot of pretzels, chips and other super-salty foods, you are unlikely to eat more salt than your body can handle—unless you're salt-sensitive (see below).

I do advise people to avoid processed foods—mainly because these foods tend to be high in sugar, which can increase the risk for high blood pressure, diabetes and obesity. Most processed foods also lack fiber, and a lack of fiber can cause sugar spikes. It's much better to indulge your salt cravings with foods that are naturally salty—for example, sea vegetables (kelp, seaweed and algae), seafood, cheese and olives.

ARE YOU SALT-SENSITIVE?

There are no readily available tests to determine whether a person is salt-sensitive. So how do you know whether a low-salt diet would help you or hurt you?

Try this: With your doctor's OK, for two weeks, reduce your sodium intake to less than 2,300 mg of sodium per day. If your blood pressure drops by 5% or more, chances are you are

salt-sensitive. If your blood pressure does drop, be alert for dizziness, fatigue, nausea, muscle spasms/cramps and blurred vision—signs that your blood pressure may be too low. In these cases, you may be better off listening to your body's salt cravings and eating the salt that it demands rather than adhering to a strict low-sodium diet.

Important: Discuss this with your doctor, and monitor your blood pressure closely.

Cardiac Arrest Alert

Romergryko G. Geocadin, MD, professor of neurology, anesthesiology–critical care neurosurgery, The Johns Hopkins University School of Medicine, Baltimore.

When a cardiac arrest patient is resuscitated, less permanent brain damage occurs if the patient's body is cooled by several degrees for 24 hours—either with special cooling blankets or with a device that cools the blood inside the vessels.

New recommendation: Ask if body cooling, known as therapeutic hypothermia, is appropriate and available if your loved one experiences cardiac arrest.

Fewer Hospital Readmissions but More Deaths

Ankur Gupta, MD, research associate, Brigham and Women's Hospital, Boston, and leader of a study of 115,245 people, published in *JAMA*.

Medicare penalties for hospitals that readmit patients with heart failure have had their intended effect of reducing the frequency of readmission…30-day readmission rates dropped from 20% before the penalties were instituted to 18.4% afterward. But this has not translated to better patient outcomes—it has had the reverse effect. The 30-day mortality rate for heart-failure patients rose from 7.2% to 8.6%. And one year after an inpatient stay, mor-

---

Squeeze Away High Blood Pressure

Squeeze a handgrip at one-third of your strength in your nondominant hand for two minutes…rest three minutes…repeat three more times. Do this three times a week to drop your systolic blood pressure.

Based on a study by researchers at University of New England, New South Wales, Australia, published in *Medicine*.

Better Heart Surgery

Afternoon heart surgery may be safer than morning surgery. Patients who had open-heart surgery for aortic valve replacement in the afternoon had fewer heart attacks during surgery—and, over the next 500 days, fewer major adverse cardiac events, such as heart attack or heart failure. In a separate study, those operated on in the afternoon had much lower levels of troponin, a measure of heart-muscle damage.

Possible reason: Natural circadian variations in the genetic mechanisms that protect tissue under stress.

Bart Staels, PhD, professor of pharmacology, University of Lille, France, and senior author of two studies, one of 596 patients and one of 88, published in *The Lancet*.

tality rates rose from 31.3% before the penalty program to 36.3% afterward. Medicare officials say that they are monitoring the readmission penalty program.

Tai Chi May Aid Cardiac Rehab

Elena Salmoirago-Blotcher, MD, PhD, assistant professor of medicine, Brown University Alpert School of Medicine, Providence, and leader of a study published in *Journal of the American Heart Association*.

More than 60% of heart attack victims refuse cardiac rehabilitation, often because of financial concerns or difficulty getting to a rehab center. But some refuse because they regard physical exercise as unpleasant, painful or impossible after a heart attack. For those patients, tai chi's slow, gentle movements may be an option. Researchers found tai chi to be safe, with no adverse effects except minor muscle pain, and well-liked by participants. Patients who went through an extended tai chi program involving three classes per week for 12 weeks (plus maintenance classes for 12 more weeks) engaged in greater weekly physical activity after three and six months than patients who did not do tai chi or who did a shorter tai chi program of two classes per week for 12 weeks.

Heart-Stopping Plays

Canadian Journal of Cardiology.

The average heart rates of fans who watch hockey games live more than double during the games. Those who watch on TV show an increase of 75%.

Implication: Increased stress on the heart, particularly during high-stakes moments, could be risky for those with cardiovascular disease.

Nondrug Clot Fighter

Kousik Krishnan, MD, cardiac electrophysiologist, Rush University Medical Center, Chicago.

For patients with atrial fibrillation (Afib), blood-thinning drugs such as *warfarin* (Coumadin) help prevent clots but can have serious side effects.

New option: A quarter-sized device inserted into the atrium of the heart to prevent clots from forming allows patients to be gradually weaned off blood thinners. The WATCHMAN implant is FDA-approved and covered by insurance.

Are You Stroke-Ready?

Michael Frankel, MD, professor of neurology at Emory University School of Medicine, and chief of neurology and director of the Marcus Stroke and Neuroscience Center at Grady Memorial Hospital, both in Atlanta. His team played a major role in the DAWN trial, published in *The New England Journal of Medicine* in January 2018. This study provided critically important data showing the benefit of thrombectomy within 24 hours of stroke onset.

Of course, no one wants to have a stroke. But about 800,000 times a year someone in the US has one. Most often, it's an acute ischemic stroke—blood flow to the brain is interrupted, starting a cascade of damage that can lead to death or disability.

The good news: Today's stroke is not your grandfather's stroke. Your chances of surviving and thriving have increased dramatically, thanks to recent advances. To have the best chance of recovering from a stroke, you need to act quickly—and smartly. *Here are four mistakes that can make the difference between life and death...*

MISTAKE #1: Not recognizing stroke symptoms. A stroke often causes multiple symptoms, but some people have only one. However, to spot one or more stroke symptoms, you need to recognize them.

Most people can name at least one of the many stroke symptoms. Classic symptoms include a droopy face on one side...numbness or weakness of the face, arm or leg (especially on just one side)...and trouble walking or balancing. *But there are other symptoms that are also important to watch for...*

- Trouble seeing in one or both eyes.
- Sudden confusion.
- A severe headache with no known cause.
- Sudden, unexplained dizziness.

Helpful: If you think someone near you may be having a stroke, think FAST. *The letters stand for...*

F: Face. Ask the person to smile to see if one side of the face droops.

A: Arms. Ask the person to raise both arms to see if one drifts downward or can't be moved at all.

S: Speech. Ask the person to repeat a simple phrase and listen for slurring or other difficulties.

T: Time. If you see any of these signs, call 911 right away—and make note of the time. Medical personnel will want to know when the symptoms started.

MISTAKE #2: Ignoring a stroke symptom that lasts only a few minutes. You may have had (or witnessed) a transient ischemic attack, a so-called TIA or "ministroke." That can be a warning that a bigger stroke is coming. You should still call 911.

Important: If you witnessed a person who had possible stroke symptoms, be sure that the hospital team has your cell phone number so

you can be reached to confirm what you observed in the patient.

MISTAKE #3: Getting a ride to the hospital. In a medical emergency, you may be tempted to wait to see what happens or have someone drive you to a hospital or doctor's office. With a possible stroke, this is a very bad idea. Instead, call 911 and tell the operator you are seeing or having possible stroke symptoms. Don't worry about being wrong.

Emergency medical workers will assess you and look for other conditions (such as low blood sugar, low blood pressure or a seizure) that could mimic a stroke. They can start treating such conditions right away. If the emergency crew suspects a stroke, they will call ahead to the nearest appropriate hospital so the medical team can prepare.

MISTAKE #4: Going to any hospital. With a stroke, it does matter what hospital you go to—and that's another reason to call 911.

Under an accreditation system maintained by The Joint Commission, hospitals can get certifications ranging from "acute stroke ready" for those with basic supports in place...to "primary stroke centers" for those offering more advanced care...to "comprehensive stroke centers" for those offering the most advanced state-of-the-art care.

A new approach: According to new guidelines from the American Heart Association/American Stroke Association (AHA/ASA), if the patient is having severe stroke symptoms, emergency personnel can travel an additional distance (up to 15 minutes) to reach a comprehensive stroke center. In some regions, the distance may need to be longer. And in some states, medics are required to take patients to the hospital of their choice, while other states leave this decision to emergency personnel. Medics are trained to make the best hospital choice for the patient's needs.

GETTING THE RIGHT TREATMENT

If you are taken to the hospital as a possible stroke patient, ideally you will arrive with a loved one who can describe the onset of your symptoms and share your medical history. Important: Keep a cell phone number for a family member in your wallet—this is critical so that someone who knows you well can give medical information if you are alone and cannot speak for yourself.

If the hospital team determines that you may be having symptoms of an acute stroke, you will receive brain imaging—most often in a CT machine, ideally within 20 minutes of arriving at the hospital.

If your scan rules out bleeding in or around your brain (a hemorrhagic stroke) and you meet other criteria—including onset of your stroke no more than three to four-and-a-half hours earlier—you will get immediate intravenous treatment with a clot-busting medication called a tissue plasminogen activator, or tPA, to break up the clot in your brain, limiting damage and potential disability.

BEYOND TPA

There's now an alternative to tPA called mechanical thrombectomy. This procedure physically removes the blood clot. It is sometimes done after or instead of clot-busting drug treatment. In some cases, you will need to be transferred to another hospital, by ambulance or helicopter, to get it.

Under guidelines from 2015, the procedure had to start within six hours of your initial stroke symptoms. This was a problem for people far from well-equipped and well-staffed hospitals or who woke up with symptoms (a so-called "wake-up stroke") or had stroke symptoms of uncertain duration.

Now: The treatment window has been expanded. Studies show that some patients with blockage in a major artery leading to the brain can benefit from thrombectomy 16 to 24 hours after the stroke began.

Again, doctors will try to determine whether you are in that time window by asking when your symptoms started (or when you were last seen symptom-free). Patients also are screened with advanced brain-imaging tests to find those who still have large areas of brain tissue healthy enough to benefit from restored blood flow.

The Stroke Treatment You May Need to Ask For

Sameer Ansari, MD, PhD, associate professor of radiology, neurology and neurological surgery at Northwestern University Feinberg School of Medicine, Chicago. NM.org

A surgical procedure called thrombectomy dramatically improves the odds that many stroke victims will survive and return to independent lives.

Problem: Many hospitals don't offer it. Compelling evidence for its effectiveness is so new that many aren't geared up for it yet. But there are ways to make sure you get it if you need it.

Background: Every year, about 800,000 people in the US have a stroke and 130,000 die. The vast majority (87%) of strokes are ischemic—caused by a clot that blocks blood flow to the brain. The go-to treatment offered by virtually every hospital is the clot-dissolving drug tissue plasminogen activator (tPA), given as soon as possible intravenously.

But if the clot is large—a kind often resistant to tPA treatment—a neurosurgeon can do a thrombectomy, a procedure that physically removes the clot. A surgeon uses a device called a stent-retriever to remove the clot from a blood vessel in the brain. This procedure is not brand new, but only in the past few years have studies made it obvious that it often is the best treatment option when a large clot blocks blood flow to

New Stroke Risks

Even accounting for longer average life spans, more US women than men die from stroke.

New study: Some women face two unique risks—starting monthly periods early (before age 10)…and having a low level of DHEA-S, a naturally occurring hormonal building block of testosterone and estrogen. This finding, which needs further study, reinforces the importance of controlling known risk factors such as high blood pressure.

Kathryn M. Rexrode, MD, associate professor of medicine, Harvard Medical School, Boston.

the brain. Compared with standard stroke care, this reduces the death rate from 26% to 14%—and patients who survive score 26% higher on a post-stroke independence scale, on average. Recent improvements to the surgical tools used in thrombectomies likely are increasing survival rates as well. New research finds that the procedure can be effective as long as 24 hours after a stroke—not just six hours, as previously believed—although the sooner, the better.

What to do: Before you or a loved one has a stroke, get familiar with the "thrombectomy-capable stroke center" nearest to you. This hospital will have undergone a rigorous certification process for stroke care, including this procedure. You can do this by calling area hospitals or searching the database at StrokeCenter.org/trials/centers.

If you or a loved one experiences potential stroke symptoms, call 911. The EMS team should transport the patient to the nearest stroke center if one is close enough, but you can always ask to be sure. Wherever you wind up, ask if the patient is a candidate for a thrombectomy. If the answer is yes but the hospital can't perform it, ask how quickly the patient can be transferred to such a hospital—by helicopter, if necessary.

Recover Faster from a Stroke

Steven R. Zeiler, MD, PhD, head of stroke research at Johns Hopkins Bayview Medical Center in Baltimore.

You already know that the most important thing you can do if you are having a stroke (or suspect that you are) is to get to an emergency room as fast as possible. Every second that you save may stop precious brain tissue from dying.

But what you and your care team do in the days immediately after a stroke also is critical—especially for recovering from motor deficit and regaining control of your muscles.

Two important new findings…

First finding: In animal studies in a lab, waiting just one week to start rehab led to significantly worse outcomes.

Second finding: A certain medication can prevent that stroke recovery window from closing so quickly.

The overall window for stroke recovery in people continues well past the first week, of course. Many people who have had strokes can continue to improve for months, even years. So never give up! *But here's what to do immediately after the emergency phase…*

•**Start rehab quickly.** Take advantage of that early recovery period—the sooner you begin, the greater your recovery. If your doctors don't start your rehab in the hospital a day or two after the stroke, ask about it and push for it—even if there are medical issues that make it difficult.

•**Ask about the drug fluoxetine.** Other recent research has shown that this antidepressant, aka Prozac, started within one day after a stroke, not only improves recovery but also extends the length of the recovery window. An earlier randomized clinical trial showed that patients with moderate-to-severe motor deficit after ischemic stroke (the most common kind, caused by a blood clot) who took fluoxetine every day for three months, starting five to 10 days after a stroke, had significantly greater improvement than patients who received a placebo. Other drugs in the same class also seem to improve stroke recovery, but the most data exist for fluoxetine—and the new research adds to the urgency of that prescription. While more and more physicians are prescribing fluoxetine, it is not yet a standard of care—so ask.

•**Engage your brain right away.** What you do matters, too—so don't rely solely on rehab services. Do your best to stimulate your brain by playing games on a tablet or working on a puzzle. When people visit you in the hospital, rather than just watching TV together or exchanging pleasantries, have a real conversation about current events or a book you recently have read. In animal studies, mice kept in enriched and stimulating environments after stroke had greater recovery than those kept in simple cages. You want as much of your brain back as possible…so use it as soon as possible!

CHAPTER 5

Consumer Health Alerts

Generic Drugs: Shortages, Price Gouging and Other Crimes

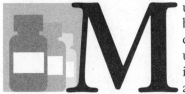

Much attention has been paid in recent years to the unfortunate reality of drug shortages and wild price inflation in the United States. The reasons for this serious problem are complex but the bottom line is (as always in these types of things) money. Almost everyone who has had a need for chronic or even short-term drug therapy has experienced the frustration and upset of having to pay unreasonably high prices for prescribed treatment. Many of these same patients have been told that there is a shortage of medications that have been in existence for decades.

Before I can speak about what you can do to help yourself when drugs are too costly or unavailable, let's understand how this dilemma came about...

First, it is important to realize that prescription drugs are either available as brand name or generics. Over 85% of the prescriptions written in our country are for the generic, or "off-patent," version of a medication. Since the majority of prescribed medications are generic, many of these agents have been on the market for decades. One would think that since these medicines have been used for so long, and their safety and effectiveness has stood the test of time, they would be the least costly. In many cases that is true. But in some critical areas of treatment, such as in cancer care, antibiotic therapy, anesthetics and even something as simple as intravenous salt solutions, forces have conspired to create shortages that have led to price gouging by certain large generic suppliers.

In 2007, the FDA said that 154 drugs had become scarce or no longer on the market. By

David Sherer, MD, practices anesthesiology in the suburbs of Washington DC, and has held two US patents in the fields of critical care medicine and telecommunications. He is author of *Dr. David Sherer's Hospital Survival Guide: 100+ Ways to Make Your Hospital Stay Safe and Comfortable*. His blog at BottomLineInc.com is titled "What Your Doctor Isn't Telling You."

2012, that number had grown to more than 300. What is causing this? Recently, a report in the journal *Global IT* quoted the National Center for Biotechnology Information, saying that…

•**Manufacturing difficulties caused a decrease in production of updated drugs.**

•**Shortages of raw materials cause delays in crucial materials.**

•**Natural disasters caused shortages in inventories.**

•**FDA regulatory issues tied up production and distribution.**

•**Simple supply-and-demand issues disrupted the stock of necessary medication.**

But there are other, more sinister reasons behind the alarming shortages and increase in prices that have resulted in staggering increases in medicines for gout (*colchicine*, up 50-fold), heart failure (*digoxin*, up six-fold) and arrhythmias (*isoproterenol*, up five-fold) over the last five decades. (One 62-year-old treatment for the parasitic disease toxoplasmosis is up over 5,000%, from $13 to $750 per tablet!)

Health Affairs Blog has recently reported that it is the sharp rise in generic drug prices that has affected the consumer most. In February 2016, that journal stated, "…Stronger generic manufacturers…absorbed numerous competitors…For many drugs…a combination of supply-chain disruptions, manufacturing problems, FDA compliance problems, and business failures…reduced the number of suppliers. As a result,…generic products were left with only 2 or 3 active suppliers…creating a natural monopoly…While generic drugs are still…less costly than brand-name…in 2013 one-third of generic drugs had a price increase, with about 10% of generics posting an increase of 50% or more…"

The article goes on to say that this caused "…President Obama to issue an Executive Order…directing the FDA to take steps to alleviate 'a serious and growing threat to public health…'"

So what is the patient to do about the fact that, according the US Department of Health and Human Services, 22% of the top generics reviewed in the decade prior to 2014 rose faster than inflation? How can we all get a handle on this ever-growing concern?

I have a few ideas…

•**Always ask your doctor for the least-expensive alternative for your medication.** If he or she does not know the answer, check with your insurance plan to see what blood pressure, blood thinner or diabetic medication is most cost-effective AND meets with your doctor's approval for your treatment plan.

•**Better yet, take better care of yourself with good health habits!** Restrict saturated fat, sugar and refined carbohydrates from your diet. Exercise. Lose weight. Stop smoking. Think of the freedom you'll have (as well as the extra money) by not having to take as many medications.

•**ALWAYS ask your doctor if you need to be on medications that a former practitioner had put you on.** Oftentimes, conditions improve or resolve altogether, but patients are still on medication for conditions that are no longer problems. *Americans are overmedicated!* I can't stress this enough.

•**Get politically active.** I know it seems like an impossible task, but if enough citizens got on their senators and congressmen and women about the predatory monopolies in the drug industry, there might be some improvement.

•**Shop for health plans that are large enough and strong enough to have negotiated better pricing** for necessary medication.

•**Consider acupuncture, yoga, meditation, herbal, psycho- or physiotherapy** or other non-drug modalities for some of your medical issues. They are almost always better for you than pills.

Melatonin Can Be Dangerous

Michael J. Breus, PhD, clinical psychologist and a fellow of The American Academy of Sleep Medicine. Based in Los Angeles, he is author of *The Power of When.* TheSleepDoctor.com

More than three million Americans take the hormone melatonin to help them sleep. Most people assume it is safe. But this supplement can reduce the effectiveness of certain medications, and it has potentially dangerous side effects. What's more, many people who take melatonin do so at the wrong times or for problems that it will not solve.

Contrary to popular belief, a melatonin supplement will not help you fall asleep—but it could help you sleep through the night if you chronically wake up way too early and cannot fall back asleep. (This sleep pattern is particularly likely among people in their 50s or older—our natural melatonin production decreases as we age.) A melatonin supplement also can help shift your sleep schedule following travel between time zones, reducing jet lag.

Melatonin supplements are safe for most people, but they have been shown to decrease the effectiveness of certain crucial medications including blood pressure drugs, seizure-prevention drugs, antidepressants and birth control medications. They can increase blood sugar levels, too, making them potentially dangerous for diabetics.

Other potential side effects include headaches, dizziness, stomach irritation, irritability, short-term depression and grogginess. These side effects are most likely when people take excessive doses—but almost everyone takes excessive doses. An appropriate initial adult dose typically is 0.5 milligrams (mg), but most melatonin supplements contain three, five or even 10 mg per pill.

What to do: If you have trouble remaining asleep through the night or want to head off jet lag, take a 0.5 mg dose of melatonin 90 minutes before bedtime to give it time to be released into the bloodstream and reach the brain. If you wait until bedtime, you might still be groggy in the morning.

If this proves ineffective, gradually increase the dosage on future nights until you find a level that works for you, but do not exceed 5 mg. (If you have diabetes or are taking medications for any of the health conditions mentioned, consult with your doctor.)

If your problem is falling asleep, not remaining asleep, try the herbal sleep inducer valerian root instead.

Antibiotics Are Turning Up in Fish

Study by researchers at Arizona State University, Tempe, published in *The Journal of Hazardous Materials*.

Both farmed and wild fish from 11 countries, bought in Arizona and California, had detectable amounts of antibiotics. All levels were below limits set by the Food and Drug Administration, but even very low levels could increase the development of antibiotic-resistant bacteria.

A Chef's Strategy for Buying Seafood at the Supermarket

Aliza Green, a Philadelphia-based chef and author of more than a dozen books about food including *The Fishmonger's Apprentice* and *Field Guide to Seafood. The Philadelphia Inquirer* inducted Green into its Culinary Hall of Fame in 1988. She currently leads culinary tours and serves as chef manager of Baba Olga's Kitchen in Philadelphia. AlizaGreen.com

The key to preparing delicious seafood occurs before you set foot in your kitchen—you must buy a great piece of fish. If the seafood you start with is not high quality and fresh, the meal you make will fall flat.

Unfortunately, many areas do not have top-notch seafood stores. That means most Americans must buy their seafood at supermarkets. This is not necessarily a bad option—some supermarkets have excellent seafood departments—but quality can vary dramatically.

How to decide where to buy seafood and how to pick the best seafood…

WAYS TO EVALUATE A MARKET OR SEAFOOD DEPARTMENT

Before buying from a supermarket seafood department or stand-alone fish market…

•**Take a whiff as you approach the counter.** You should smell ocean brine or nothing at all. If instead you get a low-tide–like fishy odor, walk away—the store does not pay sufficient attention to freshness or cleanliness.

•**Examine whole fish on display—even if you intend to buy a fillet.** The fishes' eyes should be bright and clear, not cloudy...scales should be shiny and metallic-looking, not dull. If you can touch the fish, gently press its flesh—if it is fresh, the depression you create will quickly disappear. It speaks poorly of the store if there are past-their-prime whole fish on display.

•**Look for liquid in packaged fish fillets.** Tip a few packaged fish fillets to one side. If you see liquid sloshing around, the fillet has been sitting around too long—those are juices that have escaped the fish as it aged and dried out. You could simply select a different fillet, but the smarter move is to not buy seafood there at all—liquid in fillet packages is a red flag that a store is not sufficiently focused on freshness.

•**Eye the ice in fish display cases.** This ice should look clear. If it is cloudy or yellowed, it likely is not changed very often—another sign of inattention.

•**At a supermarket, ask to speak to the fish-department manager.** I always consider it a warning sign if this manager is summoned from the meat department—supermarkets that take seafood seriously tend to have specialists running their seafood sections. The main point of asking for the manager is to see who he/she is. To that end, you can ask about his background with seafood...and you might also ask, "What's the freshest fish you have today?"

•**Notice fish-department traffic.** The more customers a seafood department or seafood store has, the faster it will turn over its inventory and the fresher its seafood is likely to be. Be wary if you've been to a store several times and rarely see anyone buying fish.

•**Seek out markets that cater to immigrant groups from coastal, seafood-loving nations.** I have found that if there's a market in the area that has a large clientele of people from Portugal, Korea, Vietnam or Italy, for example, it likely is a great place to buy excellent seafood for reasonable prices. Members of these communities tend to be savvy seafood shoppers. And because these groups tend to eat lots of seafood, inventory turnover often is high.

WAYS TO SELECT SEAFOOD

Even at a well-run seafood store or supermarket seafood department, some pieces of fish inevitably will be fresher and better than others...

•**Look for a slight blue tint in white-flesh fish.** A white, flaky fish such as cod, flounder or haddock should be translucent or such a brilliant white that it seems to have a slight bluish tint. If there's a slight yellowish tint instead, the fish has begun to oxidize and won't taste very good.

•**Seek a distant sell-by date.** Prepackaged fish should include a sell-by date on the label. But it's not sufficient that a packaged piece of fish hasn't passed its sell-by date—you want to find fish that is at least two days away from this date.

Warning: If seafood has a far-off sell-by date but seems past its prime, don't buy it—disreputable stores occasionally repackage fish as it nears its original sell-by date.

•**Don't be afraid of the word "frozen."** When it comes to seafood, fresh is best only if you live very near where that fish was caught. Otherwise you may be better off buying frozen, particularly when the frozen fish is vacuum-sealed and the packaging says it was "flash frozen"—that is, frozen almost immediately after coming out of the water.

Warning: When you choose frozen fish, avoid packages that have frost on the fish inside the packaging...and/or where sections of the frozen fish's flesh appear discolored. These are signs that frozen fish has been sitting around too long.

•**Lean toward seafood that is sold in thick steaks.** The higher a piece of seafood's ratio of volume to surface area, the better it likely will hold up over time, whether fresh or frozen. All else being equal, that means the best bet for freshness often is large fish that's cut into thick steaks, which might include tuna, swordfish, salmon or Chilean sea bass. (Be aware that swordfish—and to a lesser extent tuna and Chilean sea bass—sometimes have high mercury levels, so they should not be eaten very frequently, especially by children and pregnant women.)

•**Avoid seafood imported from Southeast Asia.** Fishing industry standards and quality controls are not as reliable in Southeast Asia as they are in North, South and Central America. Among other issues, fish imported from Southeast Asia—including from large exporters such as Vietnam, Thailand, Indonesia and China—might not have been frozen promptly and properly, increasing the odds of flavor and safety problems.

Warning: Virtually all the tilapia sold in the US is imported from Southeast Asia. Much of the shrimp sold in the US comes from Southeast Asia, too, but it is possible to find shrimp from Mexico, Venezuela or the US Gulf Coast instead.

•**Don't automatically skip the fish that's on sale.** Buying bargain fish might sound like a bad idea—because fish sometimes is marked down because it is about to go bad. But sometimes the fish that's on sale is the freshest fish in the store because there have been big recent catches of a certain type of fish and distributors must temporarily slash prices to move this inventory.

•**Avoid exotic or obscure fish unless you have great trust in the store.** Some people find it fun to try new foods—but most don't, which means unusual types of fish tend to sit around in stores longer than well-known types of fish. It's fine to buy unusual fish if a store you trust assures you that it's fresh, it's a fish that is popular in the community that frequents the store (such as whiting in an Italian market or monkfish in an Asian market) and/or you have faith in your fish-selection skills.

•**Buy shellfish that grew in northern waters, especially if you're planning to enjoy it raw.** These are less likely than warm-water shellfish to harbor dangerous parasites, and they often have more flavor, too.

Examples: Oysters and mussels from Atlantic Canada or New England are excellent options.

AFTER YOU BUY YOUR FISH...

It might not be the store's fault when a piece of seafood tastes less than fresh. *How you transport and store seafood after you buy it matters, too...*

•**Ask for ice for the trip home.** Seafood can significantly degrade in the time it takes to get it home from the store, especially on hot days. Most seafood stores and departments will provide a bag of ice upon request.

•**Store seafood on ice in your fridge.** Unless you're cooking seafood as soon as you get home, fill a container with ice and put the seafood on this bowl in your fridge. (Wrap the seafood in plastic wrap first if it is not already sealed well.) This ice provides additional cooling—I find that seafood is best stored at around 28°F, which is colder than a fridge on its own.

•**Defrost frozen seafood in the fridge.** This takes longer than defrosting it at room temperature, but it's safer—there's increased risk for contamination when you defrost seafood at room temperature. Defrosting in the fridge leads to tastier seafood—too much liquid often drips out when seafood is defrosted at room temperature, taking a lot of the flavor with it.

Helpful: The ideal time to cook a piece of seafood that has been frozen is when it is no longer rigid but you can still feel tiny ice crystals in its flesh. If you wait until these ice crystals melt, some flavor will be lost even if you do defrost in the fridge.

•**Don't let seafood languish, even frozen.** Even frozen, most fish should be kept tightly wrapped and positioned in the back of the freezer where it's coldest and used within one month for the best flavor.

What the "Natural" Label on Beef Really Means

Karen Lewis DeLong, PhD, assistant professor, department of agricultural and resource economics, University of Tennessee, Knoxville, and corresponding author of a study published in *Applied Economic Perspectives and Policy*.

T he beef label "natural" is misleading. The USDA label simply means that meat is minimally processed and contains no artificial ingredients or added color. But many consumers think that it means much more—

for instance, that the meat was raised without antibiotics or growth hormones.

This directly affects consumer costs: Beef consumers who did not know the official meaning of "natural" were willing to pay $1.26/pound more for meat with the label—and $2.43/pound more for meat also labeled as having no growth hormones. But consumers who were made aware of the FDA label's definition were not willing to pay more for beef labeled "natural" unless it had other positive labels, such as "no growth hormones." In these cases, consumers were willing to pay $3.07 per pound more.

The Truth About Organic Foods

Sharon Palmer, RDN, a Los Angeles-based registered dietitian nutritionist and author of *The Plant-Powered Diet* and *Plant-Powered for Life.* Palmer also is the editor of the newsletter *Environmental Nutrition* and nutrition editor for *Today's Dietitian.* SharonPalmer.com

Organic food is on a roll. Sales have doubled in the last decade, and organic foods are now available in three out of four conventional supermarkets.

Rather than being relegated to the "organic produce bin," there is now a wide assortment of organic foods and beverages. You can not only toss organic apples in your cart but also add a few organic gummy bears from the candy aisle, for example, and then pop over to the liquor store for organic vodka!

We are willing to pay more for organics, mostly because we think they are healthier for us. But are they really? What does "organic" on a food label really mean, anyway?

Let's explore a few common myths—and truths.

6 ORGANIC FOOD MYTHS

For such a popular (and pricey) part of our everyday food-buying habits, organic foods are surprisingly misunderstood…

1. Belief: Organic foods are more nutritious. Not exactly. The science is mixed. In 2012, a meta-analysis of 17 studies done by Stanford University found very little difference in vitamin content between organic and conventional produce. However, other studies have found that organic dairy and meat products contain more heart-healthy omega-3 fats, and organic fruits and vegetables are richer in antioxidant compounds than conventional produce.

The bottom line? While there may be some nutritional merits, the main reason to buy organic is not to get more nutritious fare but to support systems of cultivation that are good for the environment (see What "Organic" Really Means on the next page).

2. Belief: Organic foods are less likely to cause food poisoning.

Sorry, not true either. An organic chicken or hamburger meat that you buy from a farmer's market is no less likely to cause food-borne illness than conventional products.

3. Belief: Organic foods improve health. Maybe. Organic produce is significantly lower in pesticide residues than conventional. Both adults and children who eat more organic foods have lower levels of pesticides in their bodies compared with those who eat little or no organic foods. But whether that translates to healthier lives isn't known.

4. Belief: Organic foods are always local and sustainable. Sometimes, but not always. The standards do promote "sustainable practices," but do not require foods to be produced locally. The US imported $1.65 billion worth of organics in 2016, both fresh and processed, mostly from Turkey, Mexico, Italy, Peru and Ecuador. Transporting foods long distances means greater use of fossil fuels, which is not a sustainable practice.

5. Belief: Organic foods are pesticide-free. Not necessarily. It's true that farming practices that promote biodiversity, natural borders, soil health and natural pest predators lessen pest problems, so there's less need for pesticides.

But while most synthetic pesticides are not allowed in organic produce, there are a few exceptions—25 are allowed (compared with about 900 in conventional produce). In addition, "natural" pesticides are allowed, such as soaps or lime sulfur.

6. Belief: All organic producers are the same. Not by a long shot. Some farms practice techniques that go well beyond the standards—avoiding even "allowed" pesticides and selling locally—while other farms barely squeak under the minimum compliance to standards.

So you may want to seek out local organic producers who are more in tune with the spirit of organic, such as caring for the environment and supplying a local food source. The moral of the story? If buying organic matters to you, do some homework on organic producers before you buy.

WHAT "ORGANIC" REALLY MEANS

The main reason to choose organic is to support a kind of food cultivation that preserves the soil and promotes a cleaner environment. Nutrition and safety aren't the primary goals. Organic cultivation isn't so much about the end product as it is about the process.

The USDA's National Organic Program (NOP) maintains standards for organically produced agricultural products. The purpose is to support a system of farming that encourages recycling of resources within a farm, protects the environment, enhances soil and water quality and conserves ecosystems and wildlife. Most synthetic fertilizers, sewage sludge, irradiation and genetic engineering can't be used.

Only products that have been through a rigorous certification process to show that they meet these requirements may carry the USDA organic seal. Foods with the seal may be labeled "100% organic" (everything in it is organic)…"organic" (at least 95% of the ingredients are organic)…or "made with organic ingredients" (at least 70% of the ingredients are organic). This includes both whole foods (for example, an apple) and packaged foods (such as applesauce).

BEST FOODS TO BUY ORGANIC…AND WHAT TO SKIP

According to data analyzed by the nonprofit Environmental Working Group (EWG), these are some of the foods that should be at the top of your organic shopping list…

•**Leafy greens.** Crops such as these, which grow close to the soil, are prone to pests. Spinach samples had twice as much pesticide residue as any other crop.

•**Strawberries,** which also grow close to the soil, had up to 20 different pesticides.

•**Peaches and nectarines** tested positive for at least one pesticide in nearly all samples.

•**Cherries and apples** tested positive for pesticide residues in nearly all of the samples tested.

•**Dairy foods, eggs and meat.** Organically raised beef cattle, dairy cows and chickens are not treated with synthetic growth hormones or antibiotics. Plus, organic dairy, meat and eggs have higher levels of omega-3s, and organic eggs have more vitamins A and E.

If your food budget is limited, don't waste your organic dollars here…

•**Candy and soda.** Organic sugary foods are just as bad for your health as conventional sugary foods.

•**Baked treats, such as cookies, cakes and pies.** A few organic ingredients in a decadent treat won't make it any healthier.

•**Nuts, melons and avocados.** The outer shells of these foods protect them from pests, so few pesticides are needed. They tend to have low residue levels.

•**Carrots and sweet potatoes.** These root vegetables, which grow in the soil rather than above it, can absorb some pesticides through the soil but are usually peeled before eating.

•**Citrus.** Citrus fruit, especially grapefruit, registered among the fruits with the lowest levels of pesticide residues, according to EWG. Thank the thick rind!

Egg Labels That Matter

Consumer Reports.

"Organic" means that eggs were laid by uncaged hens that have access to outdoors and are fed grains grown without synthetic pesticides. "Free Range" and "American Humane Certified" mean that the birds were not caged—the two labels mean that the chickens had access to outdoors.

Egg labels that do not matter also are sometimes used on eggs and cartons: "No hormones" is irrelevant because all egg-producing chickens must, by law, be raised without hormones. "Farm fresh" means eggs come from a farm—all of them do—and the eggs have not been frozen, which they should never be. "Natural" means nothing—all eggs are natural foods.

avoiding sourcing meats from farms that use inhumane or unsustainable practices such as crowding and overusing antibiotics. Restaurants that pass the certification process display a window decal with "REAL Certified."

More information: EatReal.org.

The Truth About Coffee Labels

Consumer Reports.

Ethically/sustainably farmed, shade grown and direct trade have no legal definitions or specific standards. But some seals do indicate coffee-growing conditions. "USDA Organic" means that synthetic fertilizers and synthetic pesticides that may harm farmers and wildlife are not used. "Fair Trade" means that beans come from small-scale farmers who were paid a fair price. "Fair Trade Certified" means that beans were grown on small or large plantations that meet standards including protecting workers from unsafe conditions and paying at least the local minimum wage. "Bird Friendly Habitat" means that the farm meets the term as defined by the Smithsonian Migratory Bird Center—the environment must protect biodiversity and maintain native trees. "Rainforest Alliance Certified" means that the beans come from farms that meet standards promoting sustainability.

An Easy Way to Find Ethical Eateries

USA Today.

An independent program that certifies restaurants and packaged-food companies for meeting health and nutritional standards now is including a certification for animal welfare. Washington, DC–based nonprofit Eat Real has certified about 500 food-service companies as

Is Raw Milk Safe?

Michelle Dudash, RDN, nutritionist, Carmel, Indiana. MichelleDudash.com

Raw milk has not been pasteurized (heated at a high temperature) to kill harmful bacteria, such as campylobacter, E. coli and salmonella, which can cause stomach cramping, vomiting and diarrhea. Young children, pregnant women, the elderly and people with weakened immune systems are at highest risk for illness.

Some farmers test their raw milk for bacteria, but these tests do not always detect low levels of contamination, and bacteria will continue to grow in the milk each day.

My advice: Look for local dairies that sell pasteurized milk…it's likely to have been pasteurized at a lower temperature and will taste fresher.

Don't Eat Raw Cookie Dough

Uncooked flour, like uncooked eggs, can make you sick. In a recent report, 56 people got sick from the uncooked flour in cookie-dough products. The flour was contaminated with E. coli bacteria. While dry flour is not a high risk, it's best not to taste any raw dough or other batter—which also may contain eggs contaminated with salmonella.

Bill Marler, JD, is an attorney specializing in food safety, Seattle. The study of E. coli contamination in dry flour was recently published in *The New England Journal of Medicine*.

Bacteria Grow in Bagged Salads

Study by researchers at University of Leicester, UK, published in *Applied and Environmental Microbiology*.

Even slight damage to the leaves releases juices that encourage the spread of salmonella bacteria, a cause of food poisoning.

Self-defense: Choose salad with minimally damaged leaves, rinse before eating and consume before the "best by" date.

Beware: Toxic Lead and Cadmium in Decorated Drinking Glasses

Andrew Turner, PhD, associate professor in environmental sciences, University of Plymouth, UK, lead author of study titled "High Levels of Migratable Lead and Cadmium on Decorated Drinking Glassware" published in *Science of the Total Environment*.

It may seem like harmless fun to sip a smoothie, beer or cola from your favorite superhero glass. But unless you, too, can be felled only by kryptonite, you'll be much healthier if you drink your beverage from a plain glass. *Here's why…*

Background: Popular decorative glassware, such as drinking glasses that have characters, logos or colorful patterns painted onto them, have come under scrutiny again for their potential danger to health. This isn't the first time. For example, in 2010, Coca-Cola voluntarily recalled 88,000 glasses marketed to kids after tests found the toxic metal cadmium in the decorative paint. Now a new study shows evidence that the problem may be more widespread.

Study: A team from the University of Plymouth in England ran 197 tests on 72 pieces of decorated glassware. Researchers tested both new and secondhand beer mugs, shot glasses, tumblers, jars and wine glasses decorated with enamel paint or glaze in a variety of colors, including gold leaf, that had been made in China and Europe.

Results: Regardless of paint color used, more than 70% of the drinkware tested positive for lead. About the same amount also tested positive for cadmium, with the highest concentrations found in red enamel finishes.

Worse: When the researchers used a reagent that replicates acidic drinks, such as fruit juices, sodas and wine, metals from the rim area where the lips are in direct contact with the glass were easily dissolved. Also, flakes of paint came off when researchers put the glassware through tests that duplicated regular use, such as cleaning or stacking—further increasing the likelihood of mobilizing and ingesting these dangerous metals. And even though lead and cadmium were found on only some of the rim areas, having them anywhere on the surface of drinking glasses can potentially lead to ingestion if people touch their faces and/or mouths after holding the painted glassware.

Exposure to lead above four parts per million (ppm) and cadmium above 0.4 ppm from glass products that come into contact with food is considered unsafe, according to the US Food and Drug Administration. Alarmingly, lead concentrations on the tested glassware were as high as 400,000 ppm…and cadmium concentrations as high as 70,000 ppm.

Both lead and cadmium are highly toxic. Cadmium can damage the kidneys and increase the risk of lung, kidney and possibly pancreatic cancer. Unsafe levels of lead can cause high blood pressure, joint and muscle pain, memory problems, anemia and kidney disease, and are particularly damaging to young children. If you've been regularly drinking out of a glass that has enameled decoration near the rim, mention it to your doctor. A simple blood test is one way to detect cadmium or lead poisoning. A blood level above five micrograms per deciliter for lead and/or above five nanograms per milliliter for cadmium is considered elevated. If your levels are very high, your doctor might recommend medication that will bind with the metal so you can excrete it in your urine.

Note: All plants absorb cadmium from the soil, but tobacco is especially efficient at doing this—which makes smokers at increased risk for high levels of the metal in their blood.

Bottom line: The researchers did find that organic inks, more common in newer glassware, tested negative for lead and cadmium. But since there's no way to tell by looking whether the decorations on a particular glass are made with organic ink, stick to plain, undecorated glass bottles, glasses and food-storage containers.

Adults and Lead Paint

Hyla Cass, MD, a psychiatrist and integrative medicine practitioner in Los Angeles. She is author of *The Addicted Brain and How to Break Free.* CassMD.com

Although most information about lead paint toxicity concerns exposure in children, lead can be dangerous for adults, too. Even though lead paint has been banned in the US since 1978, the dust from old paint can become airborne when you scrape down surfaces to repaint.

Lead that is inhaled or ingested accumulates in the bones and is released through the blood (especially as we age and bones thin), increasing risk for anemia, high blood pressure, nerve damage, decreased kidney function and reproductive issues. Lead toxicity can contribute to memory loss, too.

If you live in or are moving to a living space built before 1978: Use a test kit (such as the 3M LeadCheck, less than $25) to test for the presence of lead paint.

If you detect lead paint and plan to remodel, make sure you or your contractor follows all safety guidelines, such as sealing the room, covering vents with plastic and wet-washing surfaces instead of dusting.

Get a blood test after the remodel. If lead levels are high, you may need further blood testing or urinalysis. With very high levels of exposure (over 80 ug/dL, for example), your doctor may recommend chelation therapy (a process that removes metals from the blood). The typical blood lead level for adults is under 10 ug/dL.

Paint Strippers Can Kill You in Minutes

Katy Wolf, PhD, director of the Institute for Research and Technical Assistance, a nonprofit organization that identifies safer alternatives for industrial and consumer solvents and other products, Los Angeles. IRTA.us

A 21-year-old Tennessee man died recently while refinishing a tub in an unventilated bathroom. Fumes from methylene chloride, a chemical in the paint stripper he was using, caused carbon monoxide to build up in his blood, and within minutes his heart stopped beating.

Most paint strippers sold in hardware stores and home centers contain methylene chloride, yet few people who use these products understand the danger. These products are known to be responsible for at least 56 accidental-exposure deaths in the US since 1980, and the true death toll is no doubt higher—some methylene chloride fatalities are likely recorded as heart attacks, with no one realizing that this chemical is to blame.

Methylene chloride also is known to cause cancer, though that's a risk mainly for people who have prolonged exposure to it because they use paint strippers in their professions, not for consumers who use them only occasionally.

What to do: Choose a benzyl alcohol–based paint stripper rather than one that contains methylene chloride. It's safer and does a good job stripping paint, though it does not work as quickly as methylene chloride.

If you do use a methylene chloride paint stripper, do so outdoors or in a large, well-ventilated area, never in a small and/or enclosed space. Do not use methylene chloride to strip the inside of bathtubs, storage tanks or similar objects even if they are not fully enclosed—its fumes are heavier than air, so they can quickly build up to lethal levels inside these, even outdoors.

Water Purification Concern

Jessica Fairley, MD, MPH, assistant professor of medicine and global health, Emory University, Atlanta.

Devices, tablets and liquids that filter and/ or purify water are effective, though some are better than others for specific needs. For example, filtration devices (pump or gravity-drip devices) can remove bacteria and parasites such as Giardia, but only those devices that also use chlorine, iodine or a microfiltration process can remove viruses such as enterovirus. These cost $20 and up. Devices using ultraviolet light cost under $100 and can disinfect small amounts of water (about 25 ounces) quickly, though you may need to filter the water first. Some pocket-size, battery-powered units use a technique called salt electrolysis in which briny water is electrically charged to kill pathogens. And boiling water for 60 seconds is a tried-and-true way to purify water, although it may still look discolored.

Visit CDC.gov/travel and click on "Destinations" to find precautions for each country before selecting a device to buy. Or opt for sealed bottled water.

Caution: Use iodine in the filtration devices mentioned earlier for no more than a few weeks, and avoid it if you are pregnant or have a thyroid condition.

Are Old(er) Microwave Ovens Safe?

Devra Davis, PhD, president of the Environmental Health Trust, Teton Village, Wyoming.

Is your older microwave oven still safe to use?

Make sure the door isn't warped and the hinges are not bent…the mesh window screen is not damaged…and the seal around the door is not loose. If you are able to turn on your oven while the door is open, the FDA recommends that you immediately stop using it. Any of these issues could signal that the oven is leaking radi-

ation in excess of safe limits. It's safer to replace your oven than to fix it.

Helpful: Limit exposure to all forms of radiation by putting distance between you and products that emit radiation. Opt for wired products, such as corded headphones, over wireless. Use the speaker mode on your cell phone…don't carry your cell phone in your pocket unless it's on airplane mode…and don't stand next to your microwave while it's on—even new ovens emit some radiation.

Avoid These 4 Nasty Chemicals in Your Skincare!

Ginger Hodulik Downey holds a BS in foods and nutrition, an MS degree in nutrition and a CNS (Certified Nutrition Specialist). She is currently the co-owner and vice president of R&D for DermaMed Solutions.

Your skin is this super-absorber of substances both good and bad, and the products you put on your skin end up in your body. On average, consumers use about 10 personal care products containing 126 ingredients in total per day!

The government doesn't require health studies or pre-market testing for these products. The FDA has a GRAS (Generally Regarded as Safe) list, but almost every chemical is included in that list! They focus on things like softness or wrinkle reduction, not the unintended consequences. Of the 7,000 ingredients on the list, only 6 have been tested for long-term safety. This means that consumers need to be extra-vigilant about evaluating their skincare products for themselves since the government is not watching out for us.

I'm going to discuss the top offenders and why you should avoid them. It's going to get a little technical but I'll try my best to break it down!

CHEMICALS IN SKINCARE

Parabens are preservatives found in many skincare products. You can spot them easily on the product label because they end with the

89

word paraben. [*Ingredients to look for*: methyl-paraben, proplyparaben, isopropylparaben, isobutylparaben, butylparaben, and sodium butylparaben.]

Although the FDA has determined that parabens are safe for inclusion in skincare products, many scientists agree that they are not a wise choice. Why is this? Well, one reason has to do with the chemical structure of a paraben, which is close to that of estrogen and can fit into estrogen receptors at the cellular level. Basically what that means is that your delicate endocrine (hormone) system is disturbed and may eventually lead to breast and other forms of cancer.

THE NITTY-GRITTY

The body of evidence against parabens is growing.

Recently, a 2015 study conducted at the University of California Berkeley looked at parabens in their interaction with estrogen receptors in the body, specifically HER. Researchers said that previous tests potentially missed the "real world" effects of parabens by only considering them in isolation, rather than factoring in interaction with other molecules in cells, as the parabens in this setting stimulated tumor growth significantly.

There are numerous research studies like this which are mostly suggestive, however, the suggestion is strong enough for me to avoid parabens until further research is done to tell me they are safe. Better safe than sorry, right?

CHEMICALS IN SKINCARE

Phthalates are chemical compounds that are used as plasticizers—ingredients that give plastics their elasticity and change the texture and quality of skincare products. [*Ingredients to look for*: di-2-ethyl hexyl phthalate (DEHP), diisodecyl phthalate (DIDP), butylbenzyl phthalate (BBP), dibutyl phthalate (DBP), di-isononyl phthalate (DINP), and diethyl phthalate (DEP).]

Now these probably look like a lot of confusing chemicals that you don't understand, but just check the ingredient labels in your skincare products. You're more than likely to find them!

Phthalates are considered estrogen disruptors and the cause of reproductive problems. They also have been indicated as causing fat-related health risks.

A University of Rochester Medical Center study connected common chemicals to rising obesity rates. The analysis found men with the highest levels of phthalates in their urine had more belly fat and insulin resistance. Who wants their skincare products adding to the already difficult task of battling weight gain?

SULFATES

These ingredients generally act as detergents or foaming agents and are found in cleansers and shampoos. [*Ingredients to look for include*: sodium lauryl sulfate (sls), sodium laureth sulfate (sles), ammonium lauryl sulfate, sodium myreth sulfate.]

Tests show that sodium lauryl sulfate can penetrate into the eyes as well as systemic tissues (brain, heart, liver, etc.) and show long-term retention in those tissues, especially when used in soaps and shampoos. This is especially important in infants, where considerable growth is occurring. SLS also changes the amounts of some proteins in cells in eyes, even of all ages.

SLS forms nitrates. Why does this matter? When SLS is used in shampoos and cleansers containing nitrogen-based ingredients, it can form carcinogenic nitrates that can enter the bloodstream in large numbers. This can cause eye irritations, skin rashes, hair loss, scalp scurf similar to dandruff, and allergic reactions!

One rule of thumb to remember—if it foams, it may not be your friend.

CHEMICALS IN SKINCARE

Petroleum is used by many skincare companies because it's a cheap ingredient that can be used as a moisturizing agent. In many European countries it is banned as an ingredient in skincare products. Petroleum can contain known carcinogens (cancer-causing chemicals). Additionally, these products block moisture from escaping the skin, and clog pores. They offer a false sense of hydration, when actually they prevent the action of your skin's natural fats to act to provide a moisture barrier.

CHEMICALS IN MAKEUP

Artificial dyes and fragrances in lotions, shampoos, and many other cosmetic products are composed of aromatic hydrocarbons. What does that mean for you? Perfumes and products containing fragrance can contain many hundreds of chemicals to produce a distinct scent. A significant number of these aromas are derived from petroleum. These chemicals have been associated with allergic reactions and hormone disruption. Some fragrance chemicals have not been assessed for safety. Until all fragrance ingredients are disclosed on the label, consumers cannot know what is in a particular fragrance. Therefore it's best to avoid synthetic fragrances altogether.

Certain artificial colors and dyes can cause allergic reactions. It takes up to 25 chemicals to create the synthetic color purple for example. That's a lot of chemicals just to add some visual appeal to a product! (If you think purple cream is attractive that is…) This puts a great deal of stress on the body's detoxification system. There's simply no need to add artificial colors to skincare products.

THE BOTTOM LINE

There's really no need to sacrifice safety for clinical efficacy! There are safe alternatives to the ingredients discussed here, even though it may cost us a little more.

Hair Dye and Breast Cancer Risk

Adana Llanos, PhD, MPH, assistant professor of epidemiology with Rutgers School of Public Health, New Brunswick, New Jersey, and leader of a study of more than 4,000 women, published in *Carcinogenesis*.

The use of brown or black hair dyes by black women was tied to a 51% greater risk for breast cancer. White women who used dark dyes had 31% higher risk. The study found an association between using hair products and the risk of being diagnosed with breast cancer, but it does not prove cause and effect.

FDA Warning on MRI Dye

Janet Woodcock, MD, director, Center for Drug Evaluation and Research, FDA, Silver Spring, Maryland.

A recent FDA warning notes that the metal *gadolinium*, commonly injected during an MRI scan to improve image quality, can linger in the brain, skin and bones for years. While it has not been directly linked to adverse health outcomes in people with normal kidney function, some patients have complained of pain, burning sensations and weakness after injection.

If you're scheduled for an MRI, especially if you get repeated scans: Don't avoid the dye, but do ask whether it is required.

The Legal Fight Over Marijuana's CBD

James Anthony, Esq., an attorney in Oakland, California, who has practiced cannabis-related law since 2006.

You can buy CBD—cannabidiol, the therapeutic yet noneuphoria–inducing marijuana component—online and in some health-food stores even if your state doesn't allow it. But is it legal to do so?

That's now being battled out in federal courts. While a US law makes it legal to sell marijuana-plant products such as hemp and hemp oil that have only trace amounts of THC (the compound in marijuana that makes people high), the Federal Drug Enforcement Agency still classifies CBD (the marijuana compound that doesn't make people high) as an illegal narcotic—like heroin.

As a consumer, though, you're almost certainly safe—it's highly unlikely that you'd get into legal trouble for buying or using a CBD product. The real target of the federal prohibition seems to be sellers, not buyers.

If your state allows the sale of medical marijuana—you can find out by going to Governing. com and searching for "marijuana map"—go to a state-licensed dispensary. If your state doesn't allow medical marijuana and you want to try using CBD, you still might be able to find it for sale…if not, you always have the option of ordering online.

Medical Marijuana Can Be Dangerous to People with Compromised Immune Systems

George Thompson III, MD, associate professor of clinical medicine, University of California, Davis, and leader of a study published in *Clinical Microbiology and Infection*.

Researchers have found infectious bacteria and fungi in some samples—pathogens that would not harm an average user but could be fatal to someone whose immune system is suppressed by disease or chemotherapy. One death has been reported—of a man using raw, blended cannabis inhaled as a mist to try to cope with the side effects of cancer treatment.

Health Care Is (Finally) Going to Pot—with Medical Marijuana

David Sherer, MD, practices anesthesiology in the suburbs of Washington DC, and has held two US patents in the fields of critical care medicine and telecommunications. He is author of *Dr. David Sherer's Hospital Survival Guide: 100+ Ways to Make Your Hospital Stay Safe and Comfortable*. His blog at BottomLineInc.com is titled "What Your Doctor Isn't Telling You."

Almost every consumer of health services today has heard that medical marijuana is in clinical use. Indeed, 30 states and the District of Columbia now have laws on the books that allow for the use of marijuana for medicinal purposes. Incredibly, these states are still in violation of federal law but, for now, the United States government has decided to look away. The federal government's policy of not prosecuting states that allow for medical marijuana might cause one to think that there must be some benefit in the use of this controversial agent. But first, some history.

Marijuana, or cannabis (as it is commonly called), has been used as a medicine for a variety of purposes for thousands of years. Ancient cultures in China, Egypt, Greece and certain Arab populations used cannabis for everything from wound healing to hemorrhoids to insomnia and anxiety. It is actually one of the 50 essential plants used in traditional Chinese medicine. Until the advent of aspirin and the wider use of both naturally occurring and synthetically made narcotics (opiates and opioids), marijuana enjoyed some degree of notoriety in the medical community. It wasn't until its criminalization in the US in the 20th century that marijuana use for medical and recreational purposes went underground. However, with increasing opiate addiction and a growing populace of older and sicker people, scientists have turned in recent decades to the potential benefits of this most interesting of plants.

The science of marijuana as medicine can be plainly put. Our bodies contain billions of natural receptors that are stimulated by the many chemicals in marijuana that cause various beneficial and not-so-beneficial effects. Two of these chemicals, tetrahydrocannabinol (THC, the mind-altering component) and cannabinol (CBD, the major therapeutic part) are what we are concerned with most in discussing pot as medicine. Scientists have been able to alter the ratio of these chemicals in medical marijuana, whether in pill, vapor, tincture, edible or dermal patch formulations, to best affect a number of medical conditions. *So far, medical marijuana shows promise in…*

•**Reducing eye pressure from glaucoma.**

•**Improving appetite in cancer patients and patients with AIDS.**

•**Relieving chronic pain from a variety of causes,** such as from arthritis (both osteo and rheumatoid) and neuropathy.

•**Limb spasticity in patients with multiple sclerosis,** Parkinson's disease and other neurologic diseases.

•**Children with uncontrolled seizures.**

•**Reducing nausea and vomiting in patients receiving chemotherapy.**

•**Helping people with insomnia to sleep better.**

There are other applications that are actively being studied. They include using marijuana in the treatment for cancer, diabetes, asthma, fibromyalgia, chronic fatigue, depression, post-traumatic stress disorder (PTSD), Tourette's syndrome, Crohn's disease and many other illnesses. This truly is an exciting time in medical marijuana research. Bear in mind there are some side effects from the use of medical marijuana, but they are usually mild. *Most often they are…*

•**Dizziness**

•**Feeling tired**

•**Hallucinations**

•**Drowsiness**

•**Vomiting**

If you live in a state that has a medical marijuana program, I have the following suggestions…

•**Do research on the web about your state's medical marijuana program,** or simply call your state's Board of Health or Medicine.

•**Always deal with a reputable and licensed physician and dispensary.** Do research on the web or ask to see licenses or certificates from the state to verify compliance.

•**Ask friends and relatives** if they have experience with a certain provider of medical marijuana services.

•**Ask your personal physician if he/she knows of a licensed marijuana practitioner.** Ask if other patients have benefitted from such a regimen.

•**Contact your local university medical center** (if there is one in your community) to see if they have a medical marijuana program or do cannabis research.

Always remember that you should not carry marijuana across state lines—even if for medicinal purposes and even if it is legal in both states. (This is because marijuana is still illegal at the federal level.)

Medical marijuana may not be for everyone. It is not a cure all. Nor is it, I feel, snake oil. It still, unfortunately, carries the stigma that "pot" has had for decades, even centuries. However, if you have tried other therapies for your medical issue and they have failed or you can't tolerate the side effects, strongly consider trying this most fascinating and potentially beneficial of plants. You might be pleasantly surprised.

8 Mistakes to Avoid If You Get Bad News

Steven Z. Pantilat, MD, a palliative-care physician and the Kates-Burnard and Hellman Distinguished Professor in Palliative Care, University of California, San Francisco School of Medicine. He is author of *Life After the Diagnosis: Expert Advice on Living Well with Serious Illness for Patients and Caregivers.*

Sooner or later, it happens to most of us: We find ourselves sitting in a doctor's office hearing some very bad news. The diagnosis is heart failure, cancer, dementia, kidney failure, Parkinson's disease or some other serious (and possibly terminal) illness. At that moment, we are scared and vulnerable. It's easy to make mistakes when we're in a frantic quest to beat back illness. *Here's how to avoid or overcome these common mistakes…*

MISTAKE #1: **Making rash decisions.** Even when a diagnosis is dire, jumping right into treatment can be a mistake. So slow down, and make sure you have all the information you need. That means asking how your illness and the treatments you are considering will affect your day-to-day life…how likely it is that treatments will work…and what "working" means. To truly understand the answers, you need to also (politely) insist that doctors cut the jargon—so you won't end up thinking, for example, that a "response rate" is the same as a "cure rate."

Cancer patients often are surprised to learn that they can wait a bit before starting chemotherapy or other treatments—it is almost always safe to wait two to three weeks, but the doctor can tell you if it's not. These days, this short pause will often include waiting for a genetic analysis of the tumor, which might point to a more effective, targeted treatment. Getting extra information like that can make a wait worthwhile.

MISTAKE #2: Believing everything you read online. By now, everyone knows that all online information is not created equal. But many people cannot resist reading everything they find—and, in the process, they stumble across a lot of information that is scary, wrong or not relevant to their personal situation.

Best approach: Ask your doctor for reputable information sources, and discuss what you find with him/her.

MISTAKE #3: Not focusing on what you really want. Let's say you might benefit from a cutting-edge treatment, but you learn that getting it will mean frequent trips or a long stay in another city.

Those trips might be worth the hassle if your goal is to explore every avenue for treating the illness and taking any chance, no matter how small, to find a cure or at least manage an illness—but not if your primary goal is to enjoy the comforts of home and family in what might be precious remaining weeks or months.

The right question to ask is: Will this procedure or medicine help me to get back to my home and family? If it won't, what will?

MISTAKE #4: Focusing on death instead of living. It's important to think and talk about the end of life, but not at the expense of planning for the weeks, months or years that might still lie ahead. What will you need to do to keep up cherished hobbies and habits for as long as possible? Can you take a long-delayed trip, reconnect with long-lost friends or reach other personal goals?

To do that planning, you need to know the truth, so do not be afraid to ask your doctor how much time you have left, even if he has to estimate. You might have a lot more (or less) time than you assume.

Helpful: Regardless of your prognosis, ask about "palliative care"—care aimed at helping you function better, with less pain and stress and more emotional and spiritual support.

MISTAKE #5: Keeping your illness a secret. It might come as a surprise in this age of online over-sharing, but many people still keep serious illness a secret from family members, friends and others. That's a mistake. At the very least, you want a support person to go with you to important medical appointments to act as a second set of ears.

But you also may find a wider network of people eager to help with everything from meals to rides to lawn-mowing. Let them help. Share your hopes and fears with people you love and trust to help keep your stress levels in check.

Helpful: If you are wondering whether to tell someone close to you, try turning the table. What if you learned that this person had a serious illness and had not shared it so that you could help him? If you wish this person had told you, then you should think about sharing your news with this person.

MISTAKE #6: Assuming that the most aggressive or newest treatments are best. Even if your main goal is to live as long as possible, the most aggressive treatments are not always the best choices. You might sacrifice both quality and quantity of life by going ahead with a treatment that has little chance of helping you and a high probability of harming you.

For example, for some people with heart failure, a left ventricular assist device (LVAD), a pump surgically implanted into your heart to help pump the blood, might seem like a great idea. But there are serious complications, such as bleeding and stroke. Many people who have an LVAD implanted feel better, but some never get over the operation or have complications early and may feel that they are worse off with the LVAD than without it.

Helpful: Ask your doctor what is the best case, worst case and likely case with a particular treatment…and ask for the same assessments if you don't get that treatment.

MISTAKE #7: Limiting your care to alternative treatments. Complementary therapies—especially yoga, meditation, acupuncture and others that have been shown in research to have benefits—can be helpful when combined with standard treatments or when the benefits of standard treatments are exhausted. But patients who rely only on unproven approaches, including those pitched by pricey foreign clinics and online hucksters, sometimes wait too long to get evidence-based treatments that could have made a difference in how well and long they live.

MISTAKE #8: Beating yourself up. Many people blame themselves for getting sick—a woman may have forgotten to get a mammogram, for example, and developed breast cancer. Give yourself a break. It's true that there are risk factors for serious diseases. But generally speaking, the development of illness is more complex than that.

Also, don't beat yourself up for not staying positive enough. While cultivating joy, hope, gratitude and love will help you face your illness, blocking off all sadness, worry and grief will not help. Find a balance.

Helpful: Talk about things that are real, meaningful and personal with those who care about you.

MRIs Misdiagnose the Cause of Chronic Pain

Mitchell Yass, DPT, a specialist in diagnosing and resolving the cause of pain and creator of the Yass Method for treating chronic pain. He is the author of *Overpower Pain: The Strength Training Program That Stops Pain Without Drugs or Surgery* and *The Pain Cure Rx: The Yass Method for Diagnosing and Resolving Chronic Pain* and host of the PBS special *The Pain Prescription*.

If you ask 1,000 people "Does arthritis, a herniated disc, stenosis or a meniscal tear cause pain?" all would say "yes." Not because they have a full-factual understanding of these structures and whether it is even possible for them to elicit pain, but simply because this view has been programmed into our brains for the past 30 years. Since the advent of the magnetic resonance imaging technique (MRI) in the 1980s, arthritis and herniated discs have become so commonly diagnosed as the cause of pain that as soon as one of these conditions is identified on an MRI, people automatically assume it is the cause of their pain.

These ideas have been promoted by the medical establishment and pharmaceutical industry—and promoted in massive doses in direct-to-consumer advertising on television, radio and other media outlets. People are now so desensitized to the idea of these structural variations existing that they are happily willing to undergo surgery when they find that "all other methods have failed."

But the fact is that there is absolutely no theoretical, clinical or scientific evidence to prove that these structural variations are the cause of pain in almost any case. I will now provide you some details and you can make up your own mind about whether these are causing your pain and warrant any treatment.

Let's start with a historical review...

If arthritis, spinal stenosis, herniated discs, meniscal tears and every other structural variation identified on the MRI were the cause of pain, then why wasn't the number of people suffering from chronic pain overwhelmingly higher before the MRI was invented? Clearly nobody is going to make the argument that these structural variations began in the 1980s just at the time they could be identified by the MRI. So if they have existed through the history of mankind, why wasn't roughly the entire population of mankind having chronic pain before the very cause of the chronic pain was identified by the MRI? And if the MRI is identifying the cause of pain, why isn't the number of people suffering from chronic pain or those addicted to prescription pain medication falling at a rapid rate? In fact, the numbers simply continue to rise the more treatment is provided.

Now let's look at pain based on the time frame of those suffering with it versus the time frame of these structural variations...

Most people get their first MRI within weeks or a couple of months of when their pain began. And this is when they find out they have a herniated disc, spinal stenosis, arthritis, a meniscal tear or the like. Since the abnormalities are discovered at the same time that individuals are having pain, the assertion is that the structural variations are the cause of the pain. The next common assertion is that if the structural variation is the cause of pain, then the structural variation didn't exist before the pain began.

95

This view is insane to me. These structural variations take years or even decades to develop. If you knew that the structural variation existed long before you had pain, then how could anyone conclude it is the cause of the pain?

Finally, let's look at the relationship between those who have pain and those who do not. If these structural variations cause pain then, simply, those who do not have pain should not have structural variations. Yet 90% of people over age 60 with no back pain have bulging or degenerative discs, according to a study published in the journal *Spine* by researchers at University of Delaware and University of Pittsburgh. This statistic does not at all match up with the theoretical idea of structural variations causing pain.

Sometimes the biggest constraint to healing is clinging to what you "know." Allow yourself to try a different approach that runs counter to your beliefs and decades of programming from the medical establishment. Let go of the MRI fairy tales, and open yourself up to break free from chronic pain.

Your Biopsy Results Might Not Actually Be Yours

John D. Pfeifer, MD, PhD, professor and vice chair for clinical affairs in the pathology and immunology department at Washington University School of Medicine in St. Louis. WUSTL.edu

It's no secret that biopsies occasionally produce inaccurate results. But what if the biopsy result you get is accurate—but the tissue sample came from someone else's body?

Yes, it happens. A study of more than 13,000 prostate biopsies found that switched or contaminated samples caused the wrong patient to be told he had cancer approximately three times in 1,000. Additionally, three times in 1,000, a patient is told he doesn't have cancer when in fact he does. And there's no reason to assume that such mix-ups are limited to prostate biopsies.

Lab mix-ups such as these can have catastrophic consequences. A healthy person might be subjected to life-altering treatments, including surgery, chemotherapy and/or radiation, for someone else's medical problem. Meanwhile, the person who actually has this major medical problem might be told that he is fine, delaying potentially lifesaving treatments.

What to do: When the stakes of a biopsy are high, ask your doctor, "Does it make sense to do a DNA test to confirm that the tissue that was tested originated from me?" Some private labs that do DNA testing for criminal investigations also test to make sure that biopsied tissue samples truly came from the patients who received the results. This type of DNA test typically is covered by health insurance—contact your insurance provider for details. If not, expect it to cost several hundred dollars.

Example: Strand Diagnostics, a reputable DNA-testing lab that is accredited by the FBI and CLIA, charges $295 (KnowError.com).

How to Cope When Only One Hand Is Working

Jeanine Beasley, EdD, OTR, CHT, FAOTA, an occupational therapist, certified hand therapist and past board member of the American Society of Hand Therapists. Dr. Beasley is a professor at Grand Valley State University's occupational science and therapy department and a hand therapist at Mary Free Bed Rehabilitation Hospital, both in Grand Rapids, Michigan. She has authored and coauthored book chapters and journal articles on hand therapy and speaks in the US and internationally on the subject.

It would take far more than 10 fingers to count all the tasks we use our hands to accomplish each day. From eating to typing to driving to combing our hair, we rely on our hands nearly every waking moment. But what if one hand is out of commission—either temporarily from a broken wrist, torn tendon or other injury…or permanently, because of a bigger setback such as a stroke, rheumatoid arthritis or an auto accident?

When you lose the use of one of your hands, it becomes difficult or impossible to button a shirt, for example, tie your shoes, wash a glass or cut your food...in other words, to function normally.

Good news: There are several effective—and simple—ways to fight back and regain your independence.

2 QUESTIONS TO ANSWER

When only one hand is working properly, answering two key questions will give you the best possible combination of coping tips for your particular needs...

Is your dominant hand affected? As you might expect, it's generally a much larger problem when your dominant hand—whether you're a righty or a lefty—is the one that's out of commission.

Is your hand problem temporary or permanent? Before buying any adaptive equipment, consider how long you may need it. Someone with a wrist fracture may be one-handed for only a few weeks. Those who've suffered a stroke or traumatic brain injury may be challenged long-term. Some insurers may cover the cost of certain assistive products if they are considered a medical necessity. Check with your insurer.

TRICKS AND PRODUCTS

Tricks and products (widely available online) for one-handed tasks...*

•**Typing, texting or writing.** Speech-to-text tools, such as voice-recognition computer software or smartphone options, can reduce the need for bilateral hand involvement when typing or texting.

Or you can try the one-handed Matias Half-QWERTY Keyboard ($575). With this keyboard, your functional hand does traditional touch-typing. Letters that would ordinarily be typed with the nonfunctioning hand are accessible by holding down the space bar with your working thumb so you can then use the same finger movements you would normally use with the other hand.

*An occupational therapist or hand therapist can also help with exercises and strategies. To find one near you, ask your doctor for a referral or contact the American Occupational Therapy Association at AOTA.org or the American Society of Hand Therapists at ASHT.org.

For people with wrist fractures, a "fat pen" is easier to grip while your wrist is in a cast. These pens can be found for just a few dollars.

Another option: You can make a pen "fatter" by taping pipe insulation or layers of tape around it. Find out by trial and error the thickness that is most comfortable for your limited grip.

•**Cutting food.** A pizza cutter can help stabilize meat as you cut it. Another option: "Rocker knives," such as the Ronco Rocker knife ($8.99).

If you're chopping vegetables, a nonskid polyurethane cutting board with aluminum spikes that secure the food can be found for about $40. And when eating out, ask to have the chef cut your meat before it leaves the kitchen.

•**Cooking.** Dycem makes a non-slip mat (starting at $14) that stabilizes mixing bowls while stirring.

•**Opening jars.** A variety of one-handed jar openers are available for less than $10. You can also try this: If you have a stable drawer, place the jar in it and lean into the drawer to stabilize the jar, then open the lid with one hand.

•**Playing cards.** One-handed cardholders (starting at less than $10) make it easy to play your favorite card game. For do-it-yourselfers, cardholders can be made from a block of wood or even a trimmed, flattened pool foam noodle with a narrow slit cut out for the cards.

•**Washing dishes.** A brush with a suction cup that can be secured to the sink (starting at just a few dollars) allows you to wash dishes with one hand. If you'll be one-handed only temporarily, you may prefer to use paper plates/cups and plastic utensils...or order in so you won't need to worry about washing pots and pans.

•**Bathing.** A long-handled brush can help you wash under your arms and reach farther. You can find an 18-inch-long brush with natural bristles starting at about $10.

When it comes time to dry off your back, slip on a cotton terry cloth bathrobe (put the weaker arm in the robe first). Use a towel on the floor to dry off your feet and a reacher or dressing stick to pull the towel up onto your legs. A dressing stick is made by securing a rubber-coated hook on the end of a dowel rod. Dressing sticks are also available online.

•**Hair drying.** Mount your hair dryer on a wall. With a hands-free hair-dryer holder that's mounted with suction cups, you don't need to hold the dryer at all. Models are available for less than $10.

•**Dressing.** Always dress the weak arm first. A good way to remember this is "in first" and "out last" when dressing the weaker extremity.

Fastening a bra can be challenging, so donning a sports bra instead can help, especially if you place the weaker arm in first. When removing the bra, take the stronger arm out first. This makes it easier to remove the bra from the weaker arm. Or you could try the Buckingham Bra Angel Dressing Aid (available online for about $25) to help stabilize one end of the bra fastener.

Slip-on shoes or those with Velcro fasteners eliminate the need to tie shoes.

When putting on socks, insert all the fingers of your stronger hand into the open end of the sock and spread to enlarge the sock opening. Then slip the sock over your toes and pull up with your stronger hand. Or you can try a "pull-on sock aid," available for around $20.

Pants and skirts with elastic waists can ease dressing.

Buttons or zippers on your clothes can be replaced with Velcro. You can also try a zipper pull and button hook, available for less than $10.

Get Acute Care at Home

David M. Levine, MD, a clinician-investigator at Brigham and Women's Hospital and Harvard Medical School, both in Boston, and lead author of a study of 20 patients, published in Journal of General Internal Medicine.

Some acute care that once required hospitalization for conditions such as serious infections or asthma can now be provided at home just as effectively and at half the cost. Adults who have home-based care also are more active and receive fewer tests. While acute home hospital care is not common in the US, some Medicare Advantage plans now offer it.

Too Many Medical Tests Can Be Bad for Your Health

Dennis Gottfried, MD, an associate professor of medicine at University of Connecticut School of Medicine, Farmington, and a general internist with a private practice in Torrington, Connecticut. He is the author of Too Much Medicine: A Doctor's Prescription for Better and More Affordable Health Care.

Getting all the health screening tests possible sounds like a great idea. After all, frequent screening tests help detect diseases early and help you live longer, right? *Not always…*

DO YOU NEED THAT TEST?

People who are sick obviously need medical attention and appropriate tests. So do those at high risk for certain diseases. If you have a family history of melanoma, for example, I believe an annual skin check is wise. But many tests administered to millions of healthy people every year have no clear benefits. So why, then, do doctors order unnecessary tests? According to a 2014 physician survey, more than half admitted that they do it to protect themselves from malpractice lawsuits…36% said they recommend these tests "just to be safe"…and 28% said they do it because patients insist.

My advice: Before getting any medical test, ask your doctor why he/she is recommending it and what he will do with the information. Will the test reveal a problem that needs to be fixed? Is it likely that you will live longer if your doctor confirms a tiny thyroid nodule? If the answer is no, the test might be unnecessary—and needlessly risky.

Common tests you may not need…

LATE-LIFE COLONOSCOPY

Most people are advised to have a colonoscopy every 10 years, starting at age 50. The benefits seem obvious. Colonoscopy allows doctors to detect early-stage cancers and remove precancerous growths. Overall, the test has reduced the risk for death from colorectal cancer by about 40%.

Exception: For those who are age 75 or older, the risks of colonoscopies usually outweigh their benefits. A Harvard study looked at data from more than 1.3 million Medicare patients between the ages of 70 and 79. The researchers found that while colonoscopy slightly reduced cancer death rates in those who were under age 75, the test made little to no difference in those who were older.

Why: Between 30% and 50% of Americans will eventually develop polyps in the colon, but the vast majority of polyps will never turn into cancer. This is particularly true in the elderly because cancers take a long time to develop. Someone who's age 75 or older probably won't live long enough for the polyps to become cancerous.

Routine colonoscopies are generally safe but not totally risk-free. Bleeding and perforations can occur, and in rare cases, there have been deaths as a result of complications of colonoscopy. Plus, the test is expensive, and the "bowel prep" can be very unpleasant.

My advice: Get a colonoscopy every 10 years starting at age 50 (or as directed by your doctor), but if nothing serious is ever found, you can skip the test after age 75.

SKIN EXAMS

Millions of Americans ask their dermatologists to perform an annual head-to-toe skin exam. The early detection and removal of melanoma skin cancers is critical. More than 80,000 cases are diagnosed annually, and almost 10,000 people will die from melanoma. But only about 1% of all skin cancers are melanomas. The vast majority of skin cancers are basal and squamous cell carcinomas, which are slow-growing and present little health risk.

The US Preventive Services Task Force (USPSTF), an independent group of national experts that makes evidence-based recommendations about tests and other medical services, concludes that the evidence is insufficient to recommend for or against annual dermatological screening for melanomas. According to the group, the downsides of screening include overdiagnosis (the detection of diseases that are unlikely to ever be a threat) and the possibility of disfigurement caused by needless biopsies. There is also the expense of procedures and visits to the dermatologist. The USPSTF consciously did not address screening for basal and squamous cell carcinomas because of their relative medical insignificance.

My advice: An annual skin screening by a dermatologist doesn't make sense for everyone—particularly individuals who don't have a personal or family history of melanoma or those who are not severely immune impaired, such as people who have HIV. However, do be sure to see a dermatologist if you notice a mole, growth or "spot" that meets the ABCDE criteria—Asymmetrical…Border irregularity…Color that is not uniform (often with shades of black, brown or tan)…Diameter greater than 6 mm (which is about the size of a pencil eraser)…and Evolving size, shape or color, or new symptoms such as bleeding or itching. These are the changes that are most likely to signal melanoma.

PROSTATE-SPECIFIC ANTIGEN (PSA) TEST

Before this blood test was developed, about 70,000 men in the US were diagnosed with prostate cancer every year. With the advent of PSA testing in the 1990s, that number has increased to about 161,000 per year, and at the same time, the number of men dying from prostate cancer has decreased slightly. Is this due to early diagnosis using PSA testing? Many experts believe that the decline in prostate cancer death is from improved treatment of advanced prostate cancer, not early detection.

The vast majority of cancers that are discovered by routine PSA tests are indolent, meaning that they grow so slowly that they're unlikely to ever threaten a man's health. In fact, prostate cancer is typical in aging men. By age 80, about 60% of men have cancer in the prostate gland, but most never know it and go on to die from something else. Finding these cancers early is of no value and even may cause harm.

PSA test findings can lead to treatments that are not risk-free. For example, men who have elevated PSA levels will often be advised to undergo biopsies, which carry risks, such as bleeding and infection. Others will have radiation therapy, which can cause fatigue and frequent urination…or surgery, which can cause incontinence, impotence and, in rare cases, death.

Plus many men will have to live with the scary knowledge that they have cancer, even though most of the cancers pose no risk at all.

The USPSTF recommends that men ages 55 to 69 discuss the benefits and harms of screening with their doctors to make the best decision for themselves based on their values and preferences. But for men age 70 and older, the group has concluded that the risks of routine testing outweigh the likely benefit and that PSA testing should not be done.

The USPSTF does not address PSA screening in men under age 55, but the American Cancer Society recommends that men at average risk for prostate cancer discuss screening with their doctors beginning at age 50 and that men at high risk consider screening at age 45. The American Urological Association recommends that men discuss PSA screening with their doctors before age 55 if they are at high risk for prostate cancer...between the ages of 55 and 69 if they are at average risk...and at age 70 or older if they have a greater than 10-year life expectancy.

Bottom line: Men should be sure to discuss the pros and cons of PSA testing with their doctors.

THYROID SCREENING

Ultrasound technology has made it easier to find and evaluate growths in the thyroid gland. As a result, there has been a threefold increase in the diagnosis of thyroid cancers, but there hasn't been any change in the thyroid cancer death rate.

A study from the Department of Veterans Affairs Medical Center and Dartmouth Geisel School of Medicine concluded that the apparent increase in thyroid cancer was mainly due to improved detection. About 87% of the cancers measured were just 2 cm or smaller and were unlikely to ever pose a threat. Yet patients were treated surgically with the risk for bleeding, vocal cord paralysis and disfigurement. They also had to deal with the psychological trauma of being told they had cancer. Radiation is also standard treatment for thyroid cancer and can cause side effects. Additionally, radiation exposure presents a cumulative lifetime risk of developing cancer.

My advice: Don't get routinely screened for thyroid cancer. However, if you have a neck mass or lump...you notice changes in your voice...or have a family history of medullary thyroid cancer, an ultrasound of your thyroid may be advised.

Remember: At the proper age and appropriate intervals, screening tests, such as colonoscopy, mammograms and Pap smears, are necessary. Also be sure to get a cholesterol test every five years and blood pressure checks annually...and regular dental and eye exams.

Wide-Awake Surgery

David Sherer, MD, practices anesthesiology in the suburbs of Washington DC, and has held two US patents in the fields of critical care medicine and telecommunications. He is author of *Dr. David Sherer's Hospital Survival Guide: 100+ Ways to Make Your Hospital Stay Safe and Comfortable.* His blog at BottomLineInc.com is titled "What Your Doctor Isn't Telling You."

It's becoming more common—even for fairly complex operations. Instead of general anesthesia, which makes you unaware and immobile during surgery, you stay awake.

Why it's happening: "Regional anesthesia," such as nerve blocks and epidurals, are now more accurate, effective and safe.

Why it's a good thing: Recovery time is generally faster, with fewer side effects, so you get to go home sooner. There may be less postoperative pain as well, which can reduce the need for opioids during recovery.

Here's why: Regional anesthesia blocks painful stimuli completely. So you wake up in less pain and need less acute pain relief.

Bonus: Costs are lower, too.

THE DOWNSIDES OF GOING UNDER

Let's be clear—overall, general anesthesia is safe and getting safer. Fewer than one in 100,000 US surgical patients die from general anesthesia. But many patients wake up with side effects, such as nausea, vomiting and sore throats (from the breathing tubes). An unlucky few suffer breathing problems that can lead to infections, even pneumonia. Plus, studies show that many patients feel less anxiety if they can remain at least partially awake during surgery.

ALTERNATIVES TO GOING UNDER

The primary forms of regional anesthesia are…

•**Nerve block.** A local anesthetic medication is injected near nerves that affect specific body parts. Anesthesiologists use ultrasound to guide the needle to exactly where it will reach the right nerves.

•**Spinal anesthesia.** Anesthetic medicine is injected into spinal fluid inside the lower back, quickly numbing the lower half of the body.

•**Epidural.** Anesthetic medicine is injected outside the spinal fluid sac. It takes longer to work, but a tube can be left in place to give you pain relief after the operation.

•**Sedative.** Since the regional anesthetics will not affect the central nervous system—meaning you'll stay awake—you'll be offered a sedative drug to relax you and ease anxiety.

SURGERY WITHOUT GOING UNDER

So can you just say, "No thanks, doctor"? Not always. *Example*: In nearly all cases, open-heart and other chest surgeries require general anesthesia. So do nearly all abdominal and brain operations.

But a growing list of surgeries can now be performed without general anesthesia if you and your doctors agree. *Here are several common ones…*

JOINT REPLACEMENT

Nerve blocks, which work very well for individual body parts such as legs and arms, can be ideal for joint replacement. For hip or knee replacement, a spinal or an epidural may be used instead.

ACL RECONSTRUCTION

Anterior cruciate ligament (ACL) reconstruction is similar to joint replacement and can now be done with various regional anesthesia techniques. These options are often preferred by the generally younger, fitter patients who frequently require this surgery.

PROSTATE SURGERY

Spinal or epidural anesthesia can be ideal for these surgeries. If the surgery is for cancer, you are likely to need heavy sedation as well because such procedures can be extensive. Less sedation may be needed for transurethral resection of the prostate (TURP), a technique used to reduce an enlarged prostate gland.

FACE-LIFT

Here, your choice of anesthesia will most likely be guided by your choice of plastic surgeon. Some prefer an alert patient who can make facial expressions during the procedure, so they offer patients nerve-blocking injections along with light sedation. Others feel they can do better work with unconscious patients. If you have your own preference, choose your surgeon accordingly.

THE RISKS OF REGIONAL ANESTHESIA

While safer overall than general anesthesia, regional techniques do have some risks…

•**Sedatives.** Drugs such as *propofol, fentanyl, midazolam* and *ketamine* are generally safe when used during surgery but can leave you woozy and muddleheaded for a while afterward. Make sure you have someone to drive you home.

•**Nerve blocks.** Nerve injuries are very rare but can occur. Overdoses and misplaced needles can allow drugs to get into the bloodstream, which might cause confusion and even seizures.

•**Spinal and epidural anesthesia.** Risks include nerve injury, infection, bleeding and headache. These are rare.

To lower your risks: Thoroughly and honestly answer all the questions your anesthesiologist will ask about your medical history. But also ask questions. Not all anesthesiologists are trained in using ultrasound to guide a nerve block, for instance. Ask about your surgical team's experience with using these regional techniques for your specific surgery.

What if you still want general anesthesia? That's not uncommon or wrong. The idea of being even partially aware during surgery makes some people extremely anxious. Others are poor candidates for regional anesthesia because of medical problems. But if it's right for you, you'll likely recover faster and get home sooner.

HOW AWAKE DO YOU WANT TO BE?

If you choose regional anesthesia for surgery, you also may face a second choice—just how sedated do you want to be?

Some people want to remain awake and fairly aware…others want the oblivion of "twilight sleep." The less sedated you are, the more you'll be aware of your surgical team talking, as well as sensations such as tugging and pressure (though not pain). It's a good topic to discuss with your doctor.

Can't Remember What Your Doctor Said?

Glyn Elwyn, MD, PhD, professor, physician and researcher at The Dartmouth Institute for Health Policy and Clinical Practice in Lebanon, New Hampshire, and at the Scientific Institute for Quality of Healthcare, Radboud University Nijmegen Medical Centre, in the Netherlands. He leads an international team examining shared decision-making among patients and providers. GlynElwyn.com

---

So how did your doctor visit go? We've all heard that question from family and friends, but it can quickly lead to a frustrating exercise in trying to remember exactly what did happen during those precious minutes you spent with your doctor.

Perhaps you recall something about needing to return for some tests…but you're not quite sure what the tests are for. Or maybe your doctor suggested a better way to monitor your symptoms…but you don't remember what it was.

Luckily, most of us have a cure for this common ailment right in our pockets or purses—our smartphones. Pull it out and press a recording app the next time you sit down with your doctor, and you never have to wonder again about what happened at your appointment. It's easier to make a recording than to take notes. Plus, you can relisten to what was discussed during the appointment…and share it with others electronically.

Sounds easy, right? It is—but there are some important points to consider before you hit "record."

A COMMONSENSE SOLUTION

Very few people are blessed with perfect recall, and our memories tend to become less efficient as we age. Add on the possibility of hearing loss—a common problem for adults over age 50—and you've got a recipe for miscommunication.

Throw in the overall stress of a medical encounter—especially one where you may be receiving new or distressing information—along with the high probability that your doctor may have lapsed into medicalese while explaining a complex concept, and it's no wonder that so many of us struggle to remember and understand what we hear under those conditions.

Among patients who have access to recordings of their doctor visits, studies suggest that there are benefits. One review, published in *Patient Education & Counseling*, found that about 72% of patients took the time to listen to the recording after the appointment…and 60% shared it with caregivers, including family and friends. Just knowing that a conversation is being recorded may also encourage patients and doctors to express themselves more clearly.

IMPORTANT CONSIDERATIONS

Before you whip out your smartphone at your next doctor visit, keep these key points in mind…

***POINT #1:* Know the law.** In 38 states and the District of Columbia, you can legally record a conversation with another person—even a medical provider—with or without the other person's consent. In the following 12 states, you do need consent from both the patient and the physician (verbal consent is acceptable)—California, Connecticut, Florida, Illinois, Maryland, Massachusetts, Michigan, Montana, New Hampshire, Oregon, Pennsylvania and Washington.

So if you ask a doctor for permission to record your visit in one of these 12 states, he/she could refuse. If you went ahead and made a recording without permission and the doctor finds out, you could be reported to legal authorities. You could also get into legal trouble for sharing the recording.

As mentioned above, in the 38 states and District of Columbia that don't require permission, you could record and share the doctor visit secretly, but there are good reasons not to do that (more on that shortly).

Important: If you use a recording to damage the reputation of a doctor—by posting a damning conversation on Facebook, for example—you could face legal consequences. If you sue a doctor for medical malpractice, a recording may or may not be admissible as evidence. An attorney would need to advise you.

POINT #2: **Don't jeopardize your relationship with your doctor.** Even if you are in a state where it's legal to secretly record a doctor visit, it's a bad idea.

Here's why: Good patient/doctor relationships are built on trust. If your doctor finds out that you are secretly recording him, that's going to undermine trust. And even if your doctor doesn't find out, many patients will find themselves feeling anxious about the deception.

Better idea: Let the doctor know that you would like to record the visit, emphasizing the potential benefits to you. You might say: "You know, sometimes I have real trouble recalling everything. Would you mind if I recorded this conversation so I can review it later and perhaps share it with my relatives?"

We don't have much data on how doctors respond to such requests. In some states, as noted earlier, they can legally say "no." But as more patients ask, it will be interesting to see what happens.

Ideally, groups representing medical providers and patients will get together to develop guidelines for recording doctor visits so that eventually it will become common practice. Until then, doctors might be reassured by preliminary evidence suggesting that patients rarely set out to use a recording against a doctor—as evidence in a malpractice case, for instance.

POINT #3: **Know the technical details.** Don't own a smartphone? A simple digital recorder will work fine, and it costs a lot less (prices start at about $20). If you still own an old-fashioned cassette tape recorder, that will work, too.

But if you do have a smartphone, making a recording is easy. On an iPhone: You can just tap the Voice Memos icon and then press the red button to record. You can download other recording apps, for both iPhone and Android phones, and many are free. Some come with bells and whistles—like the ability to type in notes as you tape or convert audio to text.

To make the process even more user-friendly, some providers are experimenting with secure online systems that are specially designed to record and store audio from medical visits and make key exchanges easier to find and play back.

WHAT ABOUT PRIVACY?

One law that patients do not need to worry about if they are recording and sharing a doctor visit is the Health Insurance Portability and Accountability Act (HIPAA). This health-privacy law limits what health providers, insurers and other professionals can do with your medical information, but it doesn't stop you from making or using your own audio medical recordings.

Get Set for the "New" Hospital

Charles B. Inlander is a consumer advocate and health-care consultant based in Fogelsville, Pennsylvania. He was the founding president of the nonprofit People's Medical Society, a consumer advocacy organization credited with key improvements in the quality of US health care, and is the author or coauthor of more than 20 consumer-health books.

You may—or may not—have noticed it, but there are more hospitals closing these days than new ones opening. With fewer patient admissions, shorter stays for those who are admitted and new, highly innovative ways that treatment can be delivered in less costly, more comfortable and safer settings (with fewer infections and better-trained staff), a new world of hospitals has emerged. Over the past several years, hundreds of procedures and treatments (from cataract removal to treatment for pneumonia) that formerly were available only in hospitals are now delivered in outpatient facilities, doctors' offices and sometimes even in your home. *What all this means for you…*

•**Get in and out quickly.** Hospital owners—both for-profit and nonprofit—are making concerted efforts to embrace new technologies and transfer care closer to the patient in settings that are less costly and, in many cases, safer and more specialized. The latest trend is what the industry terms "micro-hospitals." These are usually newly constructed, two- or three-story buildings popping up mostly in urban and suburban areas. They offer emergency care, ob-gyn services, rehab programs (such as physical and occupational therapies), primary-care practices and, in some cases, outpatient surgical facilities all at one site. Many also have a small number of beds (eight or fewer are typical in the current model) to keep a patient overnight if he/she needs more observation or help in starting a treatment. But typically, patients arrive, get treated and are sent home with a treatment plan that may include home-care services, such as a visiting nurse—often with real-time monitoring through the patient's computer Wi-Fi or telephone line.

Insider fact: Studies show that this type of care is as effective—or even more so—than being treated as a hospital inpatient, and it can be far less costly for the patient.

•**Use the "old" when it's needed.** Most major hospital companies are gradually converting their older buildings to new uses. The traditional hospital is not going away…it is chang-ing. Some are being used strictly for critical-care patients who need intricate surgeries (including coronary bypass surgery, major back surgeries, such as spinal fusions, or organ transplant) or intensive care. Others are being converted to specialty facilities such as orthopedic surgical centers or women's health clinics. And still others are being used for transitional-care services or reconfigured to nursing home or hospice facilities.

Insider fact: These specialized facilities often bring better quality care to patients, since teams of doctors, nurses and other medical professionals focused on one medical specialty are concentrated in one setting.

•**Take advantage of telemedicine.** Given today's high-speed Internet and cell-phone technology, medical experts in one locale can offer guidance and even direct care to patients and other practitioners almost anywhere in the world. Large hospital chains, with facilities throughout the country, have assembled specialists in centralized hubs who can monitor surgical procedures (even by video) or advise your local physician about a course of treatment or procedure in real time. This is especially useful in more rural areas, where there are fewer practitioners and facilities.

Insider fact: Telemedicine allows doctors to share MRI scans and other test results with doctors throughout the world, to aid in making a better diagnosis and plan a course of treatment. Ask whether the center where you're being treated offers telemedicine.

CHAPTER 6

Diabetes Care

Got Prediabetes?

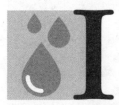

If you're over age 45 and you get regular checkups, your doctor will probably test you for diabetes. But only about half of doctors, according to recent research, raise the alarm when those same tests indicate prediabetes, characterized by slightly elevated blood sugar that hasn't yet progressed to full-blown clinical diabetes.

Why that's a dangerous omission…

•**Prediabetes now affects 38% of American adults.** The risk increases substantially over age 60.

•**Unless you treat prediabetes as a wake-up call to change your lifestyle,** your chance of progressing to clinical diabetes is a whopping 70%.

•**Prediabetes hurts your health now—** even if it doesn't progress to clinical diabetes. Years of higher-than-normal blood sugar can cause some of the same damage as full-fledged diabetes.

•**It's much easier to reverse prediabetes than full-blown diabetes.** In prediabetes, your body is developing insulin resistance so that you need more insulin to regulate blood sugar. But if producing that extra insulin overtaxes your pancreas so that you can't keep up with the demand for insulin, you've got type 2 diabetes—and reversal is much harder to achieve.

•**America's doctors are missing the boat on treatment of prediabetes, too.** Even when patients are diagnosed with prediabetes, only 33% get counseling about nutrition…only 32% get counseling about exercise…and a mere 26% about both.

My advice: As a patient, you need to take prediabetes seriously. *Here's how…*

Gerald Bernstein, MD, an internist and endocrinologist, who is program director of the Friedman Diabetes Institute at Lenox Hill Hospital in New York City. Dr. Bernstein was president of the American Diabetes Association and has served on its national board of directors and on the editorial board of Clinical Diabetes.

GET TESTED

Prediabetes is a stage between a normal blood glucose level and one that's so high that it triggers the "big" diagnosis. It's measured with the same blood tests that doctors use to identify diabetes.

My advice: Given the enormous number of people who develop prediabetes, every adult should get tested—without exception.

There are three common tests—any one of which is sufficient to diagnose prediabetes, so you'll need only one…

•**Fasting plasma glucose (FPG).** This is the standard blood test for diagnosing both diabetes and prediabetes. Take the test first thing in the morning (since you have to fast for at least eight hours). A reading of less than 100 milligrams per deciliter (mg/dL) is normal…100 mg/dL to 125 mg/dL is prediabetes…and 126 mg/dL or higher means you already have diabetes.

•**A1C (glycated hemoglobin).** This blood test measures the percentage of glucose that's attached to the hemoglobin in blood. It indicates your average blood sugar level over the last two or three months. I recommend this test because it's fast, inexpensive and doesn't require fasting. A normal reading is below 5.7%. A reading between 5.7% and 6.4% indicates prediabetes. A reading of 6.5% or higher means diabetes.

•**Glucose tolerance test.** This test is more cumbersome but more accurate. Instead of eating a meal, you consume a standard amount of glucose, and then your blood glucose is measured at 30 minutes and at least one hour and two hours afterward. If your blood sugar tests high (between 140 mg/dL and 199 mg/dL) two hours after drinking the glucose solution, it means that you have prediabetes. If your blood sugar tests 200 mg/dL or higher, then you have diabetes.

How often should you get tested? If your result is normal but you also have two or more diabetes risk factors (such as being overweight and sedentary), get tested annually…otherwise, every three years is fine. But if the test shows prediabetes, you should embark on a program to reverse it—and make sure your doctor retests you more frequently, such as every six months, to see if your changes are working.

HOW TO REVERSE PREDIABETES

Most people with slightly high blood sugar can lower it with basic lifestyle changes, along with medication in some cases. Make sure you discuss various interventions with your physician, and, if possible, work with a diabetes educator, especially one associated with a diabetes program. *The basics…*

•**Start with weight loss.** Not everyone with prediabetes is overweight—but most patients are. Often, losing just 10 pounds is enough to improve insulin sensitivity and bring blood sugar into the healthy range.

•**Take a daily walk.** A daily 30-minute walk reduces your risk of developing diabetes by 30%, according to the Harvard School of Public Health's Nurses' Health Study and the Health Professionals Follow-Up Study. Exercise increases insulin sensitivity. It also increases metabolism and muscle mass, which lower glucose even more.

•**Eat whole grains.** Research has shown that people who eat two to three servings of whole grains daily, compared with those who eat little or none, are 30% less likely to develop type 2 diabetes. Processed grains—such as white rice and most breakfast cereals, etc.—are digested quickly and cause a faster rise in glucose.

•**Minimize red meat.** Red meat (especially fatty cuts) is high in saturated fat, which can increase diabetes risk. Be especially sparing with processed red meats, such as bacon and bologna. In one large Harvard study, people who ate as little as two ounces of processed red meat daily had a 19% increased risk of developing diabetes.

•**Say no to sugary soft drinks.** A Harvard study found that women who drank one or more of these beverages a day, compared with those who drank them rarely, had an 83% higher risk of developing diabetes. Beware of any sugar-sweetened drink, including sugar-sweetened teas and sports drinks.

My advice: Sugary drinks should be avoided altogether.

WHAT ABOUT MEDICATION?

Nearly 10 years ago, the American Diabetes Association updated its guidelines to include *metformin* (Glucophage) for treating high-risk patients with prediabetes. Research shows that it cuts the risk of developing diabetes by 31%. Yet it's still prescribed for only a small fraction of these patients. The drug can cause diarrhea and gas, but the side effects usually go away within a week or two. It can also diminish appetite, which is sometimes a benefit for people trying to lose weight. I recommend it for people who can't get their blood sugar under control with lifestyle measures alone. If you tolerate it well, you can stay on it indefinitely.

Can Whole-Body Vibrations Help Prevent Diabetes?

Meghan E. McGee-Lawrence, PhD, department of cellular biology and anatomy, Medical College of Georgia, Augusta University, and lead author of a study titled, "Whole-Body Vibration Mimics the Metabolic Effects of Exercise in Male Leptin Receptor Deficient Mice," published in *Endocrinology*.

Standing still—or better yet, lying down—in a gym or at home on a machine that does all the work for you seems like a cheater's vision of exercise. But for many people who are obese and/or have a lack of stamina or other issues that make it difficult to exercise, it may be a realistic vision.

Good news: These folks may be able to get many of the benefits of exercise—including reduced blood sugar and increased insulin sensitivity—in a different way.

It's called whole-body vibration.

Background: Whole-body vibration (WBV) —standing, sitting or lying on a machine with a vibrating platform—causes muscles to contract and relax repetitively, placing a "biomechanical load" on the body that is similar, in some ways, to what exercise does. Although it's been around for decades, new technology has revived interest in it. But does WBV provide the same protective effects on the body—including preventing diabetes—as traditional physical exercise? Researchers from the Medical College of Georgia decided to find out.

Study: This was an animal study, but it sheds light on basic physiology. Researchers used obese mice with diabetes. Half of the mice exercised for 45 minutes a day on a treadmill. The other half were given whole-body vibration for 20 minutes a day.

Results: After 12 weeks, the two groups showed similar improvements. Muscle fiber increased 24% in the vibration group compared to 29% in the treadmill exercisers. The size of fat cells went down by 15% (vibration) versus 21% (treadmill). Both groups had similar improvements in insulin sensitivity, which reduces the severity of diabetes, and similar reductions in fat deposits in their livers—a risk factor for both fatty liver disease and for diabetes. Overall, treadmill exercise was more effective than whole-body vibration at improving blood sugar control and reducing weight—but only slightly.

Surprising finding: The whole-body vibration mice experienced a mild bone benefit, too. Just like the treadmill exercisers, they had small increases in blood levels of *osteocalcin*, a marker for bone formation.

Bottom line: Whole-body vibration does indeed provide some of the same physical and metabolic benefits as more strenuous physical exercise. To be sure, this study doesn't prove that standing on a vibrating platform is as good at preventing or controlling diabetes as running, swimming or riding a bike. But the findings are encouraging—and other research on people has found that whole-body vibration can improve muscle strength and coordination while improving the flexibility of blood vessels and reducing high blood pressure. You can find whole-body vibration machines (often referred to as vibration trainers) at some gyms. They are also available in stores that sell fitness equipment, as well as online. If you know someone who just can't or just won't exercise, these "good vibes" may be a good alternative.

Beware: Artificial Sweeteners Are Not a Safe Alternative to Sugar

John La Puma, MD, a member of Bottom Line's Diabetes Center panel of experts, is a board-certified specialist in internal medicine, a professionally trained chef and culinary medicine pioneer. He is cofounder of the popular video recipe series "ChefMD" and *The New York Times* best-selling author of *Refuel: A 24-Day Eating Plan to Shed Fat, Boost Testosterone and Pump Up Strength and Stamina.* DrJohnLaPuma.com

If you're borderline diabetic, you may have started using artificial sweeteners to help cut back on sugar.

Not so fast.

If you're borderline diabetic—aka, you have prediabetes—you should cut back not just on sugar and starches but also on artificial sweeteners. Use them rarely—no more than once a month.

Why? Since the 1950s, when tiny tablets of saccharin became available to shake into your morning coffee, artificial sweeteners have promised dulce…but for people with blood sugar concerns they are more likely diablo.

Recent evidence: An 18-year study of 61,440 women showed that those who "always or almost always" used artificial sweeteners of any kind had an increased risk of developing type 2 diabetes. Nor was the link based on the likelihood that people who are overweight may be using artificial sweeteners. It was independent of body weight.

New research is uncovering just how artificial sweeteners may contribute to diabetes—or make it worse if you already have it.

Example: *Aspartame* (NutraSweet, Equal) can alter the activity and composition of the microbes in your intestine, creating glucose intolerance. It may also increase levels of the stress hormone cortisol and increase systemic oxidative stress—both contributors to metabolic diseases including diabetes. Aspartame may also interfere with the N-methyl D-aspartate (NMDA) receptor in nerves, which can cause insulin deficiency or resistance. It's not the only artificial sweetener that's troubling—*Sucralose* (Splenda), although considered safe for most people, has been report-

ed to raise blood sugar levels in people with diabetes.

The truth is, artificial sweeteners are bad for everybody, not just for people with prediabetes or diabetes. Healthy people who drink more diet soda, compared with those who drink little or no soda, are more likely to become obese… and have big bellies. That, too, may have something to do with interference with a healthy gut microbiome. Plus, by tricking your palate into thinking that you are eating something with calories (sugar) when there are no calories, you may stimulate your appetite, making it easier to overeat. A recent review of 37 studies found that long-term use of artificial sweeteners was associated with weight gain, diabetes, high blood sugar and heart disease.

Small amounts of stevia, a natural sweetener derived from a South American plant, are likely safe for daily use. But I wouldn't use large amounts of stevia extracts, which may disrupt hormones in large doses according to some reports. Extracts are different from the whole unprocessed leaf, which is likely the safest choice—you can boil the leaves in water and then keep the sweetened water in the refrigerator to use by the teaspoon.

You can also reeducate your sweet tooth. Gradually cut back on natural sweeteners such as sugar, honey and maple syrup to reprogram your "sugar meter" so you crave sweetness less. Fruit, which is naturally sweet, has a place in a balanced diet. Dried fruit is often high in sugar, but you can learn to use small amounts to

Berries Fight Diabetes

Recent finding: A daily no-calorie drink that contained extracts of strawberry and cranberry antioxidants called polyphenols (equivalent to the amount found in about one-half cup of fresh fruit) improved insulin sensitivity by 14% in overweight men and women with prediabetes.

Note: Whole berries, fresh or frozen, are believed to be most helpful because they are rich in many beneficial nutrients, including fiber.

Hélène Jacques, PhD, professor of nutrition, Laval University, Quebec City, Canada.

sweeten dishes. For cooking, especially whole grains and whole-grain salads, I like "sweet" herbs and spices such as cinnamon, anise, clove, fennel and allspice. And you know what? Your gut bacteria will come back in balance shortly after you stop the synthetics.

Kidney Disease Boosts Diabetes Risk

Ziyad Al-Aly, MD, assistant professor of medicine, Washington University School of Medicine, St. Louis.

It's well known that diabetes increases risk for kidney disease. Now it appears that the reverse is also true.

Recent study: Among 1.3 million nondiabetic adults, those with higher levels of blood urea nitrogen (a sign of reduced kidney function) were 23% more likely to develop diabetes over the five-year study period than those with normal urea levels.

Why: Blood urea nitrogen results in increased insulin resistance and impaired insulin secretion—both hallmarks of diabetes.

Glucose Dips Are Common

Shuyang Fang, MD, endocrinology resident, Mount Sinai St. Luke's and Mount Sinai West, New York City.

People with a history of heart disease who are hospitalized for any reason have a greater likelihood of hypoglycemia (low blood sugar) episodes—even if they are not known to have diabetes, a review of 1.2 million hospital patients has found.

Details: Patients developing hypoglycemia had almost four times the risk for death as those who did not develop hypoglycemia.

Takeaway: Blood sugar should be monitored daily in heart disease patients who are hospitalized (more often if the patient has diabetes).

Diabetes from Your Mouthwash?

Marvin Fier, DDS, Pomona, New York, about a study titled, "Over-the-Counter Mouthwash Use and Risk of Pre-diabetes/Diabetes," published in *Nitric Oxide.* Smile Rockland.com

Using mouthwash twice or more a day may keep your breath "minty fresh," but it also may increase your risk of developing type 2 diabetes.

A recent study observed 945 adults for three years. The people studied, ages 40 to 65, were overweight or obese, so they already were at increased risk for diabetes—but the results may be important even for people who are not overweight.

Findings: Participants who used a mouthwash twice or more a day typically had 55% higher risk for prediabetes or diabetes than those who used mouthwash less frequently or not at all.

This kind of study can't show cause and effect, and it leaves many questions open—especially about the kind of mouthwash people used. But there are reasons to avoid excessive use. Most mouthwashes contain alcohol or other ingredients, either synthetic or essential oils, that kill microbes indiscriminately—including beneficial ones that help the body make nitric oxide. But you need nitric oxide—it's a remarkable compound that is important for everyone's health, protecting against not only obesity and insulin resistance but also high blood pressure.

The truth is, you don't need to use mouthwash at all. It's not particularly effective at improving oral health anyway. For example, brushing and flossing are much better at disrupting plaque, the biofilm that sticks to teeth and causes cavities, gum disease—and, often, bad breath.

Tip: Thin, unwaxed floss is best at physically dislodging plaque. (If you still love the mouthwash habit, choose alcohol-free products to avoid drying the delicate mucous membranes of the mouth.)

Finally, don't ignore persistent bad breath. It could point to a health problem. If you are using mouthwash several times each day to get rid of bad breath or a bad taste, speak with your dentist or other health-care provider.

For Better Blood Sugar, You Can't Beat Beets

Christopher Bell, PhD, department of health and exercise science, Colorado State University, Fort Collins, and coauthor of the research article "Concurrent Beet Juice and Carbohydrate Ingestion: Influence on Glucose Tolerance in Obese and Nonobese Adults," published in *Journal of Nutrition and Metabolism*.

"10 Best Juicing Recipes for Diabetics." iFocusHealth. com

If your blood sugar is too high and you're fighting the battle of the bulge, there's an easy way to enhance your insulin sensitivity and better regulate your blood sugar.

Drink a long cool glass of beet juice before a meal.

Background: The idea that drinking beet juice has a positive effect on general health is hardly new. Beet juice is rich in dietary nitrate, which the body uses to make nitric oxide, a compound that helps widen blood vessels, improving circulation. Drinking beetroot juice has been shown to reduce blood pressure, improve blood flow to the brain, improve athletic performance and even prevent altitude sickness. Improving circulation also helps the body deliver glucose to the tissues more efficiently so that the body needs to produce less insulin to metabolize food and control blood sugar. But obese people tend to have low nitric oxide levels. Could beets help boost their nitric oxide and improve their insulin sensitivity? To find out, researchers gave people beet juice and a large amount of sugar to digest. It's a way to simulate the effects of a meal in a lab.

Study: Twelve nonobese men and women and 10 obese men and women took part. Being obese is a significant risk factor for developing diabetes, although none of the participants actually had diabetes. They all were asked to not eat any nitrate-rich foods such as beets or greens the day before. They were also asked to not brush their teeth, floss or use mouthwash for 18 hours before the test. On the day of the study, they each drank a 17-ounce glass of beet juice and then were given a large amount of glucose sugar to consume.

On another day, they rinsed with mouthwash—which prevents the body from turning beet's nitrates into nitric oxide—before consuming the beet juice and sugar. It may seem odd to study this—after all, who rinses with mouthwash before a meal? But the researchers had a reason. They knew that the healthful bacteria in the mouth are needed to convert beet's nitrates into nitrites, the first step for the body to make nitric oxide. When you kill the bacteria in your mouth with mouthwash, they aren't around to do the necessary work.

Result: For the obese beet-juice drinkers, insulin resistance was improved and blood sugar didn't go up as much in the 60 to 90 minutes after consuming the sugar—compared to when they rinsed with mouthwash first. Their insulin resistance and blood sugar still were slightly higher than in their nonobese counterparts—but it was a big improvement for them. That's a key benefit, since elevated insulin resistance plus high blood sugar, over time, increase the risk of developing type 2 diabetes. For the obese, who likely started with low nitric oxide levels, drinking beet juice apparently boosted nitric oxide levels high enough to help them better metabolize sugar.

Buddy Up Against Diabetes

When Dutch researchers asked 3,000 study participants age 40 and older to count the people, including family and friends, in their social networks, those with type 2 diabetes reported having seven or eight people in their networks—two to four members fewer than their peers without diabetes.

Theory: A larger network may encourage more healthful eating and more physical activity.

Miranda T. Schram, PhD, associate professor, department of medicine, Maastricht University Medical Centre, the Netherlands.

But the beet juice didn't have the same effect on participants who weren't obese—their insulin sensitivity and blood sugar response to eating sugar was normal when they drank beet juice and when they negated the benefits of beet juice by rinsing with mouthwash. Why? One probable reason is that their nitric oxide levels were already sufficient to help their bodies metabolize sugar, so boosting it a little extra with beet juice didn't have any practical effect.

Bottom line: Obese adults at risk of developing insulin resistance may benefit from adding healthful nitrate-rich foods—including a glass of beet juice—to their meals.

What about the sugar naturally contained in beet juice itself? It's true that there's a lot of sugar in beets—and even more in beet juice. But evidence suggests that the physiological benefits outweigh the sugar—just make sure you skip less healthy sources of sugar such as soda, candy and other sweets. You can also experiment with other nitrate-rich foods, such as spinach.

Try this nitrate-rich homemade beet/apple/celery/spinach juice at breakfast: The night before, cut up one medium-sized beet into cubes and freeze it. The next morning, put the cubes in your juicer along with one sliced and cored apple, two chopped celery stalks, one-half cup of spinach and the juice of one small lemon. Like your beets at lunch or dinner instead? Nothing beats roasted beets!

Caution: Before consuming beet juice regularly, ask your doctor whether there's any reason you should avoid or limit foods such as beets, beet juice and spinach. These foods may not be safe for people who are at risk for kidney stones or who are taking certain medications for heart conditions or erectile dysfunction.

Don't Fear Diabetes! Straight Talk for the Newly Diagnosed

Theresa Garnero, RN, MS (nursing), a member of Bottom Line's Diabetes Resource Center expert panel and an advanced-practice registered nurse (APRN), board-certified in advanced diabetes management (BC-ADM), certified diabetes educator (CDE) and instructional designer in the Family Health Care Nursing division at University of California, San Francisco. She is the author of *Your First Year with Diabetes: What to Do, Month by Month.* DiabetesCatalysts.com

If you've recently been diagnosed with diabetes, you may be in shock for a bit…that's normal. But if you're afraid or panicked, try not to give in to those feelings or let your imagination run wild. It's easy to jump to conclusions based on the worst outcomes you've heard about or seen within your family or friends, such as amputation and blindness—but the reality, with today's know-how, is usually nothing like that.

Key insight: For most people with well-managed diabetes, the most common complication is…no complication at all! And even though you will have to make some lifestyle changes, you're not doomed to a lifetime diet of no treats and no carbs.

As a diabetes educator, the first thing I do with new patients is to help them face their fears. Doing so not only helps them feel better but may motivate them to take the manageable small steps that will help in so many ways. *Let's get started…*

WHAT'S GOOD ABOUT A DIAGNOSIS

Think of a diagnosis of type 2 diabetes as a bit of good fortune in one way. As many as 40% of people with type 2 diabetes are walking around unaware that they have it, which means the disease is doing damage to their bodies unchecked. With a diagnosis in hand, you're a step ahead—and you can stay ahead by employing some smart management strategies.

Can you look at the glass-half-full side of your diagnosis?

Here's the first benefit: You can take action. I see people every day who amaze me in their ability to take control of their condition rather than the other way around.

This means managing your blood glucose... which in turn reduces your risk of getting many diabetes-related complications. And if you do have complications, taking action means tackling those problems head-on and early so they don't progress. Your diagnosis also can be the inspiration you need to tweak some habits that may have needed it anyway, such as eating a healthier diet and exercising.

Though it's normal to be overwhelmed at first, remember...knowledge is power. It's also the best way to counter anxiety and remain in control. Ready to face your fears, one by one? Here are the top five worries that people newly diagnosed with diabetes ask me about, the reality behind them—and how you can take action.

FIVE COMMON DIABETES FEARS

•**I'll need amputation.** The thought of losing a foot or leg is terrifying. But there's typically a long chain of events that would have to happen before you'd need an amputation, and most of them are avoidable. First, blood glucose would have to be very high for a number of years...think, a wildfire burning out of control. Next, you would need to injure your foot and not notice it and not get it treated. Finally, a rip-roaring infection would have to take hold.

Take action: The key to avoiding all diabetes complications, including the prospect of amputation, is doing your best to monitor and manage your blood glucose, blood pressure and cholesterol or "lipid" (blood fat) profile.

Why are all three important? Think of your blood vessels as like the plumbing in your house—it is a closed circuit. The water should stay in the pipes. If your water pressure is high (the analogy being high blood pressure) or filled with years of debris (think fat deposits built up along the inside of your arteries), then the water flow changes (think of blood circulation with less flow). Now add uncontrolled high levels of blood glucose, which can block the mechanisms that the body enlists to fight infections. If your blood is "sweet" and doesn't flow well because it is under a constricted, high-pressure

system and full of debris, that all combines to increase your risk for foot infections after an initial injury or small skin cut occurs.

Uncontrolled high glucose, blood pressure and cholesterol can also lead to a decreased sensitivity in your feet. If left unchecked, it can lead to damage of the nerves, called neuropathy. This is a significant factor for people with diabetes who are faced with an amputation. You might not even realize your foot has a cut if you can't feel it. That is why you need to take good care of your feet! Check your tootsies daily for any cuts or scrapes, and protect them by wearing closed shoes. See a podiatrist if you have a problem, such as an ingrown toenail...don't attempt "bathroom surgery." If you get a pedicure, bring your own tools to avoid being exposed to bacteria from the shop's tools.

•**I'll go blind.** While it's true that the risk for blindness is higher in people with diabetes than in people who don't have the disease, most people with diabetes don't go blind...and even more modest vision loss, when it does occur, doesn't happen overnight. It's usually the result of a trifecta—unchecked high blood glucose, high blood pressure and high cholesterol.

Here's what happens: High blood glucose causes damage to the blood vessels in the retina. That in turn makes the tiny vessels in the eye prone to bleeding or leaking fluid. It is the tiny hemorrhages in the eye that over time can block vision. Unhealthy levels of cholesterol in your blood further gum up the works. And high blood pressure puts a lot of strain on the vessels in the back of the eye. Over time, and unchecked, these factors may lead to vision loss.

Take action: Schedule an eye exam with dilation at least once a year to check for problems. If it is discovered that you have retinopathy, several treatments exist including injections in the early stages (Anti-VEGF therapy or corticosteroids) or laser surgery in the late stages.

•**Taking insulin is scary or dangerous.** Plenty of people hate the very idea of sticking themselves with a needle, and that's natural. Most believe, wrongly however, that insulin itself is somehow harmful. Insulin is simply a hormone your body is missing and that needs to be replaced. Some believe that going on insulin is a sign their disease has just become serious. The truth is that by the time most people get a type 2 diabetes diagnosis, they've already lost 50% to 80% of the function of insulin-producing beta cells, as well as some of the cells, in the pancreas.

Take action: Remember that diabetes is a progressive disease…nearly everyone who lives long enough with the disease eventually needs insulin. You might need it now, or you might not for a few years or even decades. Don't think of it as a punishment or a sign of failure but as another step in managing your condition and living your life to the fullest. You haven't failed—your pancreas has. Many patients end up saying, "I wish I had started insulin earlier because I feel so much better." And if you fear needles…take heart. If you participate in a diabetes-management program, you'll learn about the latest and greatest equipment, including insulin pens. These needles are really tiny—I can't tell you how many times people trying them have said, "I didn't even feel that."

●**I'll need dialysis.** Dialysis is necessary when your kidneys can no longer do the job of filtering waste from your blood. While kidney problems are a known complication of diabetes, dialysis is not a given by any means. As long as you get the recommended screening tests, you'll be warned of any potential kidney problems so you can take lifestyle steps—and if needed get appropriate medications—to help protect your kidneys.

Take action: All of the things that are good for your health in general—such as focusing on whole, fresh foods…watching your blood pressure and cholesterol…not smoking or being around secondhand smoke—are also good for your kidneys. The tiny blood vessels in the kidneys, just like the ones in your eyes, don't do well if your blood glucose or blood pressure is high. Exposure to tobacco smoke also constricts vessels.

●**I won't be able to eat anything fun.** Hold on! The key to managing diabetes isn't cutting out entire categories of foods, such as fat or carbs. It's eating more mindfully and with more planning. You can still have some bread, pasta—even sugar. While no one food is "for-

bidden," though, you do have to think about the timing of meals and snacks and how much you eat. You'll also learn how to balance out carbs with protein and to figure out which foods have the biggest impact on your blood sugar.

Take action: Follow some basic rules, such as relying more on fresh, whole foods and less on packaged or processed items. Do a "food inventory" of your kitchen to see how you can better stock your fridge and cupboard for success. Discover what inspires you. Get the help of a registered dietitian who specializes in people with diabetes. You can ask your local hospital or search the website of the American Association of Diabetes Educators. With that expert help, you'll learn diet strategies that work for you.

NOTES FOR THE JOURNEY

Taking small steps is the best advice for conquering any fears you have when you're first diagnosed with diabetes. Letting yourself be consumed by stress can lead to burnout or fatalism. Start by realizing that this is a journey, not a destination, and that there are measures you'll be taking daily to remain healthy. Get ready for bumps in the road—and for successes and opportunities.

A few final thoughts…

●**Pay attention to your numbers**—blood glucose, cholesterol, blood pressure and others. Knowing these stats helps you stack the deck in your own favor and avoid complications.

●**Focus on overall health.** If other health issues come up as a result of your diabetes, there are many things that can be done to minimize or stop their progression. It all starts with being aware, engaged and involved.

●**Don't rely only on one doctor.** People with diabetes have better results with a health-care team that includes (ideally) an endocrinologist… and if that's not possible, a primary care provider with a focus on diabetes. Your team should also include a diabetes educator, who may be a nurse or a registered dietitian, to whom you can turn with questions. You'll also need an eye specialist, podiatrist and dentist—all part of ongoing maintenance to keep you tuned up.

•**Don't go it alone.** You might also want to find a support group, either online or in person, to get and share tips from others in your shoes. That may be more meaningful than what the person in the white coat says! People with diabetes who participate in support groups have lower glucose levels, on average. You can find a community to connect with by searching the American Diabetes Association support community or the Diabetes Hands Foundation. You may also find it helpful to use an app for your phone like MySugr, which has more than a million users worldwide, or a new app called KingFit that offers free diabetes education from national experts.

•**Most important...try to focus on the positive.** Swap negative thoughts (about what you have to stop doing) for positive ones (about changes that will be good for you). Having diabetes is a challenge, and your efforts are worth the energy it takes to maintain your health. You've got this!

Wireless Blood Sugar Monitor Now Available

Gerald Bernstein, MD, program coordinator of the Friedman Diabetes Institute at Lenox Hill Hospital, New York City.

The FDA has approved the Dexcom G5 Mobile Continuous Glucose Monitoring System, which uses a tiny sensor inserted under the skin and a transmitter worn on the skin to measure glucose. The data is then sent wirelessly to a dedicated receiver or smartphone. The Dexcom G5 requires the user to do only two finger-sticks daily—to calibrate the device. It is eligible for Medicare and other insurance.

The 4 Best Nondrug Remedies for Diabetic Nerve Pain

Michael Murray, ND, naturopathic physician and educator, based in Scottsdale, Arizona. He serves on the Board of Regents of Bastyr University in Seattle, and is author of more than 30 books, including *How to Prevent and Treat Diabetes with Natural Medicine* and *The Encyclopedia of Natural Medicine*. DoctorMurray.com

If you have diabetes, there's a seven-in-10 chance that you will eventually develop diabetic nerve damage, or neuropathy. It's just one of the many consequences of poorly controlled blood sugar, which is why controlling your blood sugar through diet and exercise is the best way to prevent—or at least slow—the often painful condition.

While neuropathy doesn't always cause symptoms, over time most people who have it will develop uncomfortable tingling, numbness and even chronic pain in the extremities—feet, legs, hands, arms. Other symptoms of neuropathy can include nausea, indigestion, constipation and dizziness. Unfortunately, there's no medical treatment that can cure diabetic neuropathy, only medications, including antiseizure drugs and some antidepressants, that help the pain.

But if you have diabetes, or even prediabetes, you don't have to accept that neuropathy is inevitable—and if you have diabetic neuropathy, you don't have to just live with its variety of terrible symptoms. Besides diet and exercise, there are certain supplements and one proven topical treatment that can help prevent, delay and even possibly reverse the cascade that ultimately causes neuropathy.

Here are four remedies—three supplements and one topical pain treatment—for diabetic neuropathy that I recommend. With the supplements especially, it's important to talk with your doctor before you start them.

ALPHA-LIPOIC ACID

My top recommendation for people with diabetic neuropathy is alpha-lipoic acid (ALA). It's a powerful antioxidant, a natural compound produced by our cells that helps convert blood glucose into energy. Yet it's often deficient within the nerve cells in patients with diabetes. By improving nerve blood flow and nerve conduction velocity, ALA is associated with improvements in pain, tingling, numbness, sensory deficits and muscle strength.

Scientific studies back this up. The strongest evidence is for intravenous ALA, which has been shown to provide substantial short-term relief from pain and numbness. But oral supplements have also had positive effects. In a randomized, double-blind study of 181 patients with diabetic neuropathy, those who took 600 mg of ALA once daily for five weeks had a 51% reduction in their "total symptom score," which measured symptoms such as stabbing pain, burning pain, a prickling sensation and foot numbness, compared with 32% in the placebo group. In a very small (45 participants) randomized study, those who took 600 mg of ALA for four weeks had a similar reduction in painful symptoms. For those who continued ALA for a total of 16 weeks, there was a further reduction in symptom severity. For those who stopped taking ALA after four weeks, however, symptoms showed no further improvement—and they wound up taking more pain medications than those treated with ALA.

In the longest trial to date, four-year treatment with oral ALA in mild-to-moderate diabetic retinopathy resulted in a clinically meaningful improvement and prevention of progression of impairment in nerve function and was well-tolerated.

The typical oral dosage of ALA is 400 mg to 600 mg daily. There are no known complications or drug interactions with the use of ALA, although at higher doses (e.g., greater than 1,200 mg per day), some people may experience nausea and dizziness. Since ALA also may lower blood sugar, if you are taking a diabetic medication, discuss taking ALA with your doctor.

BENFOTIAMINE

To enhance the effectiveness of ALA supplementation, consider combining it with 600 mg of benfotiamine, a synthetic form of vitamin B-1 that is fat-soluble and easily absorbed and may have a beneficial effect on several biological pathways that contribute to diabetic neuropathy. It has been shown in preliminary trials to be helpful in some cases of diabetic neuropathy, and one clinical trial suggests that use with ALA is an effective combination.

Animal studies suggest that another way to make oral ALA more effective is to combine it with my next recommendation—GLA.

GAMMA-LINOLENIC ACID (GLA)

Another supplement that I recommend for diabetic peripheral neuropathy is gamma-linolenic acid (GLA), one of the omega-6 fatty acids. Normally, most of the GLA that we need to maintain nerve function and other functions comes from vegetable oils that contain an essential fatty acid that the body converts to GLA. But diabetes is known to substantially disturb fatty acid metabolism. A key part of that disturbance is impairment in the ability to convert this fatty acid to GLA.

Supplementing with GLA can help bypass that disturbance.

Example: In a randomized, double-blind study of 111 people with diabetic neuropathy, those who took 480 mg a day of GLA had a statistically significant improvement in 13 out of 16 measures of diabetic neuropathy severity after one year, compared with the placebo group that didn't get ALA. Participants who had good glucose control had bigger improvements than those with poor glucose control.

GLA is found in some plant-based foods and herbs, including oils of borage, evening primrose and black currant seed. Most GLA supplements are derived from these oils. Just remember that the dosage is based upon the level of GLA, not the amount of the source oil. The GLA content of these oils is usually stated on the label—look for a GLA dose between 360 mg and 480 mg.

Important: If you are taking a supplement or medication that thins the blood or that may affect bleeding time (ginkgo biloba, aspirin, warfarin, clopidogrel, etc.), talk to your doctor before taking GLA. It may increase the risk of bleeding, so the combination can be dangerous. Don't take GLA if you have a seizure disorder, as there have been case reports of the supplement contributing to seizures in people with such disorders. It can interact with other prescription medications as well, so be sure to talk with your doctor before taking GLA.

TOPICAL CAPSAICIN

You may already know that hot peppers can provide pain relief—you can find pepper-based topical pain creams on the shelves of any drugstore. And in fact, I recommend topical capsaicin, the active component of cayenne pepper, for many patients with diabetic neuropathy. When applied to the skin, capsaicin works by stimulating and, ultimately, desensitizing, the small nerve fibers that transmit the pain impulse. Numerous double-blind studies have shown capsaicin to be of considerable benefit in relieving the pain of diabetic neuropathy. In those studies, roughly 80% of participants experienced significant—often tremendous—pain relief.

Topical capsaicin is available in both prescription and over-the-counter forms. Prescription patches with 8% capsaicin can provide surprisingly long-term relief—studies find that a single 60-minute application can reduce pain for weeks. This high-dose capsaicin works just as well at reducing pain as *pregabalin* (brand name Lyrica), the commonly used oral medication for nerve pain, and it avoids the systemic adverse effects associated with oral nerve-pain medications, including drowsiness, blurry vision, constipation and an increased risk for infection.

Capsaicin is also available over-the-counter as a cream and a patch. My recommendation is to use the cream so that it can be applied more liberally. Look for a concentration of 0.075% capsaicin, and apply it twice daily on the affected area. (Be sure to cover your hand with plastic wrap to prevent capsaicin from later coming in contact with your eyes, nose, mouth or lips, where it can be especially irritating.) It takes a few days for the nerve fibers to become desensitized, so the capsaicin cream can produce a tingling or burning sensation initially. After a few days, however, the nerve fibers will no longer transmit the pain signal. At these lower doses—as compared with the prescription patches—capsaicin works only with regular application. Capsaicin does not interfere with normal nerve function—it only affects the perception of pain.

Above all else: Although the nondrug remedies in this article can help with neuropathy, the primary goal for everyone with diabetes is to keep blood sugar in the healthy range. Reducing excess blood sugar—with a healthy diet, weight loss, regular exercise and managing stress—improves many of the consequences of diabetes, including neuropathy.

8 Tips for Living Alone with Diabetes

Judith H. McQuown, a patient advocate with firsthand diabetes experience and the author of 12 books. The tips here come from her book *1,137 Secrets for Living Well with Diabetes*, published by Bottom Line Books.

It's easy to feel vulnerable when you have diabetes and live alone. I know—I've had type 1 diabetes for more than 30 years, and I've lived alone for most of that time. Taking steps to feel safer, especially in an emergency, can reduce your stress. And when you're less stressed, your blood glucose levels stay more even. *So here are my favorite tips for living alone with diabetes—they are helpful whether you have type 1 or type 2 diabetes...*

•**Have a buddy system.** You should have someone to check in with every morning. Your buddy doesn't have to have diabetes—anyone who lives alone and might need help will benefit from this arrangement, and so will you.

Your call or text can be brief: "Hi, it's me. Are you OK? I'm OK. Do you need anything?" What counts is that you and your friend have made sure that each of you is alive and well.

•**Make blood sugar checkpoints easier with a vibrating watch.** Self-care for your diabetes is your responsibility, but living alone makes it that much more important to remember all the checkpoints in your day.

A subtle helper: Rather than sounding an alarm, a vibrating watch gives the wearer an unmistakable (but silent) reminder. Originally created for people with hearing loss, a vibrating watch can keep us on schedule, too. You'll find many brands and prices to choose from online. A smartwatch may also have this function.

•**Post medical emergency information.** Put this information on two sheets of paper on which you have drawn big red borders and written MEDICAL EMERGENCY INFORMATION. Include the same information on each paper—your name, medical problems, the drugs you are taking, any allergies or drug reactions, the name and phone number of your contact person and your blood type if you know it. Stick one of the pages onto the inside of your front door, and display the other page prominently on your refrigerator door.

•**Protect yourself from falls against sharp-edged furniture.** Why do we fall against sharp-edged furniture, especially at 3 am when our blood glucose is dropping? Because it's there! To prevent or minimize black-and-blue marks and potential fractures, pad everything. Use folded towels or movers' pads. Doorknobs can also do major damage—they are just the right height for you to hit your head on if you fall in a hypoglycemic swoon. For an easy fix, cover doorknobs with Bubble Wrap and secure with rubber bands.

•**Prepare for a power outage.** Between blizzards and hurricanes and anything else that might cause power blackouts, you must keep emergency supplies on hand, especially if you live alone. Besides extra drugs and equipment, you should have several flashlights and lots of extra batteries, a few transistor radios (one may fade out after a week of continuous use), a first-aid kit, at least five gallons of water and lots of candles with sturdy candleholders and matches. Also, keep a week's supply of canned food that you can eat cold in an emergency. My favorites are mostly 100% protein—canned chicken breast, salmon and tuna. But I also include some canned ravioli and chili in case I need some carbohydrates. And make sure you have a hand-operated can opener.

If your fuse box or circuit breakers are in your basement, paint the edge of every step with luminous white or Day-Glo paint. Then if your power goes out, you can get safely down the basement stairs to change the fuse or reset the circuit breakers. And always take a flashlight!

•**Designate a spot for important items.** One of the toughest aspects of living alone is misplacing something vital. Designate a spot in your home—the bottom of your underwear drawer, a kitchen shelf or a table in your front hallway—to be "home base" for possessions that you absolutely can't lose. When you can't find your car keys, they'll be in your "spot." You may want another space—near your bed?—for your glucose meter, test strips, lancet and glucose tablets.

•**Stay motivated with photos.** When living alone, it can be hard to stay motivated about blood glucose control and to keep your spirits up during difficult times. Keep photos of loved ones, pets and even heroes in full view. They will serve as reminders of love and courage during bad or just lonely times.

•**Dawdle over dinner.** Too many people who live alone race through their meals in front of the TV. Make your dinner last at least 45 minutes and try listening to relaxing classical music instead of watching TV. This turns eating into a pleasurable experience…and gives your body the opportunity to start feeling full, a process that takes 20 to 30 minutes, which means there's less chance that you'll overeat.

Travel Right with Diabetes

Judith H. McQuown, a patient advocate with firsthand diabetes experience and the author of 12 books. The tips here come from her book *1,137 Secrets for Living Well with Diabetes*, published by Bottom Line Books.

When you have diabetes, travel can be a wonderful way to refresh yourself and lose the stress…while continuing your self-care routine and healthy habits. I love to travel, and I've lived successfully with type 1 diabetes for more than 30 years. But before you hit the road, check out my life hacks to make traveling with diabetes both fun and safe…

GO ON A DIABETIC-FRIENDLY CRUISE

Who says controlling your diabetes can't be fun? Go online and see how many different cruises are offered for people with diabetes. Not only will you be aboard with like-minded cruising companions, you'd also be catered to by chefs cooking for your special needs. And check with your tax consultant. Some special-for-diabetics cruises also offer educational seminars aboard. See whether you can deduct a portion of the cost of your cruise, since it is medically oriented.

DON'T LEAVE HOME WITHOUT DOING THIS...

Don't even think of going out of town without giving a trusted friend or family member a copy of your itinerary. You can just email or even text it. Every single person should do this, diabetic or not. If you haven't alerted people to expect you at a certain place at a certain time, how could they know if something were amiss? Following this tip assists you and gives peace of mind to everyone who cares about you.

YOU SHOULD KNOW THIS ABOUT AIRPORT SECURITY...

Official policy: Increased security since September 11, 2001, means that you must prove that your syringes, insulin, blood-glucose meter, test strips, glucagon and other gear are for your diabetes and that it is medically necessary for you to carry them. If you are wearing an insulin pump, you must show that to airport security, too.

It's a good idea to get a letter from your doctor stating that you have diabetes and that you need to carry all these drugs and equipment. Most importantly, you will need to carry your insulin in the prescription box it came in, and at least one unopened package of syringes, as well as the syringes you need, so that airport security can verify that your loose syringes are identical to the packaged ones.

Although this is the official policy, it does not seem enforced consistently or as strongly as these paragraphs suggest. Many travelers with diabetes have never had their drugs or diabetes supplies questioned and have never been asked to produce a letter from their doctor.

IN CASE OF AN EMERGENCY...

If you think you might ever need an emergency room, pack now. A small "go" bag with your insurance information, a book or magazine, a list of all medications and vitamins or supplements you take, glucose meter, test strips, lancets, an acceptable snack and a bottle of water, $50 in small bills, important friends' or relatives' phone numbers, a disposable cell phone, an extra house key, a very warm sweater and socks (hospitals and test rooms are kept notoriously freezing to prevent the spread of bacteria) and a change of underwear are all wise inclusions. Just like an expectant mother's "It's time, honey" bag, yours should be immediately grabbable and should contain all the necessary and desirable things you'll wish you had with you—either as you're hurried into an ambulance, or as you sit and fidget in the ER.

CHAPTER 7

Digestive Disorders

Natural Ways to Beat Constipation

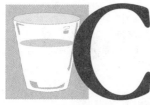

Constipation is a topic that many people are too embarrassed to discuss with their doctors. But there's no need to suffer in silence.

It's widely known that infrequent and/or painful bowel movements often have relatively simple explanations—you're not getting enough water…you're skimping on fiber…and/or you're too sedentary. If you drink more fluids, add fiber to your diet and get some exercise, you're usually good to go, right? Unfortunately, that is not the case for everyone.

What you may not know: For approximately 15% of Americans, constipation is a chronic problem. This can occur if you're taking a certain medication, such as an antacid, antidepressant or narcotic painkiller…or have a medical problem, such as low thyroid (hypothyroidism), Parkinson's disease or multiple sclerosis, that can cause constipation.

Is a pharmaceutical laxative (pill or liquid) the next best bet? Not always. These products can cause side effects, such as bloating, cramping or gas, and may even interfere with the absorption of some medications and nutrients.

A better way: Most people can beat constipation without using a pharmaceutical. *Here's how…*

START WITH THESE STRATEGIES

If you are troubled by constipation, make sure you give the strategies below a try…

•**Drink up!** A healthy bowel movement is about 75% water. Constipation can occur when the stool water content falls below 70%—this can cause the stool to become too hard for the body to evacuate easily.

Christopher Vasey, ND, a naturopathic physician who specializes in detoxification and rejuvenation in Chamby-Montreux, Switzerland. He lectures regularly about natural health in Europe, Canada and the US, and is author of *Freedom from Constipation: Natural Remedies for Digestive Health.* ChristopherVasey.ch/anglais/home.html

To avoid constipation, most people need 2 to 2.5 quarts of fluids a day. You don't need that much if you eat a lot of vegetables, fruit and other plant foods—they have a high water content that counts toward the daily total. But: If you exercise or sweat a lot, you will need more than the recommended 2 to 2.5 quarts of fluids a day.

My advice: Drink a big glass of water (or a mug of herbal tea) all at once, several times a day. Like many naturopaths, I advise against drinking fluids with meals to avoid diluting digestive juices.

•**Get your roughage.** Plant fibers take up space in the large intestine and cause the intestinal walls to stretch—the process that triggers intestinal peristalsis (contractions) and bowel movements.

Important: All plant fibers are good for constipation, but the water-soluble type—found, for example, in vegetables, fruits (raspberries, figs, dates and passion fruit are especially beneficial), flaxseed and beans—is particularly good because it absorbs water and can double or even quadruple in size in the intestine, which helps move things along.

My advice: Be sure to get enough fiber each day. For people over age 50, that's about 30 g daily for men and 21 g daily for women. Those who are constipated may need even more fiber.

•**Avoid constipating foods and beverages.** These include bananas, blueberries, fresh apricots, white rice and red wine. Generally, you would need to have these foods/drinks on a regular basis to have a problem, but sometimes having the food/drink just once causes an issue.

•**Walk the right amount.** Walking is very effective for constipation because it stimulates nerves that trigger peristaltic activity.

My advice: To work for constipation, you need to walk for at least 40 minutes a day. If it's more convenient, you can break it up into two, 20-minute sessions.

Note: Other types of exercise can also help constipation, but walking is the easiest and most convenient for most people.

FOR MORE HELP

If the advice above does not give you relief within 15 days, then it's time to step up your game. *The following tips can help—you can try all of them...*

•**Heat the liver.** According to the principles of Eastern medicine, a loss of heat from the liver—often triggered by fatigue or stress—causes blood capillaries to shrink...reduces circulation...and lowers production of bile, which you need for healthy digestion.

What to do: Place an old-fashioned rubber hot-water bottle over the liver—halfway down the right side of the abdomen, on the ribs under the right breast. The heat will increase circulation and cause the liver to expand, which has a stimulating effect on bowel movements.

Keep the bottle in place for about 15 to 30 minutes. Repeat the treatment up to three times a day, preferably after meals. People who do this for a month in addition to the steps above often find that constipation is no longer a problem. Or you can use the hot-water bottle indefinitely if you feel that it is continuing to help.

•**Self-massage.** To stimulate the peristaltic muscles that push stools out of the intestine, it helps to stretch, knead and compress the intestines with self-massage.

What to do: Using your fist or fingertips, firmly rub your abdomen (the area surrounding the navel) in a clockwise direction. This mimics the clockwise direction of intestinal peristalsis and stimulates different parts of the intestine. Once a day, rub the area for five to 10 minutes, at least two hours after a meal. You will most likely start to notice an improvement in bowel movements within three or four days.

•**Improve your bacterial balance.** There's an ideal ratio of bacteria in the gut—about 85% of the organisms should be "good" bacteria involved in fermentation (the dividing of food particles)...and the rest of the organisms should be "bad" bacteria that cause putrefaction (the decomposition of the particles). People who eat a lot of animal foods tend to have an excess of the second type and not enough of the first.

To restore a healthier balance, cut back on animal foods and eat more high-fiber plant foods such as fruits, vegetables and whole grains.

These foods have probiotic effects—they increase levels of the fermenting organisms.

Another option: A daily probiotic supplement that provides high doses (numbering in the billions) of beneficial bacteria, such as bifidus and/or acidophilus strains. Follow label instructions.*

•**Strengthen the "push" muscles.** Because of their sedentary lifestyles, many Americans don't have the strength in the abdominal and/or intestinal muscles to readily generate the pressure needed for a bowel movement. This exercise can help.

What to do: Sit on the floor with your knees bent. Recline backward and rest your weight on your forearms. Extend one leg straight out in front of you…slowly bend it to bring it back to the starting position…then do the same with the other leg. Alternating legs, extend-and-bend each leg five times, then rest and repeat the cycle two more times. Do this daily. As you get stronger, increase the number of leg extensions to 10 or 20. You can extend-and-bend both legs at the same time, but it's more challenging.

•**A better position.** Our early ancestors squatted on their heels to evacuate. This position strongly facilitates evacuation of the bowels because it relaxes the muscles of the anal sphincter, encouraging it to open, and puts the colon in a vertical position. To achieve these benefits on a toilet, raise your feet four to eight inches with a stool.

HOW DO DOCTORS DEFINE CONSTIPATION?

Depending on what's being eaten, it can take about 30 to 40 hours for food to be transformed into stools and evacuated from the body. But sometimes the body doesn't work as intended.

Doctors define constipation as having fewer than three bowel movements a week…straining or having hard stools more than 25% of the time…and/or feeling that your bowel movements are often "incomplete."

*Although probiotics are generally considered safe, anyone with a weakened immune system, including those who take corticosteroids, as well as pregnant women, should check with their doctors before taking them.

Gluten-Free Warnings

A gluten-free diet may be high in arsenic and mercury. Gluten-free foods often contain rice—not only rice itself but also rice flour, brown rice syrup and puffed rice. Elevated rice consumption can lead to higher intake of the toxic metals arsenic and mercury—rice is known to retain those metals after taking them in from fertilizers, soil and water.

Recent finding: People who ate gluten-free diets had nearly twice as much arsenic in their urine and 70% higher levels of mercury than people who did not eat gluten-free.

Self-defense: Look for non-rice–based substitutes to diversify your diet.

Maria Argos, PhD, is assistant professor of epidemiology at Chicago School of Public Health, University of Illinois.

Gluten-free pasta may raise blood sugar. *Recent study:* Researchers gave 13 healthy adults either regular wheat-based pasta or one of three gluten-free varieties. All the gluten-free pastas raised blood sugar levels over the next two hours more than wheat pasta. Rice/corn brought blood sugar levels 47% higher, brown rice pasta 18% higher and corn/quinoa 14% higher. Over time, elevated post-meal blood sugar levels increase one's risk of developing type 2 diabetes.

Carol Johnston, PhD, RD, professor and associate director, nutrition and health sciences, Arizona State University, Phoenix.

Say Good-Bye to Your PPI!

Jamie A. Koufman, MD, a laryngologist and clinical professor of otolaryngology at New York Eye and Ear Infirmary of Mount Sinai in New York City. She is also founder and director of the Voice Institute of New York and coauthor of several books, including *Dr. Koufman's Acid Reflux Diet* and *Dropping Acid: The Reflux Diet Cookbook & Cure.* VoiceInstituteOfNewYork.com

I f you watch TV, you've no doubt heard of the "little purple pill." This medication, sold under the brand name Nexium, is in a class of drugs called proton pump inhibitors (PPIs), which promise to reduce stomach acid and relieve the unpleasant symptoms of heartburn and acid reflux.

Americans spend a whopping $14 billion a year for these products, which also include brand names such as Prilosec, Prevacid, Protonix and Aciphex. Some of these drugs are available only with a doctor's prescription, while others come in over-the-counter (OTC) versions.

Here's what you may not know: While doctors have been liberally prescribing these drugs to their patients for years, there's increasing concern about the harm these drugs can cause, especially when people take them for longer than recommended—just two weeks at a time for the OTC version and up to four weeks for a prescription PPI.

For years, studies have warned that prolonged use of PPIs is linked to serious side effects, including kidney damage, severe diarrhea, bone fractures and low magnesium levels. Recently, a growing body of evidence ties the use of these drugs to even more serious conditions, including heart attack, dementia and esophageal cancer.

Latest blow: A large, six-year study of US military veterans, published in *BMJ Open*, found that those who chronically took a prescription-strength PPI died earlier (of any cause) than the group not taking the medication. The risk for death increased the longer someone took the drug.

Important: Manufacturers continue to stand behind the drugs when used as directed, and many doctors believe these medications do have a place in the long-term treatment of some patients.

Still…if you are taking a PPI and want to stop, you have lots of company. But there's a catch—people who quit PPIs often suffer a big rebound in stomach acid, triggering even worse symptoms than they had before.

For people with gastroesophageal reflux disease (GERD), a backflow of stomach contents into the esophagus, the rebound can lead to painful indigestion and heartburn. For people with respiratory reflux, a backflow of stomach acid that can reach the throat, nose, sinuses and lungs, the symptoms can include chronic cough, a burning throat, hoarseness and difficulty swallowing.

Good news: You can likely get your symptoms under control without drugs if you make the right changes to your diet and lifestyle. But first you need to wean yourself off your PPI. *Here's how…*

STEP 1: **Switch your acid-reducing medication.** Stop taking your PPI, and replace it with a histamine H2 antagonist (H2A)—the safer class of acid-reducing drugs that includes Pepcid, Zantac and Tagamet. These drugs are available by prescription and in OTC versions.

At first, you will need to take a dose four times daily, before each meal and at bedtime. If your rebound symptoms are really bad, add a liquid alginate—a product derived from seaweed that is not widely used in the US but can be found online, for sale from the UK, under the brand name Gaviscon Advance Aniseed. Follow label instructions.

Don't despair about taking more doses than you did with a once-a-day PPI—the idea is that after a week or two, you should be able to drop one mealtime pill every few days and gradually go drug-free.

Note: Some people continue to use an H2A medication and Gaviscon, as needed.

STEP 2: **Prop up your sleep.** While you are in reflux detox, you should avoid lying down for the four-hour period prior to your bedtime—and prop yourself up at bedtime to minimize nighttime reflux.

Helpful: Use pillows to get your head at a 45-degree angle and, if needed, put sofa cushions under your arms and legs to create a comfy in-bed throne. Some people sleep in recliners for the first two to four weeks of treatment.

STEP 3: **Eat early and often.** Nighttime eating is a major cause of reflux symptoms. So try to eat 75% of your calories before 5 pm and nothing after 8 pm—or even 7 pm if you can manage that.

Also helpful: Eating five small meals is better than having three big ones.

STEP 4: **Change what you eat.** The heart of your new lifestyle is a diet that is lean, clean, green and ·alkaline (the opposite of acidic)—

low in unhealthy fats and junk foods, high in healthy plants and as low as possible in very acidic foods and beverages, such as citrus and soft drinks.

Dietary acid activates the digestive enzyme pepsin, which is left on the sensitive tissue lining the throat after reflux occurs. Pepsin causes damage and is acid-activated. You will have to be strict at first, while you are getting your symptoms under control.

Over time, however, you may find some foods that are triggers for other people are OK for you…or that you can enjoy your trigger foods in very limited quantities. But make no mistake—keeping your symptoms at bay will mean sticking to a healthy, low-acid diet for life.

So say good-bye to just about all foods and drinks that come in bottles and cans, including store-bought juices, sports drinks, energy drinks and vitamin waters, as well as carbonated sodas. They are all high in acid, which will worsen your condition.

Also, cut way back on red meat, butter, fried foods, chocolate, citrus fruits and condiments and salad dressings (get these on the side so that you can add them in moderation). A salad, for example, that is bathed in too much vinegar is bad for reflux. For condiments, the same is often true. If you add them yourself, you can do so sparingly.

Alcohol—especially late at night—is often problematic. Many people find they need to give up alcohol entirely.

What you can eat: Fish and poultry (baked, broiled, sautéed and grilled are best—not fried), most nuts, grains, tubers (such as potatoes), rice, eggs and many fruits and vegetables—particularly bananas, melons, fennel, parsley and greens.

Bottled or tap water is fine.

Even better: Alkaline water, which comes in bottles (labeled with a pH of 8.0 or higher)…or it can be made with a filtration device. Good alkaline products are available from Cerra Water. Most people also can tolerate one or two cups daily of caffeinated coffee or tea.

Note: Some people can have more if it's decaf, but for others, all coffee and tea trigger reflux.

OTHER HELPFUL APPROACHES

In addition to the steps above…

•**Try sipping chamomile tea** (other herbal teas will be too acidic).

•**Chew some sugar-free gum**—it can help neutralize acid. Any flavor is fine, except for mint, which can trigger reflux.

•**Suck on manuka honey lozenges.**

•**Once symptoms are under control, try gradually adding back some foods,** such as onions, garlic and tomatoes—all no-no's at first but tasty ingredients in many common dishes. Over time, you may learn that you can't eat sautéed garlic but can tolerate garlic powder. Or maybe you can eat raw tomatoes but not canned sauces or ketchup.

If you are unsure about your triggers, keep a food-and-symptom diary for a month. When you reintroduce possible trigger foods, such as onions, garlic and chocolate, introduce one at a time so that you will know if you get reflux from that particular food. (You will know that day, that evening or the next day when you wake up.)

•**Reserve medications for as-needed use.** You may still need to take a fast-acting H2A medication before an occasional big night out.

The Best Natural Heartburn Remedies

Mona Morstein, ND, naturopathic physician and director of Arizona Integrative Medical Solutions in Tempe, Arizona.

Heartburn, a common symptom of gastroesophageal reflux disease (GERD), happens when stomach acid rises up and inflames the delicate lining of the esphagus. It's painful, uncomfortable and common.

Many people turn to proton pump inhibitor drugs such as *esomeprazole* (Nexium) or *omeprazole* (Prilosec), which significantly reduce the stomach's ability to produce digestive acid. But chronic use of such drugs can have dangerous consequences, including malabsorption of vitamin B12, iron and calcium…negative changes to the balance of bacteria in the gut "microbiome"…increased risk of food poisoning…decreased gallbladder function…possible increased risk for cognitive decline…increased cardiovascular risk. The drugs are especially risky when taken by people who also take blood thinners such as *warfarin* (Coumadin) and *clopidogrel* (Plavix), increasing the risk of uncontrolled bleeding. Although the evidence against the entire class of proton pump inhibitors is mixed, it is wise to avoid them in favor of safer alternatives. Fortunately, there are several natural remedies that can soothe your heartburn. *But first…*

GET TO THE ROOT OF YOUR GERD

Before you begin treating your GERD, I recommend that you seek care with a naturopathic or integrative physician. To find out why you have GERD, you'll need a medical evaluation, which should include a food sensitivity test. Hiatal hernias (a condition in which the upper part of the stomach pushes up into the esophagus) as well as certain prescription medications can cause GERD, and if that's true in your case, you want to know! Before you go to see a naturopathic or integrative physician, keep a diet diary for one week—writing down everything you eat and drink—and show it at your appointment. A diet diary can uncover nutrient deficiencies and inflammatory and anti-inflammatory food intake, which can have an impact on the stomach and how it functions.

MY GO-TO GERD SUPPLEMENTS

One of the best is slippery elm powder, which is mixed with water and then consumed like a thickened broth, a gruel-like "tea." Slippery elm coats and soothes the throat, esophagus and stomach, and it helps to rebuild the mucous lining. Slippery elm also contains antioxidants that can deter further damage. To make it, pour a cup of boiling water over one tablespoon of the powder and steep for three to five minutes. Try a cup in the morning and at night. That's enough for most people with heartburn to feel better. It's safe for everyone.

Marshmallow root tea also can soothe inflamed mucous membranes. Like slippery elm, it contains mucilage, which coats the lining of the throat, esophagus and stomach. It is also very safe, and you can use it by itself or alternately with slippery elm "tea." To make it, you can buy tea bags, or if you buy powdered root, pour one cup of warm water (not hot) over one tablespoon of powder. Boiling water may break down some of the mucilage that makes it effective. (Marshmallow root may reduce blood sugar, however, so if you are taking medications for diabetes, check with your doctor.)

Licorice in the form of tea or jam, capsules, lozenges or extracts can also help. It's a soothing, coating agent for the stomach. It's fine for short-term use, but long-term use can elevate blood pressure. You can avoid that risk with deglycyrrhizinated licorice (DGL).

The sleep hormone melatonin is also used to treat GERD. Melatonin is secreted by both the pineal gland in the brain and specialized cells in the gastrointestinal tract. Studies suggest that while brain-produced melatonin helps with sleep, the melatonin produced by the gastrointestinal tract protects its mucosal lining from damage caused by oxidative stress. Some research suggests that it blocks the release of acid, too. Studies show that five or six milligrams of melatonin are effective. It is usually taken in the evening, since it can make you drowsy.

PUTTING IT ALL TOGETHER

When I treat a patient for GERD, I will be sure to know the reason for it, will remove any food sensitivity, tidy up the patient's diet so that it is more nourishing and less inflammatory, and encourage eating slowly and not during stressful, rushed moments. I will then give some slippery elm powder to make into "tea" in the morning and evening. Depending on the patient, I will also recommend a GERD supplement that contains other healing, soothing agents for the stomach such as the ones listed above. They are safe to use in any combination.

Easy Way to Ease IBS

Vitamin D deficiency is common among people with irritable bowel syndrome (IBS), according to a recent review of seven studies.

Key finding: Vitamin D supplements (3,000 IU daily in one study) appear to relieve the severity of symptoms, including abdominal pain, bloating, diarrhea and constipation.

If you have IBS: Ask your doctor about checking your vitamin D levels, and discuss whether supplements would be right for you.

Bernard M. Corfe, PhD, senior lecturer, department of oncology and metabolism, University of Sheffield, UK.

What's Really Causing That "Stomach Bug"

Deborah A. Fisher, MD, associate professor of medicine in the division of gastroenterology at Duke University School of Medicine, associate director of gastroenterology research at Duke Clinical Research Institute and director of social and digital media accounts for Duke's GI division, all in Durham, North Carolina.

When stomach upset hits, if you're like most people you blame that awful cramping, diarrhea, nausea and other gastrointestinal (GI) distress on something you ate. It's true that one in six US adults do experience a bout of food poisoning every year (see next page). *But there are other culprits that are less recognized…*

•**Medications.** Certain prescription and over-the-counter medications can cause GI distress…

•Nonsteroidal anti-inflammatory drugs (NSAIDs). *Ibuprofen* (Advil, Motrin), *naproxen* (Aleve) and other NSAIDs are known to cause dyspepsia. Dyspepsia, better known as indigestion, is marked by pain and burning in the upper abdomen, below the breastbone, and queasiness without vomiting. Dyspepsia can also occur with other drugs such as some antibiotics (see below).

In one Canadian study, up to 30% of patients with dyspepsia were found to be taking an NSAID.

What helps: Try lowering your NSAID dose, but realize that some people cannot tolerate even a low dose. If this approach doesn't help, try switching to *acetaminophen* (Tylenol), which may be equally effective in treating pain but without stomach discomfort.

Note: Long-term use of an NSAID or acetaminophen can have side effects. Both types of pain relievers are for occasional use only.

•Proton pump inhibitors (PPIs). These stomach acid medications have been linked to higher rates of diarrhea caused by the dangerous *Clostridium difficile* bacterium. Chronic PPI use (generally, more than six months) reduces the diversity of bacteria in your GI tract, possibly allowing unhealthy bugs to thrive.

Commonly used PPIs include *esomeprazole* (Nexium), *lansoprazole* (Prevacid) and *omeprazole* (Prilosec). If you experience persistent, watery diarrhea, stomach pain and fever, and are taking a PPI, talk to your doctor. He/she may test you for Clostridium difficile–associated diarrhea, which can be treated with antibiotics. If PPI use causes GI distress, ask your doctor about taking *ranitidine* (Zantac) on an as-needed basis—it's less likely to cause stomach problems than PPIs.

•Antibiotics. *Azithromycin* (Zithromax, Zithromax Z-Pak) and *erythromycin* (Eryc, Ery-Tab) are among the antibiotics most likely to cause diarrhea by speeding up food's transit time through the intestine. Typically, you just have to ride it out, being sure to stay hydrated.

Helpful: Water with a splash of orange juice and a pinch of salt is an effective, inexpensive substitute for store-bought, electrolyte-infused water.

Also: Ask your doctor whether your antibiotic can be taken with food—such as crackers—to help prevent GI symptoms. Some data suggest that taking probiotics may help counteract the GI effects of antibiotics. Get them via fermented foods such as kefir, sauerkraut, yogurt, kimchi and miso soup. Never stop an antibiotic without first consulting your doctor.

•Selective serotonin reuptake inhibitors (SSRIs). This class of antidepressants, including *fluoxetine* (Prozac), *sertraline* (Zoloft) and *paroxetine* (Paxil), can cause nausea and diarrhea in some patients. This usually subsides in a few weeks.

•FODMAPs, or fermentable oligosaccharides disaccharides monosaccharides and polyols. These are difficult-to-digest sugars such as lactose, found in dairy products…fructose, in fruit…fructan, in wheat and good-for-you veggies including asparagus, onions, garlic and artichokes…and galactans, in complex carbohydrates such as beans, including kidney beans, chickpeas and soybean products.

For unknown reasons, in some people, the carbohydrates in high-FODMAP foods don't get digested in the small intestine. The undigested carbohydrates advance to the large intestine, where bacteria feast on them, causing cramping and gas, and draw excess water into the colon, triggering diarrhea. If your GI discomfort flares up when eating one of the foods above, see a gastroenterologist to find out if FODMAPs are to blame.

Helpful: The American Gastroenterological Association offers a downloadable guide for following a low-FODMAP diet.

•Stomach flu. At least 20 million Americans are hit with acute gastroenteritis (commonly known as "stomach flu") every year. It's usually caused by the norovirus, which spreads rampantly through crowded areas such as hospitals, airplanes, cruise ships and nursing homes. The virus makes its way from an infected person's feces or vomit into your mouth, usually when you touch a contaminated surface (a toilet handle or an ATM machine, for example) or eat food prepared by a person who is infected.

Symptoms such as diarrhea, vomiting, stomach pain, fever, headache and body aches usually begin within 12 to 48 hours of exposure, and most individuals recover in one to three days. There is no effective treatment. Protect yourself with thorough handwashing using soap and water. An alcohol-based hand sanitizer should not be used as a substitute for soap and water. Good handwashing is essential to avoid transmission. If you become sick, avoid preparing food for others.

Note: Stomach flu is not the same as the flu, which is a respiratory illness caused by the influenza virus. For this reason, getting a flu shot won't protect you from stomach flu. Also, stomach flu is easily confused with food poisoning, which causes similar symptoms. For more on food poisoning, see below.

•Too much fiber. Following a high-fiber diet is a healthy move. But consuming too much fiber too quickly can cause cramping, bloating and gas.

Better: Gradually increase your consumption of produce (such as broccoli, carrots, avocado, apples, pears and figs) and beans by one to two servings a day—or a fiber supplement by one tablespoon a day. As long as you experience no adverse GI symptoms, continue increasing your intake slowly for a total of 30 g of fiber per day for men…and 21 g for women. If you are taking a laxative for constipation, synthetic fibers such as *methylcellulose* (Citrucel) may be less gas-forming than natural fibers such as *psyllium* (Metamucil).

•Stress. If you've ever been stuck on the toilet due to nerves, you know that the brain and belly are linked. Numerous studies have suggested that some GI problems may have a neurological component.

Why: More than 100 million neurons (cells that carry messages from the brain to other parts of the body) line the human GI tract—creating "the second brain." Not only can stress lead to upset stomach, new research suggests that the effect may also work in reverse, possibly explaining why many people with irritable bowel syndrome and other GI disorders develop depression and/or anxiety. Cognitive behavioral therapy or hypnotherapy tailored for GI issues may help. Ask your doctor for a referral.

WHAT IF IT IS FOOD POISONING?

Food poisoning is no fun! If you consume food that has been contaminated with bacteria, such as *E. coli* or *Staphylococcus aureus*, the telltale symptoms, including abdominal cramps, diarrhea and vomiting, often come on suddenly and typically last for 72 hours or so.

Due to the "transit time" it takes food to make its way through your body's digestive system, it's likely that something you ate a few hours before symptoms began—or even a few days earlier—is to blame.

Foods that most often cause food poisoning: Undercooked meat or poultry, ground meat, unpasteurized dairy, improperly washed fresh produce and food contaminated by a sick food handler.

Note: Many fast-food chains source their meat and eggs from multiple farms, increasing your risk for exposure to bacteria.

If you get food poisoning, be sure to stay hydrated (drink enough fluids so that your urine is light colored). Dizziness when standing can be caused by dehydration. Uncontrolled vomiting requires prompt medical attention. Important: If you experience vomiting and diarrhea for more than 72 hours—or bloody diarrhea at any time—call your doctor. You may have a particularly virulent strain of E. coli that can cause kidney failure and may require IV fluids and perhaps even short-term dialysis.

Quick Fixes for a Bellyache

Jamison Starbuck, ND, a naturopathic physician in family practice and writer/producer of *Dr. Starbuck's Health Tips for Kids*, a weekly program on Montana Public Radio, MTPR.org, both in Missoula. She is a past president of the American Association of Naturopathic Physicians and a contributing editor to *The Alternative Advisor: The Complete Guide to Natural Therapies and Alternative Treatments.* DrJamisonStarbuck.com

---

Have you ever woken up with a bellyache? Or had a queasy feeling in your stomach late in the day? If you get this type of bellyache—and who doesn't?—a few simple remedies can help you feel better in a day or so. *What may be causing the problem— and the easy fixes I recommend…*

•**Indigestion.** If you've overeaten or consumed a high-fat, high-protein meal, the food could be rotting in your gut rather than being properly broken down for digestion.

Red flags: You are gassy, bloated, burping and/or still feeling full hours after a meal.

What helps: Try drinking tea made from herbs in the mint family—peppermint, spearmint, lemon balm and/or catnip. You can use just one of these herbs, combine all of them or look for a "tummy ache" mixture. Make a strong tea using two teaspoons of dried herb or two tea bags per 12 ounces of water. Drink six ounces every 15 minutes for an hour.

•**Constipation.** Medical doctors define constipation as having a bowel movement less than three times a week, but I believe this should be a daily event to help clear toxins from your body.

Red flags: You suffer from lower abdominal cramping…and/or have an urge to move your bowels but nothing happens.

What helps: Smooth Move tea (made by Traditional Medicinals). It contains senna, a botanical laxative. It also contains the herbs licorice, ginger, fennel and cinnamon—all of which soothe the digestive tract. Usually one cup, taken on an empty stomach, is enough to relieve infrequent constipation. Bedtime is an ideal time for the tea if you usually have a morning bowel movement.

Caution: Don't use Smooth Move, or any senna product, if you know you have a bowel disease, such as Crohn's or ulcerative colitis. Senna works by irritating the gut wall, which can worsen bowel disease. To be on the safe side, check with your doctor if you have any question about using senna. And do not use Smooth Move for more than two or three days—as with any laxative, you may become dependent on it.

•**Stomach virus.** Even though a stomach virus can lead to diarrhea and vomiting, sometimes these symptoms are quite mild. The only signs could be a loose stool, lack of appetite and/or not feeling quite right for 24 hours.

Red flags: Someone in your household or workplace has had the same thing…or you've recently spent time with small children, who are common carriers of these nasty viruses.

What helps: Activated charcoal capsules appear to absorb viruses and move them out of your body. Take two charcoal capsules on an empty stomach four times a day for 24 or 48 hours. Check with your doctor first if you take any medications.

•**Worry or anxiety.** Anticipating an event— whether it's a happy occasion or something that has you feeling worried and anxious—makes digestion difficult.

Red flag: You've just gone through an emotionally charged time...or you are about to enter one.

What helps: Ten minutes of purposeful walking will relax you—and promote improved digestion. While you're walking, breathe deeply so that air makes it all the way to your tight, tension-filled stomach. Listening to meditation or visualization podcasts can also be a big help!

Important: If your bellyache lasts longer than a day or two—or if it becomes a regular occurrence—see your doctor to rule out bowel disease such as diverticulitis, gastritis or irritable bowel syndrome.

Yummy Healing Soup for Tummy Trouble

Sharon Palmer, RDN, a Duarte, California–based registered dietitian nutritionist and author of *Plant-Powered for Life* and *The Plant-Powered Diet*. She is the editor of the *Environmental Nutrition* newsletter and nutrition editor for *Today's Dietitian*. Her recipes, including those in this article, appear on her website, SharonPalmer.com.

Few foods are more comforting than a piping hot bowl of delicious soup.

What you may not realize: Certain homemade soups are packed with healing nutrients that help fight chronic health problems, such as stomach troubles.

What's so special about soup? With most cooking methods, such as steaming or boiling, the liquid is discarded—along with vitamins and minerals that may have leached out of the food. Not so with soup, which uses all the liquid so that most of the nutrients are preserved, even when heated.

Bonus: Because soups are so filling and satisfying, they have also been shown to help reduce one's overall calorie intake when added to a meal!

FOR DIGESTIVE HEALTH— MISO KABOCHA SOUP

Souper star nutrient: Probiotics. Trillions of microorganisms reside in your bowels—and that's a good thing! These healthy bacteria, called probiotics, aid digestion and nutrient absorption...govern the immune system...and work to keep harmful pathogens in check.

Emerging research has linked the consumption of probiotics and probiotic-rich foods, such as miso (a traditional Japanese fermented soybean paste), sauerkraut, kimchi, yogurt and kefir, with potential health benefits, including improved immune and digestive function.

Miso is intensely flavorful and provides a note of umami—that is, a meaty, savory taste. This recipe also contains ginger, which helps fight inflammation and nausea.

Instructions: Slice a small, unpeeled kabocha squash (a round green Japanese vegetable available at farmers' markets and an increasing number of supermarkets) into large pieces. Scoop out the seeds, place in a baking dish with a small amount of water and bake at 350°F for 35 minutes (or you can microwave it with a little water for 10 minutes).

Once slightly cooled, scoop out the flesh and place it in a blender with one cup of vegetable broth...one cup of plain, unsweetened coconut, soy or almond milk...one-and-one-half tablespoons of white miso...and one teaspoon of grated fresh ginger. Process until smooth (use an immersion blender in a pot if you prefer). Heat the mixture in a medium pot until bubbly. Stir in one 14-ounce package of tofu (diced in small cubes) and one-half cup of green onions, diced. Delicious!

Herbs and More for Leaky Gut

Jamison Starbuck, ND, a naturopathic physician in family practice and writer/producer of *Dr. Starbuck's Health Tips for Kids*, a weekly program on Montana Public Radio, MTPR.org, both in Missoula. DrJamisonStarbuck.com

If you've got celiac disease, food allergies or an autoimmune bowel disease, such as Crohn's disease or inflammatory bowel disease, you probably have leaky gut syndrome. Also known as gastrointestinal permeability, leaky gut syndrome is a condition in which microscopic "holes" develop in the lining of the digestive tract as a result of medications, allergies to foods, genetics and other causes. Your digestive tract, or gut, is designed to keep food particles in your intestines and out of your bloodstream. When food is properly digested and broken down, food nutrients pass through the filter of the intestinal wall and into the bloodstream. This is how your body gets the nutrition it needs to survive.

With leaky gut syndrome, your gut wall is like a torn window screen. Insects that are meant to stay outside enter your home. When leaky gut occurs, overly large food molecules pass through these microscopic holes into your bloodstream. To the body, these large molecules are an enemy. The immune system responds protectively and makes defenders known as antibodies. If you have a lot of food-related antibodies, you have food allergies (or a food sensitivity). You'll also have an inflamed bowel and leaky gut syndrome.

One way to heal the symptoms of leaky gut syndrome, which include indigestion, irregular stools, generalized fatigue and inflammation, skin rashes and migraines, is to avoid the foods to which you are allergic. That can help. However, if you don't repair the intestinal wall, you'll continue to suffer with many of the above symptoms and may even become allergic to other foods.

How, then, do you treat the gut wall? *What I recommend...*

•**Eat the right foods.** Sauerkraut is rich in probiotics, which help crowd out pathogens that damage the gut wall. Do not use canned sauerkraut—the probiotics are killed in the heating process that is required for canning. Plant-based oils, such as olive, sunflower and borage, are nourishing to the intestine. Fish, baked or cooked on a grill, can also help heal a leaky gut. It is easy to digest, anti-inflammatory and contains helpful proteins and oils. Just be sure to avoid fried fish and fried foods generally. You may also want to try a probiotic supplement. Follow label instructions.

Caution: People with weakened immune systems (such as those using chemotherapy) should consult their doctors before eating probiotic-rich food or taking a probiotic supplement.

•**Consider these herbs.** My favorite herbs for leaky gut are slippery elm...marshmallow root...and plantain (a medicinal plant not to be confused with the banana-like food). You can use one of these herbs or combine two or more.

To treat leaky gut: You need to take herbal medicine between meals—60 minutes or more after a meal or 30 minutes or more before a meal—to ensure that the herb comes into direct contact with the gut wall.* You can take these herbs in capsules, tea or bulk powders.

Typical daily dose: Three standard-sized capsules two times a day...three cups of tea...or two teaspoons of the bulk-powdered herb. For convenience and taste, put the powdered herb in a small amount (one-eighth cup or less) of applesauce or oatmeal.

With my patients, treatment usually takes about three months to heal leaky gut. Assuming that one's diet stays healthy, the regimen above can often be discontinued when symptoms subside.

*If you use any prescription medication, have a chronic medical condition (such as diabetes) or are pregnant or nursing, consult your doctor before taking any herbs.

What Your Poop Says About Your Health

Anil Minocha, MD, professor of medicine at Louisiana State University Health Sciences Center and chief of gastroenterology at the Overton Brooks VA Medical Center, both in Shreveport. He is the author of *Seven-X Plan for Digestive Health.*

This may be a personal question...but do you ever look at your poop? *Why we ask:* The color, shape and/or smell of your stools can offer clues about your health that are more important than you may realize.

CHECK IT OUT

There's no need to obsess about your stools, but you should take a look at least every week (or more often if you feel unwell or think something may be wrong). It's a good idea to know what's normal for you so that you can report anything out of the ordinary to your doctor.

As far as bowel movements go, "normal" encompasses a wide range—healthy stools can be beige to dark brown...texture can range from firm to a little bit loose...and the average frequency is once or twice a day, but some people only go three times a week.

Most abnormalities last a few days and resolve (perhaps you've eaten something you don't usually eat, or maybe you have a virus). But do take note of anything unusual that lasts for a week or more or recurs. *What to watch for...*

•**Bright or dark red blood.** Bright red blood on toilet paper typically originates from the anus or the lower part of the intestine—it could be coming from a hemorrhoid or a slight tear in the anal tissue that comes from straining during a bowel movement.

Take note: If this happens once or twice, there's less cause to worry, but let your doctor know. If there's a lot of blood or you regularly bleed, even intermittently, make an appointment with your doctor right away, or go to the ER. Bleeding polyps in the colon can produce red blood in the stool, as can diverticula, abnormal pouches that form in the intestine. Your doctor will probably advise a colonoscopy (and possibly an upper GI endoscopy) to investigate.

•**Black poop.** Stools that are black and sticky-looking (or tarry) could indicate that there's blood in your bowel movements—possibly from an ulcer...a tear in the esophagus...an abnormal blood vessel in the colon...or colon cancer.

Important: Call your doctor right away. He/she will probably order tests (such as a colonoscopy and/or endoscopy) to see where the blood is originating and recommend a treatment plan.

Exception: Some foods and supplements—black licorice, dark berries, iron supplements and medications such as Pepto-Bismol and Kaopectate—can make stools black. But check in with your doctor if you have any questions at all.

Note: If you've eaten lots of leafy green vegetables, your poop might turn green.

•**Pale or white stools.** Bile, produced in the liver, is what gives stools their brown color. When poop is pale, the liver isn't releasing enough bile and may be diseased. Gallstones, which block the flow of bile into the intestines, are another cause of light-colored stools. Pancreatic cancer can produce pale stools, too.

Take note: Make an appointment with your doctor to get this checked out. Tests could include an abdominal ultrasound, CT scan or MRI.

•**Pencil-thin shape.** It was once thought that pencil-thin stools were a warning signal for colorectal cancer. Now doctors believe that the size/shape of stools is largely affected by what you eat. People who eat a lot of meat tend to produce smaller stools than vegetarians who tend to get more fiber.

Take note: If you have a sudden and consistent change in stool thickness, it's best to mention this to your doctor. By itself, it's not likely to be caused by cancer, but it should be checked out.

•**Foul odor.** Stools are a combination of dead and live bacteria, cells from the lining of the intestine, fiber and other undigested food...and all of this produces odor.

The intensity of the smell depends on what you've eaten. High-sulfur foods, such as garlic, broccoli or meats, tend to cause stinky stools. So does sorbitol, an artificial sweetener that's added to some medications and processed foods. Also, the bacteria in the large intestine vary from person to person with some varieties causing more odor than others. Antibiotics often cause foul-smelling stools because they temporarily disrupt bacterial balance.

Take note: See a doctor if the odor is much stronger than usual or if the smell is accompanied by other digestive symptoms, such as diarrhea, cramps, a persistent increase/decrease in bowel movements, etc.

Possible causes: Celiac disease, in which your body is unable to tolerate gluten, a protein in wheat, rye and barley...an intestinal parasite (such as Giardia)...or a bacterial or viral infection in the intestine.

Easy Solutions for Two Embarrassing Digestion Conditions

Bill Gottlieb, CHC, is a health coach certified by the American Association of Drugless Practitioners and former editor in chief of Rodale Books and Prevention Magazine Health Books. He is author of 16 health books including *Speed Healing*, recently published by Bottom Line Inc. BillGottliebHealth.com

Embarrassment can keep people from seeking solutions to their problems. And that's a shame because there are simple, fast, natural solutions for most embarrassing health problems.

Caution: If nondrug remedies don't work after a week or two, see your doctor—your health problem may have a serious cause that requires medical attention.

PASSING GAS

You need to pass gas—it's a natural part of digestion, and the average person does it anywhere from six to 21 times a day. But passing it excessively is uncomfortable and embarrassing.

Most excessive passing of gas is caused by dysbiosis—an imbalance in intestinal bacteria, with "bad" bacteria such as Clostridium difficile outnumbering "friendly" bacteria such as Lactobacillus acidophilus.

Solution: Take a daily probiotic, a supplement containing friendly bacteria.

Scientific evidence: Researchers from the Mayo Clinic and other institutions analyzed the results of six studies on probiotics involving more than 560 people—and found that the supplement "significantly improved" flatulence.

Also helpful: If you're about to be in a social situation where gas is a no-no, take a preventive dose of activated charcoal, which works by binding with toxins (including unhealthful bacteria) and ushering them out of the body. Follow the dosage recommendations on the label.

ANAL ITCHING

There are many possible causes of anal itching including diarrhea, incontinence, psoriasis, genital warts or a yeast infection. But one common cause is hemorrhoids, the swollen and in-flamed anal veins that affect half of Americans over age 50. (If you have pain and bleeding with the itching, a hemorrhoid is the likely cause. But confirm the cause of anal itching with your doctor.)

Solution: To ease itching from hemorrhoids, one vein-strengthening food factor works particularly well—hesperidin, a flavonoid (plant pigment) found in citrus fruits.

Scientific evidence: A study in *British Journal of Surgery* analyzed 14 other studies on flavonoids and hemorrhoids, involving more than 1,500 people. The scientists found that consuming flavonoids cut the risk of itching from hemorrhoids by 35%—and also significantly reduced bleeding and pain.

What to do: Look for a supplement containing diosmin, a specially processed form of hesperidin. Take 500 milligrams (mg), twice daily. Diosmin is very safe, but a few people may experience intestinal discomfort—if that happens, stop taking the supplement.

Also helpful: Other ways to help prevent and heal hemorrhoids include drinking more water (60 ounces a day is a good goal)…increasing your intake of fiber-rich foods such as fruits, vegetables and whole grains…and regular exercise, such as brisk walking.

Common Causes of Anal Itching

Mitchell Bernstein, MD, associate professor of surgery in the division of colon and rectal surgery, NYU Langone Health, New York City, quoted at MensHealth.com.

Not wiping completely or properly after a bowel movement can cause anal itching, but wiping too hard is more often the culprit. It may also help to avoid too aggressive cleaning with washcloths or using moistened tissues. Consuming certain foods—including tea, cola, energy drinks, beer, chocolate, nuts, citrus fruits, tomatoes, spicy or sugary foods and dairy—can also cause anal discomfort. If itching persists, try eliminating each food one by one for three to four weeks to see if that helps ease the symptoms.

If It's Not a Hemorrhoid... What Is This Embarrassing Lump?

Bruce A. Orkin, MD, chief of colorectal surgery, Rush University Medical Center, Chicago.

There are many reasons for lumps around the anus, and most are fairly harmless. Don't be embarrassed, be safe! Common problems include hemorrhoids, skin tags, abscesses, cysts and warts.

More than 50% of adults will have hemorrhoids (swollen, enlarged blood vessels) at some time in their lives. There are two types—internal (inside the lower rectum) and external (on the outer edge of the anus). A blood clot may develop in an external hemorrhoid, stretching out the skin and creating a painful, firm lump that feels like a marble or pea. It can cause bleeding and itching. Internal hemorrhoids may prolapse outside the rectum.

Skin tags are a painless flap of tissue, sometimes occurring with a tear in the anal canal (fissure) caused by hard bowel movements.

Perianal abscesses are pus-filled infections around the anus. They are usually very painful and develop over several days. They may drain spontaneously but otherwise should be drained promptly by a doctor.

Sebaceous cysts are lumps that form when the sebaceous glands around hair follicles get plugged up. They may also become infected.

Anal warts are growths due to infection with the human papillomavirus (HPV) and are usually spread by sexual contact. They should be removed.

Anal cancer is fairly rare but has some of the same symptoms (bleeding, pain, itching and/or an anal growth) as benign conditions.

In most cases, an anal lump will go away by itself in two or three weeks. To relieve discomfort, sit in a tub of warm water. If the lump is painful or doesn't go away or if anal bleeding continues for more than a few days, see a colorectal surgeon. He/she can evaluate the lump and remove it if needed.

CHAPTER 8

Emotional Health

Don't Let Loneliness Harm Your Health

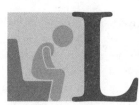

Loneliness is a miserable feeling…and generic advice such as joining a hiking club or a senior center may not help. The key to relieving your own loneliness is to understand it. Why are you lonely?

It's an important question to answer because loneliness has been linked to a variety of health problems, such as weakened immunity and hardening of the arteries. Research also suggests that the dangers associated with loneliness are on par with those related to obesity and cigarette smoking.

Latest development: Loneliness is now considered a risk factor for Alzheimer's disease according to a study published in the *Archives of General Psychiatry*. Although the exact link between loneliness and the brain is unknown, some experts hypothesize that loneliness pro-

vokes a chronic stress reaction that promotes inflammation, which accumulating evidence suggests may contribute to Alzheimer's disease, the most common cause of dementia.

How to fight loneliness and its associated health risks…

BEING ALONE VS. BEING LONELY

Many people choose to live by themselves and are perfectly content. Conversely, you can be lonely without being alone. Many lonely people are married, and some even have lots of friends.

So what is this thing called loneliness? It can include feeling that you lack companionship, feeling left out and feeling isolated. You can even be lonely without knowing it—you can have one of these feelings and not recognize it as loneliness, in the same way that some depressed people do not identify their negative moods and lethargy as depression.

Carla Perissinotto, MD, associate professor of geriatrics at the University of California at San Francisco. Dr. Perissinotto's research into the association between loneliness and health was published in *Archives of Internal Medicine*.

WHAT CAUSES LONELINESS?

Some people may be more vulnerable to feeling lonely because of their personalities. But other times, people are in situations that promote loneliness. For example, maybe they need to stay home due to an illness and miss seeing others...or perhaps they are living in a rural area where it's difficult to connect with others and they crave more daily contact with people.

Loneliness also increases with age. In one study, 43% of seniors reported feeling lonely. *Two main reasons for this...*

•**Relationships frequently dwindle with age.** Upon retirement, your career-long social network may crumble...friends and family may move away...a beloved life partner may die.

•**Our ageist, youth-centered culture tends to ignore the wisdom and experience that aging provides.** The elderly are often stigmatized as a burden on society. It's easy to believe that your life no longer has a purpose when you feel unacknowledged by a world in which you once played a productive role.

EASING LONELINESS

There's no one-size-fits-all remedy for loneliness. But if you ask yourself the important question—Why am I lonely?—you may discover a solution that works for you. The following suggestions often help people pinpoint the cause of their loneliness and allow them to overcome it.

If you feel that you lack companionship...

•**Connect with more people.** Connecting with people who share your strong interest in something may help fill that void. Try joining a book group if you love to read...or an activist group if you are passionate about politics. Consider volunteering to tutor children or serve meals at a shelter. Beneficial connections can happen one-on-one or in groups. Some people find that getting a pet is helpful.

Unfortunately, the loneliness of social isolation may have deep roots. Even if you are lonely for companionship, you may find it difficult or unpleasant to connect with others—particularly if the problem is long-standing. Dig down to find out why.

Some people never developed the social skills that foster friendships, and some hold maladaptive beliefs about themselves (a sense of inferiority or superiority, for example) or about others (such as mistrust). If this is the case, self-reflection and therapy can help.

•**Put technology to work.** Computer, tablet or smartphone applications like Skype and FaceTime allow you to talk with—and see—friends and family who aren't nearby. The apps are free (once you own the device).

If you're uncomfortable with technology, consider taking a free class at a public library or senior center. Check SeniorNet (SeniorNet. org), a nonprofit company that offers in-person classes across the country specially designed for older adults.

Useful: The AARP-sponsored website Connect2Affect.org offers valuable information and an interactive guide to local resources, such as job opportunities, volunteer programs and tax preparation services. Also, SeniorCenterWithout Walls.org enables isolated seniors to participate in groups via phone or computer.

Important: Social media, such as Facebook, provides a measure of connectedness but shouldn't displace real life contact.

If you feel left out...

•**Deepen your relationships.** Taking steps to deepen your friendships—by revealing more about yourself and listening and responding wholeheartedly to what your friends have to say—may bring the warmth of true connection into your life. Here, too, a therapist can help by giving you the tools you need to deepen your relationships.

Is it your relationship with your life partner that needs more intimacy? If your marriage leaves you lonely, you and your spouse may benefit from couples counseling.

If you feel physically isolated...

•**Overcome barriers.** Mundane difficulties can cut you off from others. Transportation is often an issue for older people who have mobility problems or don't drive. Local agencies for the aging can provide help, as can the website Connect2Affect.org (mentioned above).

Consider using a "task-sharing" service where people trade skills for what they need—for example, you help someone with balancing her checkbook and she gives you a ride to the supermarket.

Websites to try: SwapRight.com or Simbi. com. You could also take a taxi or use Uber if you cannot get a ride otherwise.

Maybe your diminished hearing or vision makes you reluctant to socialize. If that's the case, talk to your doctor about ways to improve your hearing or sight.

Magnets for Depression

Michael Banov, MD, medical director, Northwest Behavioral Medicine, Roswell, Georgia.

Transcranial magnetic stimulation (TMS) involves placing electromagnetic coils on the scalp to deliver targeted pulses that stimulate the part of the brain responsible for mood. TMS is noninvasive and has been around for several years. It can be used in conjunction with medications and traditional therapies and seems to work as well as antidepressants. Insurance may pay for TMS if other treatments have failed.

The downside: Treatment generally takes 45 minutes a day, five days a week, for six weeks. Side effects are mild and fleeting, but may include headache, scalp irritation, facial twitches and light-headedness.

Caution: Steer clear of devices sold online. Only a medical doctor can administer TMS.

Pain and Depression Link Between Partners

Andrew McIntosh, MD, chair of biological psychiatry, University of Edinburgh, Scotland.

A study of 100,000 adults found that when romantic partners lived together and one person was depressed or in chronic pain, the other was more likely to have chronic pain…and that in turn can lead to depression. The two conditions appear to have common causes, including the environment partners share.

If your partner has chronic pain or is depressed: Recognize that you may be at greater risk for these conditions.

What Surgeons Don't Talk About…Post-Surgery Depression

Charles B. Inlander is a consumer advocate and health-care consultant based in Fogelsville, Pennsylvania. He was the founding president of the nonprofit People's Medical Society, a consumer advocacy organization credited with key improvements in the quality of US health care, and is the author or coauthor of more than 20 consumer-health books.

Two days after I was diagnosed with a brain tumor, I underwent five and a half hours of surgery. Fortunately, the tumor was removed and it was benign. On the day before my operation, my neurosurgeon went over everything she would be doing during the operation. She also explained, in detail, what I might expect during my recovery, including pain, follow-up procedures I might require and what I would need in terms of physical and occupational therapy to help me regain my balance and overcome dizziness. I was pleased with the time she spent explaining everything that might occur.

If you saw me now, you wouldn't know I went through a major operation. But what you cannot see—and what my surgeon never mentioned as a potential aftereffect—is that I have been suffering from a form of depression known in medical circles as postsurgical traumatic stress syndrome (PSTSS). It really hit about three months after my operation. My symptoms were loss of appetite, anxiety, fear of recurrence and fatigue. I realized something was wrong and contacted the surgeon. She told me that what was done during the operation was not the cause but that the trauma of the diagnosis and realization of what I went through likely sparked it. She said it was not unusual and urged me to seek treatment from my family doctor. I did and have been helped by medication and by sessions I have had with a psychologist.

What you should know about postsurgical depression…

●**It is not unusual.** It has long been known that 30% to 40% of people having coronary bypass surgery suffer some form of postsurgical depression. Studies also show that patients having brain surgery, bariatric surgery or cancer surgery are at higher risk for depression. Single or widowed patients and people who have a history of depression are more prone to postsurgical depression.

●**The causes are varied.** For some people, postsurgical depression is believed to be a side effect of having been under general anesthesia during the operation. Postsurgical pain, digestive disorders, reactions to medications or chemotherapy, inability to get restful sleep and/or having restricted movement also can be causes.

The fear factor: A major cause of postsurgical depression is fear of having a recurrence, dying and/or becoming disabled. The fear factor can occur, as it did with me, many months or even years after the surgery!

●**You don't have to suffer alone.** Before having any surgery, ask the surgeon about postsurgical depression. You may not get a lot of information, but you may be told some red flags to watch out for after the surgery. Obviously, any surgery will slow you down for a while, but if you are having excessively sad feelings, fear, lack of sleep and seeing little improvement in your mood, contact your surgeon and family doctor. Don't hesitate to talk about your feelings with your doctors, family and friends. Medications (including antidepressants and antianxiety drugs) and medical professionals, such as psychologists or psychiatrists, can help. There are also many support groups, often sponsored by your local hospital, where you can talk with other people experiencing the same issues.

Remember: You are not alone—millions of other people are likely experiencing similar feelings. And there is help!

Don't Give Up

American Geriatrics Society.

Don't give up if you have both depression and metabolic syndrome (a mix of symptoms that includes high blood pressure, elevated blood sugar and excessive abdominal fat). In people with this combination, response to antidepressants may be somewhat slower, recent research has found.

Having Trouble Meditating?

Amy Zabin, DA, MT-BC, founder and director of The Music Therapy Center of Greenwich and a music therapy consultant at Greenwich Hospital and Stamford Hospital, all in Connecticut. She previously served as an adjunct professor in New York University's music therapy graduate program for 20 years. AmyZabin.com

Despite the incentive of its amazing health benefits (meditation has been shown to reduce blood pressure, improve sleep, relieve pain, minimize anxiety, ease depression and more), many people have a lot of difficulty meditating. Some people even feel anxious when they meditate—they wonder if they're doing it properly…get upset when the mind wanders…or feel like they're wasting time by sitting around and doing "nothing."

Good news: If you have tried to meditate without success, listening to music while you meditate may be the secret. And if you already meditate regularly, adding music can enhance the experience.

HOW MUSIC HELPS

For traditional meditation, you find a quiet place, remove as many distractions as possible—bright lights, cell phones, etc.—and focus on your breath or a mantra. When music is added to meditation, it offers a new and enjoyable focal point. Instead of feeling pressured to concentrate solely on your breath or mantra, you can focus on the music.

CHOOSING MEDITATIVE TUNES

Pick a genre of soothing music that you truly enjoy, but try to stick with instrumental pieces, since lyrics can be distracting. Music with a slow beat can create brain wave activity similar to that of meditation. Avoid aggressive music with a fast tempo—it can work against you by speeding up your heart and breathing rates. *Some good options…*

•**Classical music**—This type of music has been proven to slow heart rate, boost memory and more. Choose slow pieces that are captivating but not bombastic, such as Pachelbel's *Canon in D*, Bach's *Air on the G String from Orchestral Suite No. 3 in D Major* and Mozart's *Piano Concerto No. 23, 2nd Movement, Adagio*. There are many selections available for purchase online or streaming for free on YouTube or other websites.

•**New Age music**—There are lots of choices in this genre as well. An album I like is *In a Silent Place* by Eric Roberts.

•**Irish music**—Good choices include relaxing Irish and Celtic music and, my favorite, *Watermark* by Enya.

•**Guitar and flute combinations**—Various selections by Peder Helland feature guitar, violin, flute, cello and harp music. And on Music and Meditation (available at AmyZabin.com), I lead listeners into a deep meditation using guitar and flute music as well as crystal singing bowls.

Note: In my opinion, meditating to music might not be ideal at night—while the process feels relaxing, music activates so many parts of your brain that the overall effect is invigorating…you'll feel focused and alert afterward. Music meditation is best done in the morning or as an alternative to a midafternoon cup of coffee.

HOW TO MEDITATE WITH MUSIC

To start, sit or recline in a peaceful spot, free from distractions—your bed, a couch or even in your car parked on a quiet street.

Close your eyes and take a few breaths in through the nose and out through the mouth. Some people like to breathe in to a count of four and exhale to a count of eight, while others prefer to simply breathe in and out as deeply as possible.

Tune into your body and how it feels—do you notice any areas of tension or tightness? Take notice of these sensations, then release them. You can try shrugging your shoulders and releasing them and rolling your head a few times to let go of tension.

Next, turn on the music…you can play it out loud or use headphones or earbuds. Continue slowly breathing in and out as you turn your full attention to the music. Allow the music to lead the experience—to wash over, around and through you. Notice the tempo and the various instruments. Maybe you find yourself tuning into the cello in an orchestral piece or the ping of a triangle in a New Age song. Ask yourself—"How does this music make me feel?" Maybe it's relaxing you all over, or you notice your chest opening up, or you find yourself smiling.

If your mind wanders, that's fine. Think of these thoughts as clouds passing through the sky—simply notice them without judgment and gently return your focus to the music. Interesting: Some experts believe the power of meditation lies in shifting and returning to focus. The more you practice it in the soothing, controlled environment of meditation, the easier it will be for you to calm yourself during stressful times.

Remarkable: I've found that just three to five minutes, three times a week, is all you need to reap the rewards of meditating with music.

Feeling Down? That's OK!

People who acknowledge and accept feeling depressed or anxious—without berating themselves—feel better than those who ignore their emotions or judge them as negative, according to a study of 1,300 adults. Study participants, who reported feelings after journaling or delivering a three-minute videotaped test, had lower levels of distress and fewer symptoms of depression if they accepted these feelings.

Iris Mauss, PhD, associate professor of psychology, University of California, Berkeley.

Overcoming the Pain of Sexual Abuse Memories

Wendy Maltz, LCSW, DST, psychotherapist, lecturer and sex therapist based in Eugene, Oregon, who has written six books on sexuality including *The Sexual Healing Journey: A Guide for Survivors of Sexual Abuse.* HealthySex.com

A recent social movement, in which women (and some men) bravely come forth to tell their stories of sexual harassment, abuse and violence, has felled the careers of some of the most powerful men in business, politics, media and entertainment—even as it empowers the abused to stand up for their rights.

For many people, however, these stories, while inspiring, can trigger very painful memories—even bring new ones to light that you may have suppressed. To learn how to deal with these, we spoke with Wendy Maltz, LCSW, DST, a psychotherapist, lecturer and sex therapist. (*Note*: These recommendations apply to anyone—including men—who has been a victim of sexual abuse.)

The truth is, there are many paths to healing. *Here is how to find the ones that are a good fit for you…*

•**Honor your experiences.** Don't minimize your experiences or compare them with someone else's experiences that seem even worse. Each event of sexual harassment, abuse or violence—from catcalls to crude remarks to groping and beyond—is an invasion of your privacy and an attempt to diminish your dignity that can make you feel vulnerable, violated and humiliated. The appropriate response to yourself to each experience is compassion and understanding.

•**Don't overshare on social media.** The #MeToo hashtag allows anyone to make a valuable public statement without getting into the details of what happened. But sharing specifics or naming names is riskier because what goes online stays there forever, and you can't control how others might respond to your story or use it against you in the future. If your goal is to push the problem of sexual abuse out into the sunshine by saying more than "me, too" and you're willing to face potential personal consequences

of that, then sharing specifics of your #MeToo experience is an option you can be proud of. But I think it's counterproductive to expect that you'll find healing on social media.

•**Use your memories to heal.** It's upsetting to remember the painful past, but the resurfacing of old memories provides an opportunity for deeper healing. It's a chance to recognize how strong you are. Even if you feel you haven't fully resolved what happened, focus on the extent to which you withstood the incident and moved forward in spite of it.

•**Talk to someone you know who is sympathetic.** Not everyone wants to share his/her story—it's OK to stay silent forever or until you feel ready to talk—but if you do, decide how much you want to disclose and to whom. Disclosure can help dispel feelings of isolation and shame. It can feel freeing to finally receive the validation and comfort you deserve. Choose someone carefully—whether a spouse, friend, relative, clergy member or family doctor—who you know understands the prevalence and significance of sexual violence. Such a person is most likely to provide helpful support.

One way to gauge whether someone is a good person to talk to: Begin by bringing up sexual abuse in general or via a news story. Pay attention to how the person responds. Does he express sympathy with abuse victims or, instead, challenge or doubt their stories? Then you might talk in general about your own experience without going into specifics ("This kind of thing happened to me, too") and feel

Sour Foods Can Make You Bold

Sour foods can lead to more risk-taking. People who consume something with a sour taste, such as a piece of sour candy, are more likely to engage in behaviors carrying some risk. This means that people who have anxiety disorders or depression—conditions that make them especially risk-averse—may benefit from consuming sour foods.

Chi Thanh Vi, PhD, research fellow in multisensory experiences, Sussex Computer-Human Interaction Lab, University of Sussex, Brighton, UK, and leader of a study published in *Scientific Reports*.

out the response before saying more. Remember that once you share details, you can't take them back. That's why it's wiser to reveal small amounts of general information at first and then more only if it feels important and right to do so. Keep in mind that friends, family members and others are not therapists and may have difficulty hearing specifics and explicit information. You don't need to share a lot to receive some understanding and caring from people you know.

•**Find strength in numbers.** If confiding in one person isn't for you or if you feel you could benefit from joining with others in an active healing process, there are a number of support groups for survivors of sexual abuse or violence. Find local groups and resources on RAINN—the Rape, Abuse & Incest National Network (Rainn.org/statistics/victims-sexual-violence—just type in your zip code).

•**Read helpful books or listen to podcasts.** Reading about or listening to other survivors' stories can show you there's a light at the end of the tunnel. If you find the details too upsetting, you can skim over those parts to get to the recommendations. Some books to try include *The Courage to Heal* and my book *The Sexual Healing Journey.* Sometimes just listening to others' stories is therapeutic. Safe Space Radio features conversations on sex abuse and related topics.

•**Seek counseling.** I'm not a fan of digging up the past for no reason. But if the abuse you suffered in the past is affecting your mental and physical health or harming your ability to be intimate—or if you want to understand better how it has influenced your life—find a therapist. Sex abuse recovery therapists can help you undo negative thinking patterns and develop skills for self-care, self-compassion and speaking up for yourself. Ask your doctor or a rape crisis center for therapists who have worked with sex abuse survivors. It's also OK to make trial appointments with two or three therapists and see which one is the best fit.

SHOULD I CONFRONT THE ABUSER?

Counseling can be particularly helpful if the person who abused or harassed you has resurfaced or somehow still is a part of your life. A therapist can help you work out whether you want to call out this person's behavior. There's

no single right answer—unless you believe that someone else, especially a child, is in danger. Then it's your responsibility to do whatever is necessary, including calling the police, to avert future abuse.

Choosing to confront an abuser depends on your emotional strength, what you want to accomplish and who else is involved, including other potential victims, and how cooperative and safe they are. The best scenario is to confront the person with the guidance and presence of a trained professional. When therapists facilitate such conversations, they can help you prepare well and move the discussion along to a resolution. But if that's not possible, it may be appropriate to enlist a supportive friend to be there. Remember, confrontations are not always necessary or advised.

As an alternative, you may decide to confront your abuser through a letter or a phone call or by e-mail. These, too, are best accomplished with a therapist's guidance. Focus on the power of asserting your truth, rather than making the success of the interaction whether you receive a specific response.

Figure out beforehand how you'll handle your abuser's reaction. Many offenders will deny the extent of the abuse, minimize it or blame the survivor in some way. And all of that can be really upsetting, so you want to be emotionally prepared and supported.

HEALING OUR CULTURE

Finally, it's important to realize that sexual violence is a cultural problem. I challenge anyone to turn on the TV and not find a program on some channel where a woman has been or is about to be sexually intimidated in some form. Sexual aggression against women is a common feature in popular pornography, as well. It's become entertainment, and we've become desensitized to it.

We can't keep role-modeling negative behaviors and expect change or expect the victims to mop up the mess. Instead, we must change our behavior in terms of what we tolerate in the media and as bystanders. When something that is meant "as a joke" is demeaning, say so. When you see abuse, call it out—if necessary, to the authorities.

Frequent Business Travelers Suffer Emotionally

Study of 18,328 people by researchers at Columbia University's Mailman School of Public Health and City University of New York, both in New York City, published in *Journal of Occupational and Environmental Medicine.*

Those who take work trips two or more weeks per month are more likely than employees who travel one to six nights a month to have symptoms of anxiety and depression…are more likely to smoke…and report more trouble sleeping. And those who drink alcohol during business trips are more likely to develop dependency and addictive tendencies than employees who travel less often.

Self-defense: Talk to your boss about how to reduce your time out of the office and still get the same amount of work done.

Hidden Harms of Long-Ago Trauma: It's Never Too Late to Get Help

Vincent J. Felitti, MD, clinical professor of medicine at University of California, San Diego, and an expert on how childhood trauma affects adults. Dr. Felitti is coprincipal investigator of the Adverse Childhood Experiences (ACE) Study, one of the largest investigations of childhood abuse and neglect and later-life health and well-being.

If you've ever suffered physical, sexual or emotional abuse, you might think that psychological scars are the only long-lasting damage. But that couldn't be further from the truth.

A lingering threat: Volumes of scientific evidence show that these negative experiences also increase risk for chronic disease and early death…even when the incidents occurred several years earlier.

THE SHOCKING STATISTICS

The veil of secrecy regarding abuse has slowly lifted as more people have recently opened up about their past. With sexual abuse, in particular, recent allegations lodged against film producer Harvey Weinstein, actor and comedian Bill Cosby and others have prompted a renewed interest in the harmful effects of such experiences—whether the victim is a child or an adult.

Even though sexual abuse in adulthood has been linked to physical health problems, such as headaches, digestive disorders and other chronic ailments, the most extensive research has focused on the long-term effects when mistreatment occurs during childhood.

Landmark investigation: The Adverse Childhood Experiences (ACE) Study, a massive collaborative research project cosponsored by the Centers for Disease Control and Prevention, looked at the backgrounds of 17,000 adults, beginning in 1995 at Kaiser Permanente in San Diego. With more than 20 years of follow-up, the study offers crucial insights into the physical effects of abuse and mistreatment.

In the original research, two-thirds of the study's middle-class participants reported at least one incident of childhood trauma or neglect. More specifically, 28% reported physical abuse…and 21% said they were abused sexually. More than one in five people reported three or more categories of adverse childhood experiences, or ACEs. (To determine your own ACE score, see page 141.)

THE HEALTH RISKS ARE REAL

The ACE Study determined that the more of these experiences a person has suffered, the higher his/her risk is for a range of mental and physical health conditions.

For example, compared with participants who did not experience any abuses or mistreatment, those who reported four categories of adverse childhood experiences were twice as likely to be diagnosed with lung cancer and/or depression as adults. They also had a fourfold increase in chronic lung disease, such as chronic obstructive pulmonary disease (COPD), and a sevenfold increase in alcoholism. A person with six or more categories of ACEs had their life expectancy shortened by nearly 20 years.

WHY PHYSICAL HEALTH SUFFERS

It's easy to imagine how trauma would affect a person's mental health. But why would it also impact physical health? *Long-term research has identified such factors as...*

• **Coping mechanisms.** Trauma victims are more likely to use self-soothing habits, such as smoking, drinking, overeating and drug abuse, which are helpful in the short term but are known risk factors in the long term for many chronic health problems.

• **Complex brain-mediated effects.** Chronic stress due to ACEs can distort the function of brain networks, resulting in immune system suppression, which in turn can lead to a variety of diseases. In addition, it causes the release of pro-inflammatory chemicals that are responsible for additional diseases such as heart disease, pulmonary fibrosis, etc.

WHAT HELPS MOST

If you experienced trauma as a child, it is never too late to get help to reverse or at least moderate the negative physical and/or emotional effects of ACEs. The strategies below, which tend to yield positive results more quickly than psychotherapy and/or antidepressants, are likely to also be helpful for those who experienced trauma as an adult...

• **Tell a trusted person.** People who have experienced childhood trauma often carry the secret into adulthood. Victims of abuse feel shame and assume that they did something wrong to deserve the abuse. By simply telling someone, and having that person continue to accept you, the shame dissipates.

• **Try eye movement desensitization and reprocessing (EMDR).** The American Psychiatric Association recognizes this therapy as an effective treatment for trauma. Studies have found that trauma victims no longer had signs of post-traumatic stress disorder after as few as three, 90-minute EMDR sessions.

How it works: During EMDR, a clinician asks the patient to hold a traumatic memory in mind while the therapist moves one or two fingers from side to side, or diagonally, in front of the patient's eyes. This guides the eyes to move as they do during the rapid eye movement (REM) sleep phase, during which the most active dreaming occurs. Dreaming can help process trauma and move it to long-term memory,

enabling the patient to feel as if it is now resolved and only in the past.

The therapist repeats the process multiple times as needed, until the distress related to the targeted memory is gone and a positive belief replaces it. For example, a rape victim shifts from feeling horror and self-disgust to feeling empowered—I survived it and I am strong.

To find an EMDR clinician near you, visit the website of the EMDR Institute at EMDR.com. Check with your health insurer to see if your policy covers the treatment.

• **Consider clinical hypnosis.** This method helps patients identify past events or experiences that are causing problems. With hypnotherapy, a trained practitioner uses imagery and presents ideas or suggestions during a state of concentrated attention that helps bring about desired changes in thinking.

To find a certified hypnosis professional in your area, visit the website of the American Society of Clinical Hypnosis at ASCH.net. Check with your health insurer to see if clinical hypnosis is covered.

HOW TRAUMATIC WAS YOUR CHILDHOOD?

For each of the following questions, give yourself one point for every "yes" answer. *During your first 18 years of life...*

1. Did a parent or other adult in the household often swear at you, insult you, put you down or humiliate you? Or act in a way that made you afraid that you might be physically hurt?

2. Did a parent or other adult in the household often push, grab, slap or throw something at you? Or ever hit you so hard that you had marks or were injured?

3. Did an adult or person at least five years older than you ever touch or fondle you or have you touch his/her body in a sexual way? Or try to or actually have oral, anal or vaginal sex with you?

4. Did you often feel that no one in your family loved you or thought you were important or special? Or that your family didn't look out for one another, feel close to one another or support one another?

5. Did you often feel that you didn't have enough to eat, had to wear dirty clothes and had no one to protect you? Or that your parents were too drunk or high to take care of you or take you to the doctor if you needed it?

6. Were your parents ever separated or divorced?

7. Was your mother or stepmother often pushed, grabbed or slapped? Or did she often have something thrown at her? Or was she sometimes or often kicked, bitten, hit with a fist or hit with something hard? Or ever repeatedly hit for at least a few minutes or threatened with a gun or knife?

8. Did you live with anyone who was a problem drinker or an alcoholic or who used street drugs?

9. Was a household member depressed or mentally ill, or did a household member attempt suicide?

10. Did a household member go to prison?

Takeaway: If you score a four or higher, tell your doctor about your history of abuse and follow the recommendations in the main article. If these steps don't help, consult a trained therapist.

Group Singing Beats the Blues

Tom Shakespeare, PhD, professor of disability research, University of East Anglia, Norwich Medical School, Norwich, UK.

Adults with mental health conditions, including anxiety and depression, who participated in free, weekly singing workshops for six months reported improvement or maintenance of their mental health—regardless of other therapies or medications.

Why it worked: Singers of any skill level could participate, making the group inclusive and stress-free. The social aspect of the activity along with structure and peer support were also cited as important.

What to do: If you can't find a just-for-fun singing group in your community or through Meetup.com, consider starting one.

The Surprising Health Benefits of Nostalgia

Krystine Batcho, PhD, professor of psychology at Le Moyne College, Syracuse, New York. She has studied nostalgia since 1995.

We all know people who seem to dwell on the past. They are constantly bringing up memories from years or decades ago. Sometime we're tempted to shake them and yell, "Live in the present, not the past!"

Maybe it would be better to emulate them. We now know from science—not conjecture—that nostalgia is good for you. It can improve your mood, help you become more resilient and increase your motivation to tackle new challenges. To learn more, we interviewed psychologist Krystine Batcho, PhD, an expert on nostalgia.

WHAT NOSTALGIA REALLY IS

At its core, nostalgia is a sentimental affection…a yearning…for the past. We associate it with being older, but young adults often are intensely nostalgic, too—for their childhoods.

Are you nostalgic? The way researchers identify this is to ask volunteers to rate, on a scale of one to five, how much they miss things from when they were younger such as their parents and siblings…having heroes or heroines…being carefree…particular friends…school/college…a previous home…TV shows…music…pets… trips/vacations…the "way people were." The more "fours" and "fives" you record, the more sensitive you are to triggers of nostalgia. *Here's why that's a good thing…*

THE BENEFITS OF NOSTALGIA

Connecting your present and past selves can strengthen your sense of personal identity—remembering how you experienced unconditional love as a child, for example, can be reassuring during difficult times. In my research, a clear picture of nostalgic individuals has emerged, and it's largely positive. People who score high on measures of nostalgia, compared with those who score low, tend to be…

•**Empathetic.** They feel things deeply—and other people are a high priority.

•**Resilient.** They use healthy coping strategies in stressful times, including getting emotional support from others and expressing their emotions rather than burying them.

•**Stronger in their sense of self.** They have a keener sense of who they are inside while remaining respectful of other people's standards.

•**Less anxious.** The sense of continuity from connecting to the past can have a grounding effect, helping to ease stress.

•**More connected.** When lonely, nostalgic memories encourage people to reach out to others and stay socially connected. That counteracts loneliness and may help prevent depression.

•**Better at reaching goals and solving problems.** They are more likely to employ approaches such as planning, strategizing and reframing a situation more positively—and then take action to improve the situation.

•**More positive.** A study in *Psychology & Health* found that people who were asked to write about a nostalgic event rather than an ordinary event scored higher immediately afterward on measures of health optimism…and got more exercise over the next two weeks.

Nostalgia even can change how you feel physically—making you feel warmer in a cold environment.

EVOKING THE GOOD OLD DAYS

You don't have to wait for random events to trigger nostalgic memories. *You can make it happen any time you want to…*

•**Listen to songs from your early days.** Songs we loved as teenagers or young adults retain their emotional power throughout our lives. Listen to your favorites—and remember how you felt back then. And watch old movies you enjoyed when you were younger, especially those with great sound tracks.

•**Flip through your past.** Look through boxes of old family pictures. Dig out your yearbooks or souvenirs.

•**Reminisce with others.** Getting together with old friends or family can provide opportunities to bring up crazy old memories…and sometimes share stories of someone who has died.

•**Recruit your senses of smell and taste.** These olfactory cues are particularly effective

at triggering autobiographical memories, studies show. Breathe in a scent you loved…cook your favorite childhood dish.

•**Anticipate future nostalgic moments.** The next time you spend joyful time with friends or family and something memorable happens, call attention to it. Say something such as, "Let's remember this moment!" This is called "anticipatory nostalgia." You're storing up future nostalgia recollections.

STAYING ON THE RIGHT SIDE OF THE PAST

Is there ever a downside to thinking about the past? Yes, there can be. Brooding about past negative experiences (injuries, rejections, mistakes)—what psychologists call rumination—can contribute to depression. Most nostalgia, in contrast, evokes a positive feeling.

Some forms of nostalgia can be problematic, too, especially historical nostalgia—a longing for a past era. The desire to escape into an idealized world of yesteryear, say Edwardian elegance or 1960s free-spiritedness, can sometimes lead to becoming more isolated as you spend more time alone. If so, consider whether you're neglecting people or issues in your life, and work to restore healthy relationships by reaching out to others.

Personal nostalgia is more positive. It's often joyous, although it can be bittersweet and poignant. But that's good, too—it can help you integrate negative feelings, such as grief over the loss of a loved one, with positive feelings, such as memories of good times spent together.

Yet personal nostalgia can become unhealthy if it traps you in repetitive memories of the past without attempts to seek fresh positive experiences. Ask yourself, *How am I building on my past? How can the love, knowledge and skills I once enjoyed help me move forward?* At its best, revisiting a happy or healthy period from the past can help you gain strength and optimism to handle the challenges of the present.

WHEN NOSTALGIA WAS A DISEASE…

Fond memories of the past haven't always had a good reputation. The term "nostalgia" was invented in 1688 by Johannes Hofer, a Swiss physician who combined the ancient Greek words for "home" (nostos) and "pain" (algos) to make "nostalgia." He considered the phenomenon a debilitating form of homesickness, which was weakening the troops. In 1733, a Russian general whose soldiers came down with the nostalgia bug punished a few by burying them alive. Over the following centuries—even into the early-20th century—nostalgia was considered a psychiatric disorder, a form of depression or melancholia. Over the years, treatments have included leeches, stomach purges and shaming.

Don't Hate Your Body

Viren Swami, PhD, professor of social psychology at Anglia Ruskin University in the UK and lead author of several studies.

Simply looking at photographs of natural scenes leads to a more positive body image immediately afterward. Spending time in nature is even more powerful.

That matters. A negative body image—feeling that your looks don't measure up to expectations—is associated with eating disorders, depression and sexual dysfunction, as well as physical inactivity, unhealthy diets and smoking. Therapy can help, as can a regular exercise habit.

And now, the nature cure. Why does it work? One hypothesis is that natural environments lead us to think about our bodies as agents that do things—such as hiking—rather than objects to be measured against society's beauty norms. Viren Swami, PhD, professor of social psychology at Anglia Ruskin University in the UK and lead author of several studies, believes that natural images also promote "cognitive quiet," hushing the brain's background noise about everyday concerns. Over time, these experiences may lead to a more permanent change in how we think about ourselves. Says Dr. Swami, "Perhaps we will come to appreciate more important things in life than what our bodies look like." And you don't have to wander deep into the wilderness, either—a quick stroll through the neighborhood park also has this effect.

Move to Beat Depression

A little bit of exercise helps depression a lot. Just one hour of exercise weekly can reduce depression risk. People who do one hour a week of any type of exercise, at any intensity level, have a 44% lower risk of developing depression over a decade than people who do not exercise at all. More exercise or more intense exercise is not better from a mental-health standpoint. Any type of physical activity, including simple walking, had the same benefit.

Samuel Harvey, PhD, associate professor, School of Psychiatry, University of New South Wales, Sydney, Australia, and leader of an analysis of a Norwegian survey of nearly 34,000 adults, published in *American Journal of Psychiatry*.

Yoga fights depression. In a recent finding, when 21 male veterans took a twice-weekly yoga class for eight weeks, those who were depressed at the outset of the study saw a significant and clinically meaningful reduction in symptoms after the study period—regardless of whether they were in counseling or taking an antidepressant.

Theory: Yoga's stress-reducing effects help fight depression.

Lindsey B. Hopkins, PhD, research fellow, San Francisco Veterans Affairs Medical Center, California.

High-Altitude Living Is Linked to Suicide

Brent Michael Kious, MD, PhD, assistant professor, department of psychiatry, University of Utah, Salt Lake City, and leader of an analysis of 12 studies of altitude and suicide, published in *Harvard Review of Psychiatry*.

People who live in high-elevation regions, especially the US intermountain states, have increased rates of suicide and depression despite the finding that people living at higher altitudes have a lower rate of death from all causes.

Possible reason: Changes in blood oxygen levels associated with lower atmospheric pressure. If further studies confirm the findings, doctors may consider recommending supplemental use of a serotonin precursor called 5-hydroxytryptophan or use of supplemental creatinine, which can influence brain function.

Exercise and Fitness

Pain-Free Exercise: Add Intensity to Workouts, Not Impact

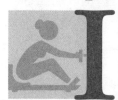

If you've been avoiding intense exercise because you're afraid the impact will cause pain, know this…impact and intensity are not the same thing. While impact can have an effect on intensity, they don't have to go hand-in-hand. Intensity refers to the amount of energy you expend, while impact refers to the amount of stress you put on your body. In fact, you can get all the intensity you need with minimal impact on your joints. And that's great news because intensity can keep your muscles young, no matter what your age.

AGING MUSCLES: THE PROBLEM IS INACTIVITY

What if much of the muscle loss commonly blamed on advancing age actually is due to inactivity, pure and simple? After all, modern men and women are not nearly as active as they were during most of human evolution, when people needed to be intensely active to survive. What if that level of activity is what our muscles still need today?

To test this theory, researchers in the UK studied muscle tissue from a group of recreational cyclists, men and women who ranged in age from 55 to 79. They were not professional athletes, which could skew the results, but people who had been very active for many years.

Their conclusion: A high level of exercise—intensity—enables muscle to maintain many of the properties of healthy young muscle that are lost when aging is accompanied by inactivity. In other words, use it or lose it applies to muscle mass, too.

Shannon Fable, certified group-fitness instructor, personal trainer and health coach in Boulder, Colorado, Shannon Fable.com. The study titled "Properties of the Vastus Lateralis Muscle in Relation to Age and Physiological Function in Master Cyclists Aged 55–79 Years" by researchers at King's College London, UK, was published in *Aging Cell*.

ADDING INTENSITY WITHOUT IMPACT

Intensity works not only your muscles but also your heart and lungs. Yes, impact is one way to add intensity but not the only way, explained health coach Shannon Fable. Even fitness pros falsely link intensity and impact, but there are many more ways to rev up intensity other than with high-impact workouts such as running and basketball. Some impact is good (if it doesn't hurt) because weight-bearing exercise is good for bone density, but it's not necessary to jump or run for an effective exercise session.

This is important news for people with knee problems, obesity or arthritis, among other conditions that make exercise a challenge, and who give up on exercise completely because it is too painful. You can get the benefits of intense exercise with no impact or low impact. Just don't opt out altogether because you assume hard means hurts.

BEST LOW-IMPACT, HIGH-INTENSITY EXERCISES

Talk low-impact, and swimming immediately comes to mind. Swimming is a great low-impact exercise. Its limitation is that it isn't weight-bearing, so it doesn't offer bone building benefits. (Realistically, many people don't have access to a pool, and not everyone likes to swim.)

As the researchers found, cycling is another great choice, and you can vary your intensity indoors or outdoors. But keep in mind that it's not weight-bearing, either. Fable's overall favorite is plain old walking. It's easy, can be done with intensity and is great for bones and balance.

Once you've chosen your low-impact activity, there are three ways to possibly increase intensity—increase range of motion, your speed or the amount of weight you're carrying. For walking, it would be best to focus on covering more ground in a shorter amount of time. Or you could add a weighted vest if you needed more intensity over time. Start with a small amount of weight—10 pounds is plenty—and add slowly over time. Fable prefers weighted vests, which more evenly distribute the weight, over hand, wrist or ankle weights that can alter your biomechanics.

You can add intensity to just about every exercise. For instance, if you're doing floor exercises or squats and lunges, make each movement wider, deeper, bigger or longer to extend your range of motion—taking up more space increases intensity. To increase speed, do more reps in your usual amount of workout time.

If you're unsure of how to start on your own, have a certified fitness trainer set up a program to fit your needs and abilities. Above all, don't let fear be a barrier to exercise or an excuse to stay on the couch. Get up and get moving!

Lots of Exercise Needed to Keep Weight Off

Jennifer C. Kerns, MD, hospitalist and co-director of bariatric surgery, Washington DC Veterans Affairs Medical Center, former contestant on *The Biggest Loser*, and lead author of a study of 14 contestants, published in *Obesity*.

In a study of former contestants on *The Biggest Loser* TV show, only those who did at least 80 minutes a day of moderate activity such as walking, or 35 minutes a day of vigorous exercise such as running, did not regain weight within six years. Significant weight loss causes the body's metabolism to slow down, so additional exercise is needed to compensate for the lower caloric needs. To keep weight off after losing it, it is necessary to increase physical activity well beyond what is recommended for people who are trying to maintain their weight without having lost a lot of it. Ask your doctor for details.

A Faster, Smarter Way to Get Fit

Martin Gibala, PhD, a professor and chair of the kinesiology department at McMaster University in Hamilton, Ontario, Canada. He has published more than 100 peer-reviewed articles and is coauthor of *The One Minute Workout: Science Shows a Way to Get Fit That's Smarter, Faster, Shorter*.

Very few of us can say that we have "extra" time. If something on our to-do list has to be eliminated, it's usually that hour spent at the gym.

But what if you could significantly pare down your exercise time?

You've probably heard of high-intensity interval training (HIIT). With HIIT, you intersperse bouts of intense exercise—say, 30 seconds of all-out pedaling on a bike—with equal or longer periods of recovery (complete rest or low-intensity exercise). Repeat that a few times, and you're done for the day.

What's new: Researchers have discovered that with HIIT, you can get significant health benefits even faster than previously thought.

HOW HIIT HELPS

Traditional aerobic workouts, involving continuous low-to-moderate intensity exercise, strengthen the heart...improve metabolism... and reduce the risk for heart disease, high blood pressure, diabetes and other chronic diseases. What's exciting about HIIT is that it offers the same health benefits as a traditional workout—but in a different way.

Here's why: Each time you push yourself into high action, you create a disturbance in your body's homeostasis, which is how the body behaves at rest. Each disturbance forces the heart to beat faster, the lungs to process more oxygen and the muscles to consume more fuel.

Very quickly, your body adapts to these changes. Muscles grow more mitochondria—your cells' powerhouses—making them more efficient at producing energy. The heart pumps more blood with each beat. You become fitter, and your cardiovascular disease risk goes down.

High-intensity workouts with frequent intervals cause more disturbances in homeostasis than traditional workouts, which push the body into a more constant state of physical exertion.

FASTER, BUT EQUAL

In a 2016 study, researchers at McMaster University compared two training protocols in sedentary men. One group followed standard exercise guidelines—they rode exercise bikes at a moderate pace for 45 minutes, three days a week.

The second group did a special HIIT workout—a 20-second all-out, hard sprint...followed by two minutes of slow cycling...repeated twice for a total of three sprint-rest cycles. Add in a few minutes for a warm-up and cooldown, and that's a sweet workout of just about 10 minutes.

Results: After 12 weeks, men in both exercise groups showed similar improvements in insulin sensitivity (the body's mechanism for regulating blood sugar) and cardiorespiratory fitness. All men also developed stronger muscles.

Bottom line: Men who followed the 10-minute HIIT workout three times weekly had the same health benefits as men who did traditional exercise for 45 minutes three times weekly.

ALMOST ANYONE CAN DO IT

You may assume that high-intensity workouts are riskier than easy ones, especially for people who are out of shape or have a high risk for heart disease. The truth is, any form of exercise, including HIIT, slightly increases cardiovascular risks during workouts...but your overall heart disease risk goes down. In fact, a wide variety of HIIT protocols have been applied to people with many different conditions, including cardiovascular disease, diabetes and metabolic syndrome.

To play it safe: If you have health problems or heart disease risk factors—smoking, high blood pressure, a sedentary lifestyle, etc.— check with your doctor before starting any new exercise program.

GETTING STARTED

Even though an HIIT workout is designed to push exercisers out of their comfort zones, you can adapt it to suit your preferences in a less strenuous way. All that's required are bursts of exercise followed by lower-intensity activity.

Do you like walking? You can do 30-second fast walks. Start slowly, then push yourself to about 70% of your upper limit—breathing hard, but not gasping for air. Then slow down for a few minutes. Alternate fast/slow for up to 30 minutes (with a short cooldown at the end), three or more times a week.

Those who are healthy, fit and have the all-clear from their doctors, may want to try this 10-minute workout that incorporates just one minute of high-intensity exercise. First, warm up for three minutes with low-intensity exercise. *Then...*

•**Blast through 20 seconds of an all-out sprint (or bike, swim, etc.).**

•**Recover with light activity for two minutes.**

•**Repeat the cycle until you've done three sprints.** End with a two-minute cooldown of light activity.

4 Balance Exercises to Keep You Steady on Your Feet

Caroline DeGroot, MPT, a physical therapist at AthletiCo Physical Therapy in Bannockburn, Illinois. DeGroot founded AthletiCo's Vestibular Program, which focuses on helping people with dizziness, balance disorders and concussions.

When you are young, you can walk confidently just about anywhere without much thought—such as on an uneven sidewalk—or while chatting at the same time. As you get older, just glancing sideways at a store window while strolling can make you wobble—and fall. *Here's what's going on…and some moves that will keep you steadier on your feet…*

WHY FALLS OCCUR

One in four Americans over age 65 falls each year. One reason is that older people are more prone to medical conditions that compromise balance—such as vertigo, dizziness, arthritis-related stiffness and weakness, stroke and loss of sensation in the feet from vascular diseases. But even without major health issues, normal physical and vision changes can affect balance.

Your eyes signal the brain where you are in space relative to other objects, which helps keep you stable. Wearing bifocals or progressive lenses requires your focus to change back and forth between lenses, making it harder to notice a loose rug, sidewalk crack or pet.

The natural age-related decline in muscle strength and flexibility also makes it harder to right yourself once your center of gravity is thrown off. That's why the key to staying on your feet is to build your muscle strength and improve your flexibility and agility. *Here's how—work up to doing each move daily to get the most benefit…*

FOOT TAPS

As we age, our pace typically slows, our step length shortens and our stance widens as shifting from one leg to the other feels less secure. To keep your strides long and confident and avert a shuffling gait, you can do foot taps—an exercise that trains your body to safely shift your center of gravity left and right.

How to do it: Stand in front of a step that is four-to-six-inches high (such as a footstool), feet hip-width apart. Slowly raise one foot to tap the step. Return that foot to the ground and then tap with the other foot. Movement should be slow and controlled. Work up to 20 taps for each foot in a session. As your stability improves, try a higher step (six-to-eight inches)…or try tapping the step as lightly as possible to further improve balance and increase muscle control.

Safety note: If needed, you can hold a railing or counter for support. If you use a cane for general walking assistance, hold it in the hand you usually use to hold it throughout the exercise, regardless of which foot you're tapping. If you're using a cane only while recovering from an injury or for a condition that affects your gait, such as arthritis, hold the cane on the side opposite to the injury or painful extremity.

HEAD TURNS

When you turn your head, a response called the vestibular spinal reflex (VSR) causes your brain to send messages to adjust postural muscles to keep you from being pulled in the direction your head turns. Your VSR can become less effective as you age, causing you to often stumble while turning your head. The following exercise helps train your VSR.

How to do it: Stand with your feet hip-width apart. If you need to, you can hold on to a railing, wall, sturdy piece of furniture or counter for support. Now slowly turn your head as far as you comfortably can to the right and then to the

---

If You Sit Too Much…

Exercise is not enough to combat the health risks of sitting too much. Adults age 60 and older spend an average of 8.5 to 9.6 hours a day sitting, and prolonged sedentary time could increase the risk for diabetes, heart disease and death from any cause.

Self-defense: Stand or exercise while watching TV, walk around while talking on the phone, stand up or walk around at regular intervals.

Statement by the American Heart Association, published in *Circulation*.

left, while maintaining upright posture. Repeat as a continuous movement for 10 repetitions.

Make sure to stay upright without leaning to one side. If you feel dizzy, pause, then continue at a slower pace.

For additional challenge: If you held on to a support, try doing the exercise without holding on to anything. Or try it with your feet only a few inches apart…or with your feet together…or with one foot in front of the other, heel-to-toe. Don't overextend your ability, though—safety first!

OVER-THE-SHOULDER WALKS

Try this exercise once you feel comfortable with standing head turns. You will look left and right as you walk—similar to what you might do when scanning shelves while grocery shopping or walking down a hallway while searching for an apartment number.

How to do it: Stand at one end of a long hallway, feet hip-width apart. Turn your head to look over your right shoulder. Maintaining that gaze, take three or four steps forward. Now turn your head to look over your left shoulder while you continue to walk forward another three or four steps. Repeat for a total of five times per side. If you feel dizzy or unsteady, stop turning your head and gaze straight ahead for a few steps. To increase the challenge, increase how quickly you turn your head.

Variation: Try head turns in a store or library. Having a stationary visual target—the items on the shelves—recruits your vision while challenging your VSR.

BALL HANDOFF

People who worry about falling often are self-conscious about walking—which is counterproductive. The more attention you pay to how you're walking, the more shuffled and fractured your gait becomes. Natural gait needs to be reflexive. This exercise uses a ball for distraction to help your gait become more fluid, increase your walking speed and improve your ability to shift weight left and right.

Safety note: This exercise is not recommended if you need to use a cane to walk.

How to do it: You'll need a partner who is comfortable walking backward and a small ball, such as a tennis ball. Start at one end of a long hallway with your partner facing you and a few feet in front of you, holding the ball. Walk forward while your partner walks backward—handing off or gently tossing the ball back and forth to each other as you go. Perform this exercise for two to three minutes or until you feel tired.

Solo variation: Stand in front of a wall, and march in place while you toss the ball at the wall and catch it as it bounces back. Repeat for 30 seconds at a time, for a total of three times.

---

4 Best Exercises to Do When You're Stuck in a Chair

Tom Holland, MS, CPT, exercise physiologist, certified sports nutritionist and certified strength and conditioning specialist. He is founder and president of the Darien, Connecticut–based fitness-consulting company Team Holland (TeamHolland.com) and author of four fitness books, including *Beat the Gym: Personal Trainer Secrets—Without the Personal Trainer Price Tag.*

If so many of us are always busy, why are our bodies getting weaker and weaker? It's mainly because we spend so much time sitting! The less we move, the more muscle mass we lose, leaving us vulnerable to injury—not to mention increased risk for obesity, diabetes and stroke. But all is not lost.

Exercise physiologist Tom Holland, MS, CPT, shared his four favorite exercises for people who are stuck in their chairs…*

EXERCISE #1: *No-Hand Get-Ups.* When we sit for prolonged periods, our powerful butt muscles or "glutes" (gluteus maximus and gluteus medius) begin to atrophy. Weak glutes can affect posture and movement, which can translate into knee injuries and hip problems as other muscles try to compensate for our deconditioned glutes.

What to do: Start from a seated position. Then…

•**Stand up from the chair—without using your hands to push off or grab hold of anything.** That's it.

*If you are wearing shoes with a heel greater than one inch, take them off before doing these exercises.

•**Stand up relatively slowly, to a count of about two seconds.** Extend your arms straight out in front of you to help your balance.

•**Then lower yourself back down even more slowly, to a count of four seconds.** This controlled movement—working against gravity—tones your muscles.

•**Repeat five to 10 times daily.**

EXERCISE #2: Butt-Pain Stretch. When people complain of a mysterious pain in their backside, the cause is often due to overuse of the piriformis, a muscle deep inside the glute that extends from the pelvis to the outer hip. Because the piriformis is a major part of our lower-body infrastructure, that "pain in the butt" is a warning that additional pains (including hip pain and low-back pain) are yet to come if this one is ignored.

What to do: To get a good piriformis stretch and eliminate the pain…

•**Cross your right leg over your left leg so that your right ankle rests on your left knee.** You may feel some tension in the upper-back portion of your right thigh.

•**Gently press your right knee toward the ground, breathing into the stretch.** You should feel a stretch in the muscle deep in your buttocks. You should not feel any stress on the knee itself—if you do, try pressing on the inside of the lower thigh just above the knee. Stretch only as far as is comfortable.

•**Lean slightly forward, and hold the stretch for 10 to 30 seconds.**

•**Switch legs and repeat.** Do two to three repetitions per side a few times a day.

EXERCISE #3: Chair Crunches. This simple exercise works your abdominal core muscles to help prevent low-back pain and other sore muscles and joints.

What to do: To build your core, lean slightly back in your chair. *Then…*

•**Lift both knees up so that you are balanced and your feet are six to 10 inches off the ground.** (If you are sitting on a couch, scoot toward the front of the cushion, lean back slightly and start from there.)

•**Hold that position for 30 seconds…or as long as you can.** This exercise is about time, not repetition. Be sure to keep your shoulders

down and relaxed, and remember to breathe normally. Do this exercise once to several times a day.

EXERCISE #4: Twist Stretch. This back stretch sounds more complicated than it is…and once you try it, you'll wonder how you ever got through a day without it.

What to do: To get started, sit up straight with both feet flat on the floor. Then…

•**Place your left hand on the outside of your right knee.**

•**Place your right hand on the outside of the right armrest of the chair.**

•**Rotate your upper body to the right.** You should feel a stretch in your lower back. Your head should follow along naturally with your upper body. Stretch only as far as is comfortable. Hold the stretch for a count of five, remembering to breathe throughout the stretch.

Note: If you feel pain, stop—this exercise should not cause any pain.

•**Then switch.** Place your right hand on the outside of your left knee…with your left hand, hold the outside of the left armrest of the chair…and rotate your upper body to the left. Repeat the cycle (turning once on each side) a total of three times. If you sit for long periods (especially in a confined space, such as an airline seat), try to do this stretch at least once every 15 to 30 minutes.

The Ultimate Workout: Two Exercises Keep You Fit!

Michael J. Joyner, MD, physician-researcher and leading expert on human performance and exercise physiology at the Mayo Clinic, Rochester, Minnesota. His research has focused on how humans respond to various forms of physical and mental stress. DrMichaelJoyner.com

If you're like most efficiency-minded Americans, you may be on the lookout for the exercise that's going to whip you into shape, keep you fit and slow down aging—with the least amount of time and fuss. For those of us looking to streamline our workouts to just the essentials, two simple exercises can do the job. They are challenging but worth the effort…and can be easily modified to suit your individual fitness level.

THE DYNAMIC DUO

Burpees and jumping rope are the dynamic duo, in my opinion. Why burpees and jumping rope? Of all the exercise choices, these maintain high vigor while promoting strength, endurance, balance and coordination all at once—precisely the capabilities that tend to deteriorate as we age, increasing our risk for falls and other mishaps. *These exercises are also…*

• **Compact.** Both can be done almost anywhere—whether you're in a hotel room…in your family room…or in your backyard.

Note: If you're indoors, you need adequate ceiling height to jump rope.

• **Quick.** The regimen can be compressed into a tidy five minutes if you're starting out and extended to a 10-, 20- or 30-minute workout when you're ready to up your game.

PERFECTING YOUR TECHNIQUE

To get the maximum benefits and reduce your risk for injuries, it's important to do both of these exercises properly…

•**Burpees.** Unless this exercise is already part of your workout, start slowly to make sure you've got the right technique. Ready?

•Stand straight with your arms at your sides.

•Squat down until you can put your hands on the ground in front of your feet.

•Kick your legs back into the plank position, straight behind you.

•Do a push-up on your toes or on your knees.

•Pull your legs back into the squat position.

•Jump up as high as you can with your arms overhead.

For a somewhat easier version: Do the same exercise without the push-up and jump. If the plank position is too difficult, modify it by kicking your legs back only halfway.

•**Jumping rope.** Maybe you haven't jumped rope since you were a kid, but it will come back to you. Keep the jump low to minimize the impact on your ankles and knees. When you feel ready, try using a weighted jump rope (which incorporates 1-, 3- or 5-pound weights) to rev up your heart rate and build upper-body strength. Skip the added weight if you have existing shoulder, arm or wrist problems. Use a jump rope that feels right to you—whether it has anti-slip handles or plastic beads strung on a nylon cord.

WARMING UP

Jumping jacks and running in place are great ways to warm up. These exercises are also good substitutes for burpees and jumping rope if you haven't been physically active in a while and/or want a gentler way to ease into your routine.

If jumping jacks and running in place don't appeal to you or you are concerned about your risk for falling or joint pain, there are other ways to modify the burpee–jump rope regimen while you increase your fitness.

Instead of burpees, try: Knee bends (also known as "squats"). If you're worried about your knees, skip the knee bends and simply stand with your back against a wall and lift up one leg with your knee bent as high as you feel comfortable. Repeat with the other leg.

Or try push-ups, either on the floor or against a counter.

Instead of jumping rope, try: Brisk walking—set a pace that puts you at the edge of being short of breath.

THE WORKOUT

To begin a burpee–jump rope regimen, do five burpees alternating with 30 seconds of jumping rope. Do each set three to five times (for a total of 15 burpees and a minute and a half of jumping rope…or 25 burpees and two and a half minutes of jumping rope). Then work up to sets of 10 burpees alternating with one minute of jumping rope. As your stamina builds, continue to alternate exercises until you work up to longer sets of up to two minutes of each. Try to do the burpee–jump rope workout two to three days a week with brisk walking or cycling on the other days.

Important: If you have any chronic medical conditions, consult your doctor before trying this workout. Stop immediately if either activity causes pain. It will take time to build up your stamina. Scale up according to your age and ability.

These Exercises Keep You Fit for Daily Living

Debra J. Rose, PhD, FNAK (Fellow of the National Academy of Kinesiology), director of the Center for Successful Aging and a professor in the department of kinesiology at California State University, Fullerton (HDCS.Fullerton.edu).

You're unloading groceries from your car trunk when—ouch!—there goes your back.

You're pulling on a sweater and—snap!—you tweak your shoulder.

Want to help protect yourself from these annoying—and often painful—everyday injuries? Functional fitness training can help you...

IN THE TOP 10

Functional fitness training is the official name for exercise that improves strength, balance and flexibility in ways that allow you to safely and effectively perform your real-life activities. It's not a new concept. It's been used for more than a decade to help patients get back to their normal daily activities after heart attacks, stroke, surgeries and other medical setbacks.

Latest development: Functional fitness training is increasingly being used preventively to stave off injury and maintain independence. In fact, it has reclaimed a spot on the top 10 list of fitness trends in the US and around the world for 2018, according to a survey of more than 4,000 exercise physiologists and other fitness professionals.

What's different about this form of exercise? Unlike traditional fitness moves that work just one or two muscle groups at a time (for example, up-and-down bicep curls or the cyclical motion of an elliptical machine), functional fitness training focuses on whole-body movements that mimic the twisting, bending, turning, crouching and reaching you do all day long.

Scientific evidence: When researchers published a review in *European Review of Aging and Physical Activity* of 13 trials looking at functional fitness training, this form of exercise beat out strength training alone (such as weight lifting) when assessing one's ability to perform daily activities.

NEW AND IMPROVED

Most signature exercises of functional training haven't gone away—they are just being supplemented by recent (and some would say improved) ideas such as introducing unstable surfaces (using Bosu balls, for example) or equipment that elevates the exercise challenge (for instance, suspension exercises, as described below).

Traditional functional fitness exercises include...

•**Chair Sit to Stand,** which engages your abdominal, back and leg muscles. This exercise, which involves rising from a seated position, helps you get out of a chair, car or bathtub.

•**Medicine Ball Low-to-High Chop** involves squatting down, picking up a weighted ball positioned next to one of your ankles, and standing up while twisting the ball overhead and then swinging it to the opposite side. This helps prepare you for unloading groceries, stashing items on high shelves and picking up an item from the floor. It also can help your golf swing!

Among the newer additions to functional fitness workouts...*

•**TRX Suspension Training.** If you've seen these black-and-yellow straps dangling from an overhead anchor point at your gym and felt intimidated, fear not. With this type of suspension exercise (TRX is short for total-body resistance exercise), the strap's handles can be gripped with your hands or looped around your feet, letting you leverage your body weight and gravity for a full-body workout. It can be a smart option for active older adults—it offers the opportunity to perform hundreds of moves that can be made increasingly more challenging as strength improves.

*Consult an exercise professional for advice on the frequency and appropriate number of repetitions for you.

SAMPLE TRX MOVE #1: **Squats.** Let's say you want to do squats, which strengthen the muscles needed to climb stairs or lower yourself into the bathtub. With this form of suspension exercise, you can shorten the straps to increase stability as you lower your body and rise back up. When the straps are lengthened, however, more strength and body control are required throughout the exercise.

SAMPLE TRX MOVE #2: **Assisted Row.** Beginning with shortened straps, hold one handle in each hand. Your hands should be chest height with your palms facing in and your elbows fully bent. Slowly lean your upper body back and away from your hands, keeping your back straight. Once your arms are fully extended, pull back up to the starting position. Increase the number of repetitions and sets as strength improves.

Note: The TRX Suspension Training System is available at more than 25,000 gyms worldwide. If you're interested in a home system, TRX Home2 System is available for $169.95. TRXtraining.com.

Important: For beginners with very poor balance or poor body awareness and control, the TRX may not offer sufficient support. To avoid injury, good body form and movement technique should be maintained throughout the exercises performed on the TRX. If you're concerned about your balance, ask your doctor if suspension exercises are right for you.

•**Resistance Bands.** These stretchy bands have been around for a while, but are now being used in fresh, new ways. With resistance band–walking, for example, a long band is tied around the user's hips while a trainer holds the other end. As the user walks far enough away to create tension in the band, the trainer then gently tugs or releases the band, forcing the user to quickly adjust to the instability.

You also can perform a number of different solo exercises by attaching your band to a post or door handle. For example, you can lower your body into a semi (partial) squat or staggered stance position and perform an alternating push-and-pull exercise with or without trunk rotation.

GETTING STARTED

One-on-one training is the safest way for beginners to start a functional fitness training program. For those who are more experienced exercisers, group classes are a more affordable option. Check your local Y or community center.

For personal guidance, look for an exercise professional with a degree in kinesiology or sports science and/or a Senior Fitness Specialist certificate from the National Academy of Sports Medicine or American Council on Exercise.

Another option: You also can use a DVD for a functional fitness workout at home. Search "functional fitness workout DVD" online.

How Not to Hurt Your Knees

Wayne L. Westcott, PhD, professor of exercise science, Quincy College, Massachusetts.

If part of your workout includes "running the stairs," can you hurt your knees?

Maybe, but you can modify your routine to reduce your chance of knee (and hip, lower back and muscular) injuries.

Your best bet is to jog up the stairs, then walk back down.

Here's why: When you're running, the fraction of time your feet are in contact with the ground and supporting your weight decreases. Add the impact of bouncing, and the average "landing force" absorbed by your ankles, knees and hips is about three times your body weight. (Walking reduces the landing force absorption by about half.) Jogging up those stairs reduces this force because your foot does not drop as far as it would on level ground. Jogging down the stairs increases the landing force because your foot has to fall farther. Walking, of course, is a lower-impact exercise and less risky.

The New, Sleeker Electric Bikes

E-bikes—bicycles that you can pedal but that also have electric motors to deliver a boost any time you want—used to be heavy and ungainly, but thanks to updated technology, they now are sleek and surprisingly light. You can rely on the electric power for up to 100 miles per charge, and you can go 20 miles per hour (mph) or faster with electric assist. You probably have at least one neighbor with an e-bike—US sales doubled last year.

These bikes are not for exercise slackers, either—most models provide electric assist only when you are pedaling, and research shows that they encourage exercise. They charge in about four or five hours from any standard household outlet. The price, though, is closer to that of mopeds than most regular bicycles. To get a reliable ride, you'll want to spend $2,800 to $3,000…and if your goal is high speed or carrying a lot of cargo, expect to spend $4,000 or more.

Before buying any electric bike, consider whether you'll primarily use it as a general-purpose recreational ride…or to commute, go on long tours, carry cargo or children or even to go off-roading. Also, think about whether you would like a model that gives you power without pedaling. *Here are five excellent e-bikes for different needs…*

Best affordable, dependable electric bike: Cannondale Quick NEO. This is the Honda Accord of electric bikes—reliable and not too expensive.

Maximum electric-assist speed/range: 20 mph/50 miles. $2,799.99.* Cannondale.com

Best for speed: Specialized Turbo Vado 6.0. The Porsche of e-bikes, the Turbo Vado 6.0 can attain speeds up to 28 mph with electric assist.

Electric-assist range: 25 miles in "turbo" (high-speed) mode, 50 miles in "eco" (battery-saving) mode. $5,000. Specialized.com

*Prices are manufacturers' suggested retail prices. Maximum electric-assist ranges are estimates.

Best for carrying cargo or kids: Tern GSD. You can carry multiple shopping bags and/or up to two young children in child seats—totaling 400 pounds, rider included. Unlike other cargo-carrying e-bikes, the Tern GSD's center of gravity is low, making it easier to pilot when loaded.

Maximum electric-assist speed/range: 20 mph/150 miles. $3,999. TernBicycles.com

Best for comfort: Riese & Muller Swing. Riese & Muller includes suspension on both wheels of most models for an impressively smooth ride, but its Swing model adds suspension under the seat as well.

Maximum electric-assist speed/range: 20 mph/100 miles. $4,209. R-M.De/en-us

Best if you don't always want to pedal: Elby S1 9-Speed. With this e-bike, you can get an assist while you're pedaling and can stop pedaling and let the motor do all the work or use the active-regeneration mode to charge the battery while you ride.

Maximum electric-assist speed/range: 20 mph/90 miles. $2,999. ElbyBike.com

Spin Class Danger

There are 46 documented cases of people developing *rhabdomyolysis* after a spin class—42 of them in people after their first class. Rhabdomyolysis is a very rare, potentially life-threatening condition in which overworked muscles start to die and their contents are released into the bloodstream, causing severe pain and kidney strain. Some soreness after exercise is normal, but see your doctor if your legs swell or become weak or if you have dark urine, nausea, decreased appetite or an overall sense of not feeling well.

CHAPTER 10

Family Health

Keep Your Love Life Alive...Despite a Health Condition

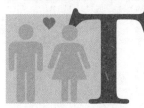There are a multitude of reasons why some couples stop having sex as they age. But a chronic health problem is definitely a big one. Fortunately, it doesn't have to be that way.

Sexual satisfaction remains within reach for just about everyone who wants it...and most people still do want it. Not only that, sexual activity has its own health benefits—for example, it helps lower blood pressure, improves sleep and relieves pain.

ADOPTING A NEW MIND-SET

If you're depriving yourself of sexual intimacy because of a health problem, the key is to start thinking about sex in a new way. Instead of viewing a sexual encounter as a pass/fail test that involves intercourse and mutual orgasm, it's time to think of it as an opportunity for sharing pleasure. How you achieve this is largely up to you. *To get started, you'll want to talk to...*

•**Your doctor.** Schedule a single consultation for you and your partner to meet with your internist, cardiologist, oncologist or other physician who is treating your health problem. Ask him/her to explain how your condition might affect your sexual intimacy and to give you any advice on what you can do medically to minimize those issues.

•**Your partner.** It's crucial for you to be able to talk about sex with your partner. Don't wait until you're in bed...or after a negative experience. Instead, bring up the subject (ideally on the day before a sexual encounter) while you're on a walk or having a glass of wine together. Avoid any blaming, and be clear that you're simply making sexual requests so that the experience is more comfortable and pleasurable.

Barry McCarthy, PhD, a psychologist, sex therapist and marital therapist who is a professor of psychology at American University in Washington, DC. He is coauthor, with Michael Metz, PhD, of *Enduring Desire: Your Guide to Lifelong Intimacy.*

In addition to what you learn by talking to your doctor and your partner, consider these specific steps to get your sex life back on track if you are affected by…

BACK PAIN

Take a man with low-back pain and have him engage in intercourse the way 70% of Americans do—with the man on top of his partner performing short, rapid thrusts—and you've got a perfect recipe for uncomfortable sex.

A better approach: The man with the bad back can invite his partner to go on top, and they can try a circular, thrusting motion. If a woman has back pain, the couple might try the side rear-entry position and long, slow thrusts. If your partner also has back problems, take lovemaking to the shower, where the warm water can loosen sore muscles.

Also helpful: If you're in chronic pain, such as that caused by arthritis, your doctor can refer you to a physical therapist, who can give you additional positioning tips.

Taking your favorite over-the-counter pain-reliever or using a heating pad about 30 minutes before sex also helps. This approach often reduces back and joint pain for an hour or more.

Even if your pain is not entirely eliminated, you may get enough relief to enjoy yourself. And after orgasm, your pain will likely be less intense for a period of time.

CANCER

Cancer treatment, such as surgery, radiation and medication, can create pain, fatigue and all kinds of psychological and physical fallout.

With breast cancer, it's common for a woman to worry about her partner's reaction to her altered body and how her breasts will respond to touch, particularly if she has had reconstructive surgery, which reduces sensitivity.

What helps: When talking about these issues, don't be afraid to get specific. Some women will not want to be touched on the affected breast or breasts, at least for a while. Others will crave that touch. Some might feel uncomfortable about nipple stimulation but fine about touching on the underside of the breast.

Cancers that affect other parts of the body, such as cervical or testicular malignancies or even mouth cancer, can also interfere with intimacy. If a man has been treated for prostate cancer, for example, he may want to focus more on pleasure-oriented sexuality rather than the traditional approach of intercourse and orgasm. Whatever the situation, talk about these vulnerable feelings and enlist your partner's help as a sexual ally.

EXCESS BODY WEIGHT

Too much body weight can get in the way—both psychologically and physically.

It's common for a person who is overweight to think: *I don't feel sexy now, but I will when I lose some weight.* While weight loss is a healthy idea, putting your sexuality on ice until you reach some ideal state is not. Learn to love and care for the body you have.

What helps in bed: Think beyond the missionary position, which can get pretty awkward and uncomfortable if one or both parties carry a lot of weight around the middle. Try lying on your sides instead. Or try a sitting and kneeling combination—a woman might sit on the edge of a sofa, supported by pillows behind her back, while her partner kneels before her.

HEART AND LUNG PROBLEMS

The fatigue often associated with heart and lung disease can douse your sexual flames. But a bigger issue is often the fear that a bit of sexually induced heavy breathing will prove dangerous or even fatal.

If this is a concern, ask your doctor whether you are healthy enough for sex. A good rule of thumb is to see if you can comfortably climb two flights of stairs. If the answer is yes, then almost certainly you're healthy enough to have sex.

What helps: If you still feel nervous, you can gain some reassurance by pleasuring yourself. A bout of masturbation produces the same physiological arousal as partnered sex. And it gives you a no-pressure chance to see how that arousal affects your breathing and heart rate.

PARKINSON'S AND RELATED CONDITIONS

People with frequent tremors, muscle spasms and other conditions in which a loss of control over the body occurs can still enjoy sex.

What helps: When talking to your partner about sex, decide between the two of you, in advance, on what you will say if, during lovemaking, your body becomes too uncooperative. It might be just a single word—"spasm," for instance—that tells your partner you need to pause.

Then agree on a "trust position" you will assume as you take a break to see if you want to return to sexual activity. For example, some people will cuddle or lie side by side.

The Sex-Starved Marriage: How to Make Both of You Happier

Michele Weiner-Davis, LCSW, founder of The Divorce Busting Center in Boulder, Colorado, which helps on-the-brink couples save their marriages. She is the best-selling author of eight books including *Healing from Infidelity, The Sex-Starved Marriage* and *Divorce Busting.* DivorceBusting.com

---

It has been two months since Janet and Mark have had sex. They're hardly speaking to each other. If you asked Janet about this, she would say that their home has become a battle zone—they fight about every little thing. Janet goes out of her way to avoid Mark to protect herself from his wrath.

Mark tells a different story. His anger, he believes, is justified. He is fed up with Janet's lack of interest in their sexual relationship. "She never initiates sex. She recoils when I try to kiss or hug her. I'm tired of being rejected." To cope with his unhappiness, Mark spends longer hours at work and busies himself on his computer at night, deepening the chasm between them.

Both Mark and Janet think that the other one is to blame for the problems between them. They have hit an impasse.

The result: A sex-starved marriage. And sex-starved marriages are surprisingly common. In fact, in about one in three marriages, one spouse has a considerably larger sexual appetite than the other. This in and of itself is not a problem—it's how couples handle their differences that matters.

Here's what you need to know to fix a sex-starved marriage and make you both happier…

YEARNING FOR CONTACT

In a sex-starved marriage, one partner is longing for more touch—both sexual and non-sexual—and the other spouse isn't interested and doesn't understand why such a fuss is being made about sex. The less interested spouse thinks, Is this just about having an orgasm? That's not such a big deal. But the spouse yearning for more physical contact sees it differently. Being close physically is more than a physical release—it's about feeling wanted and connected emotionally.

When a misunderstanding of this magnitude happens and the less interested spouse continues to avoid sex, marriages start to unravel. Couples stop spending time together. They quit putting effort into the relationship. They become more like two distant roommates. Intimacy on all levels ends, which puts the marriage at risk for infidelity or divorce.

Typically, the spouse with the smaller sexual appetite controls the frequency of sex. If she/he (contrary to popular belief, men also can have low sexual desire) doesn't want it, it generally doesn't happen. This is not due to a desire to control the relationship—it just seems unthinkable to be sexual if one is not in the mood.

Furthermore, the lower-desire spouse has the expectation that the higher-desire spouse must accept the no-sex verdict and remain monogamous. The higher-desire spouse feels rejected, resentful and miserable.

How do two people with differing sexual appetites begin to bridge the desire gap? Regardless of where you stand on the sexual-desire spectrum, it's important to keep in mind that loving marriages are built on mutual care-taking. Don't wait for your spouse to change first. Be the catalyst for change in your marriage. *Here's how…*

IF YOU ARE THE LOWER-DESIRE SPOUSE

•**Just do it—and you may be surprised.** Over the years, countless clients in my counseling practice have said, "I wasn't in the mood to have sex when my spouse approached me, but once we got going, it felt really good. I had an orgasm, and my spouse's mood really improved afterward."

Why would that be? For many people, the human sexual response cycle consists of four stages that occur in a certain order—desire (out of the blue, you have a sexy thought)…arousal (you and your partner touch, and your body becomes aroused)…orgasm…and resolution (your body returns to its normal resting state).

But for millions of people, stages one and two actually are reversed. In other words, desire doesn't come until after arousal. These people must feel turned on physically before they realize that they actually desire sex. Therefore, being receptive to your partner's advances even from a neutral starting place—when you do not feel desire—makes sense because chances are that sex will be enjoyable for both of you.

•**Give a "gift."** Let's face it, there are times when people—even people with the typical desire/arousal pattern—simply don't feel like having sex. It's perfectly acceptable to decline your partner's offer from time to time. But when "no" substantially outweighs "yes," you are creating deep feelings of frustration and rejection—guaranteed.

What's the solution to an "I'm not really in the mood for sex" moment? Give a gift—a sexual gift—or to be more blunt about it, pleasure your spouse to orgasm if that's what he/she wants, even if you're not in the mood for the same. This is an act of love and caring and completely appropriate within a marriage.

IF YOU ARE THE HIGHER-DESIRE SPOUSE

•**Speak from your heart.** If you're feeling frustrated that your spouse hasn't understood your need to be close physically, chances are you've been irritable and angry. Anger is not an aphrodisiac—it pushes your spouse further away. Press your mental-reset button, and approach your spouse differently. Speak from your heart—express your vulnerability (yes, you are vulnerable, no matter how "tough" you are!) and your hurt.

Example: Instead of saying, "I'm angry that we haven't had sex in so long," it's better to say, "When we don't have sex for this long, I miss being close to you. I feel disconnected. It hurts my feelings that you don't seem interested in me sexually."

•**Rather than complain, ask for what you want.** Complaining, even when it's justified, leads to defensiveness. Instead, ask for what you want in a positive way.

Example: Instead of saying, "You never initiate sex," say, "I'd really love it if once in a while, you threw your arms around me and said, 'Do you want to make love?' That would make me feel great."

•**Figure out what turns your spouse on.** If buying sex toys or downloading X-rated videos has failed to entice your spouse to nurture your sexual relationship, there's probably a reason. Your spouse might need to feel courted by you first. You might be married to someone who feels more connected to you when you have meaningful conversations…spend enjoyable, uninterrupted time together other than having sex…are more affirming and complimentary…or when you participate in family activities together. This is how your partner feels loved—and the truth is, there are many people who want sexual intimacy only when they feel loved first.

If you're uncertain about your spouse's way of feeling cherished by you, ask. Say, "What can I do to make you feel loved?" Believe it or not, meeting your partner's needs, though different from your own, may be a turn-on for him/her. Try it.

Warning Signs You're Having a Midlife Crisis

Michele Weiner-Davis, LCSW, founder of The Divorce Busting Center in Boulder, Colorado, which helps on-the-brink couples save their marriages. She is the best-selling author of eight books including *Healing from Infidelity, The Sex-Starved Marriage* and *Divorce Busting.* DivorceBusting.com

A woman in my therapy practice said that her grumpy 52-year-old husband complained about her incessantly. Each time she "fixed" something—lost weight or organized the house—it failed to improve his mood. His needs seemed to be a moving target.

The husband decided to move out. He told her that he wasn't sure that he wanted a divorce—he just needed some time to think about his life. He had LASIK surgery so that he could stop wearing glasses. He had plastic surgery to make his eyelids appear more youthful and liposuction to slim his belly. Shortly thereafter, he decided to quit his well-paying job to start his own company.

CAN YOU SAY, "MIDLIFE CRISIS"?

Here's how to tell if you or someone you love is going through a midlife crisis—and what to do about it…

What happens?

Although it's normal, even healthy, to question our life choices periodically, people experiencing a midlife crisis often can't think of anything else. They have a gnawing feeling deep inside that something in their lives is off-kilter and must be addressed.

This typically happens to people ranging in age from the mid-40s to mid-60s. In our 20s and 30s, we are focused on making important life decisions about career paths, where to live, life partners, whether or when to have children—and then raising those children. We're too busy carving out our niches in life to do too much reflecting about our choices.

But once we've settled into our grooves, our children have grown independent and we've had some time under our belts, we also have time to think. We ask ourselves, *Is this all there is? and Aren't I supposed to feel happier?* We obsess about the paths not taken and feel that time is running out. Failing to achieve personal, relationship or business goals and dreams can lead to deep regret or remorse, even depression.

Other problems that weigh heavily at this time…

•**Aging bodies.** Over the years, our bodies change—we gain weight, get wrinkles, lose muscle tone. We don't like what we see in the mirror. If our identity has been intertwined with our appearance, we start to feel insecure or depressed. Looking older often is difficult to accept.

•**Ailing bodies.** We begin to have more aches and pains. Activities that once were easy for us become more challenging. Additionally, our immune systems tend to weaken—when we get sick, we take longer to heal. Plus, our illnesses can be more serious and often life-threatening.

•**Ailing parents.** Another stressor for people in midlife is ailing parents or relatives who require a great deal of care. Watching loved ones deteriorate physically and mentally is emotionally draining and can create a sense of urgency to live one's life to the fullest. Plus, it's hard not to dread this unfortunate but natural deterioration in our own lives. Losing a parent exacerbates the feeling that time is running out.

To be certain, reflecting on one's life and making midcourse corrections when necessary are natural and good things. Our happiness depends on it. But unfortunately, many people going through midlife crises aren't always thinking clearly—they are overly pessimistic. Their glass-half-empty thinking can lead to remedial actions that are regrettable in the long run. They may start a completely different career or find a new life partner or embark on a completely different lifestyle. Although changes that are well thought out can make a person's life more satisfying, it's important to refrain from making irreversible changes that may be based on feelings that are merely transient.

Finally, people going through a midlife crisis often tell themselves to "grab for the gusto," and start experimenting with risky hobbies such as skydiving, bungee jumping or hang gliding, or become uncharacteristically extravagant in their spending habits. Hence, the proverbial new red convertible.

MARRIAGE: THE MIDLIFE CRISIS CASUALTY

If you're going through a midlife crisis and you're married, it's important to understand that your marriage might be at risk. When you're unhappy, you look around for the cause of the unhappiness. And sometimes the person standing closest to you—your spouse—is in the line of fire. You think about how differently your life might have turned out were it not for your spouse holding you back in some way. You tell yourself you would be better off striking out on your own or finding a new, more supportive, sexy, fun-loving spouse with whom you can spend the rest of your life.

What could be a better escape from all the thinking you're doing about what's not working in your life than to find someone with whom you can have a fresh start, who finds you fascinating and exciting?

While it's possible that your marriage has been less than satisfying and in need of a major makeover, it's important not to make any monumental, life-altering decision such as having an affair or ending your marriage while you're feeling overwhelmed with powerful emotions.

Making an impulsive decision to break up a marriage or have an affair often leads to a deep sense of regret or remorse.

IF YOU'RE HAVING A MIDLIFE CRISIS

If you think you're having a midlife crisis, here are steps you can take…

•**Try a small change.** There's a saying, "Bloom where you're planted." It is often possible to identify what you could do—without undergoing major life changes—to help you feel better immediately. Sometimes it's simply a matter of tweaking your daily routine, trying a new hobby, making a new friend or beginning a new project. Novelty makes us feel more alive. If your marriage has gotten you down, reflect on what was different when you met. Start doing some of the same activities you enjoyed early on.

•**Talk it out.** Talk to friends you trust who are able to understand what you're going through. It helps enormously to have a sounding board who knows you, has your best interest at heart and who can offer valuable feedback.

•**Stay active.** Negative thinking and emotions during a midlife crisis can lead to depression or intense anxiety. Research suggests that regular exercise is a powerful antidepressant that will help you think more clearly. It also can make you feel better about yourself.

•**Find meaning from within.** Again, without making drastic changes, it's possible to feel more purposeful in your life. Read inspirational books, keep a journal, start a meditation practice, pray, take walks in nature, listen to music. In some ways, being in the throes of a midlife

crisis is an opportunity to take a time-out from your busy life to reflect on what's truly important to you. Busyness often prevents us from pausing long enough to get in touch with our inner compass. Taking time to go inward can offer the direction we need to emerge from a midlife crisis feeling whole.

•**Hang out with positive people.** Optimism is contagious. Surround yourself with people who are joyful, upbeat and have clear visions about what matters in life. Their enthusiasm is likely to rub off on you. Conversely, it might be a good time to sever relationships with people who drag you down or don't add to your life in some way.

•**Mend your marriage.** If you're married and you believe that your relationship is problematic, do some soul searching about what's really important to you and how you might be contributing to the problem. Talk honestly to your spouse about what's troubling you. Ask for what you need rather than complain. Be specific. For example, instead of saying, "I'm feeling unappreciated," say, "It would be great if you made a point of telling me that you appreciate all the things I do to support you, such as helping you with your parents, entertaining your business associates, handling all the bills and so on."

•**Seek professional help.** If necessary, speak to a therapist who can help you sort through your feelings and help you devise a plan to feel better. He/she also can reassure you that the challenging transitional period you're experiencing won't last forever.

IF YOUR SPOUSE IS HAVING A MIDLIFE CRISIS

If you strongly suspect that your partner is having a midlife crisis, give him/her space to work things out alone. Chances are, your partner won't agree that a midlife crisis is the issue at hand. Don't debate this. Don't insist that he/she read this article. It will only make matters worse. Instead, focus on yourself for a while. Try some of the steps above such as exercising, talking to friends and finding inspiration within. Find ways to self-soothe and find peace until the haziness clears. If your spouse wants to separate or asks for a divorce, speak to a therapist either by yourself or with your spouse to focus on the real issues and chart the best possible course.

Love Hacks: Improve Your Relationship in 5 Minutes

Eli J. Finkel, PhD, professor in the psychology department and the Kellogg School of Management at Northwestern University, Evanston, Illinois. He is director of Northwestern's Relationships and Motivation Lab and author of *The All-or-Nothing Marriage: How the Best Marriages Work*. EliFinkel.com

Sure, it takes time and effort to build a successful relationship, but there are some quick, easy, surprisingly effective ways to strengthen your bond with your partner. These simple, research-based strategies are not likely to salvage a deeply troubled relationship, but they can help keep a relatively happy one on solid ground until there's time for a grander gesture. *Six of the simplest ways you'll ever find to strengthen your relationship…*

•**Make a big deal about your partner's little victory.** Listen intently and respond enthusiastically when your partner tells you about something that went right for him/her that day. Do this even if he describes something very small, such as fixing a broken appliance or receiving positive feedback from a colleague. Caring partners know that they must provide support when their loved ones experience challenging times. But research published in *Journal of Personality and Social Psychology* found that reveling in partners' victories also is pivotal for relationships, increasing trust, intimacy and overall satisfaction.

Next step: After your partner shares the story of a small success, suggest something that commemorates the accomplishment, such as, "That's worth opening a bottle of wine." This turns an everyday moment into a relationship-building shared celebration.

•**When your partner makes a misstep, picture an external, temporary explana-tion for it.** Your partner arrives late to dinner, leaving you waiting. Do you think, He doesn't care about my time…or He was probably stuck in bad traffic? If you're like most people, it often is the former, negative conclusion. We tend to blame individuals and ignore potential external factors.

This tendency is very bad for relationships—blaming our partners for everyday missteps decreases our satisfaction with our relationships, makes our partners feel persecuted and gains us nothing. When you feel let down by your partner, instead take a moment to ask yourself, *What temporary, outside factor could be to blame for this?*

Do exactly the opposite when your partner gets something right—think up a permanent, internal explanation for this success.

Example: If your partner brings home your favorite ice cream, don't think, *Oh, he did that just because he wanted ice cream, too*—instead think, *He's such a thoughtful person.*

•**Reflect on what your partner has done recently for the sake of the relationship.** Find a few minutes every month or so to mentally list two or three things your partner has done lately for you or for your relationship and note to yourself that you are grateful for these actions. They can be small things—maybe she walked the dog even though it was your turn… or he called in the middle of a busy day just to say he loved you.

Several studies have found that focusing on gratitude for even a few minutes a month is an effective way to strengthen the emotional bonds between partners. One researcher even referred to gratitude as a "booster shot for romantic relationships." It's so powerful that it can lead to a virtuous cycle—your sense of gratitude might boost your positive feelings for your partner so much that your partner senses your positivity and starts feeling and acting more positively toward you, too, encouraging kind deeds and warm feelings on both sides.

•**Be your own neutral arbitrator after arguments.** Most of us get caught up in self-righteousness after we argue with our partners—we tell ourselves that our side of the disagreement was 100% correct and our partner's side was 100% wrong. Instead, try this trick soon after an argument—mentally revisit the exchange from the perspective of a neutral third party who wants the best for all involved. What would this person think about the disagreement? How might he find the good that could come from it?

A recent study of 120 married couples in the Chicago area found that doing this significantly improved marital satisfaction—even though the couples did it for only a few minutes every few months. These couples still argued as much as ever, but their arguments did not lead to the same degree of lingering displeasure.

Next step: Attempt to take this neutral perspective during arguments.

•**Learn to accept your partner's praise.** Some people struggle to accept compliments from their partners, often because they suffer from low self-esteem and/or consider themselves unlovable. Overcoming this tendency could do wonders for their relationships—receiving kind words from a partner makes people feel much closer.

A psychologist at Renison University College in Canada found a way for people who have trouble accepting their partners' compliments to greatly improve this ability. After receiving a compliment, take a moment to silently explain to yourself why your partner admired you…and to reflect on what this compliment means to you and its significance for your relationship. Doing this will encourage you to see the praise in abstract terms, rather than only in terms of the specific, isolated item or event that was complimented. It's easy to dismiss compliments for isolated things—Sure, I got that one thing right, but it was just luck—but much more difficult to dismiss abstract praise.

•**Touch.** It won't surprise you to learn that happy couples tend to do more affectionate touching—such as holding hands, giving shoulder rubs, placing a hand on a partner's knee—than unhappy couples. What is surprising is that affectionate touching is very effective at making couples feel closer—so effective, in fact, that it's likely to work even if your partner knows that you're doing it only because it takes a lot less thought and effort than most other relationship-building strategies. In one study, psychologists at Carnegie Mellon University found that people felt more secure in their relationships and more trusting of their partners following physical contact, even when they knew that their partners were making physical contact only because the academic running the study had just instructed them to. If touch can make couples feel closer under those entirely unromantic circumstances, it's very likely to work in your life as well.

Sexual Bereavement

Alice Radosh, PhD, research psychologist and coauthor of the study "Acknowledging Sexual Bereavement: A Path Out of Disenfranchised Grief," published in *Reproductive Health Matters*.

The death of a spouse is not just the loss of a life partner. It also is the loss of a sexual partner. Unfortunately, most widows and widowers must cope with the emotional impact of that loss of sexual intimacy alone, and the isolation only deepens their suffering. Cultural taboos and personal embarrassment often prevent them from raising their feelings of what is called "sexual bereavement." But there's a way to help yourself psychologically if you are in this situation…or help a loved one who is.

Recent finding: A survey of 104 partnered women age 55 and older published in *Reproductive Health Matters* found that 72% anticipated missing sex with their partners after their partners died, and most said that they would want to discuss this feeling of loss with a friend. But the majority reported that they would feel more comfortable about the conversation if the friend raised the subject.

The problem: Most of the women surveyed also admitted that they would not raise this topic if it were one of their friends who had been widowed.

What to do: If you are the close friend of someone who has been widowed, raise the topic of the loss of sexual intimacy. If it makes you uncomfortable to ask your friend about his/her sex life, you could mention that you would grieve the loss of your sex life if you were widowed…or you could say that someone else you know who was widowed experienced these feelings. Don't assume that your recently widowed friend is too old to have had an active sex life—many couples remain sexually active into their 80s.

If you are recently widowed and are experiencing sexual bereavement, understand that these feelings are perfectly normal. Raise the topic with a friend or relative without shame. If you are not comfortable doing this, you could raise the topic with a therapist or support group…or with a friend by mentioning a recent sexual-bereavement article you read about (such as this one).

How to Remain Intimate with a Partner Who Has Dementia

Gary Chapman, PhD, author, speaker and counselor based in Winston-Salem, North Carolina. Dr. Chapman is coauthor with Deborah Barr, MA, and Edward G. Shaw, MD, of *Keeping Love Alive as Memories Fade: The 5 Love Languages and the Alzheimer's Journey.* His website offers a 30-point assessment for couples to identify which "love language" matters most to them. 5LoveLanguages.com

When your spouse has Alzheimer's disease or another type of dementia, it's natural to wonder how you can maintain your emotional bond or if, as the cruel disease progresses, it is possible at all.

The truth is, you can express love and feel connected throughout all the stages of dementia, although the disease will change the relationship—for both of you.

To learn how to better foster intimacy, we turned to marriage counselor Gary Chapman, PhD, coauthor of *Keeping Love Alive as Memories Fade: The 5 Love Languages and the Alzheimer's Journey…*

How can I show love to my spouse who has dementia?

In many ways, especially in the early stages of dementia, the way you experience intimacy remains the same for both of you.

People perceive emotional love in five distinct channels of communication—words of affirmation ("I love you"…"You look great in that

dress"…"You did a great job")…quality time (giving someone your full, undivided attention)…gifts (a visible symbol of love)…acts of service (shopping, setting the table)…and physical touch (making love, but also a hug, back rub or kiss—or even just sitting close together).

Once couples figure out how to express love to each other in the way that matters most to each of them, both will feel emotionally loved. This is especially important when one of the spouses has dementia.

What are some of the best ways to maintain intimacy in the early stages of my spouse's dementia?

One of the least talked about aspects of dementia is the fact that the disease will eventually rob the couple of their sexual relationship. In the very earliest stage of Alzheimer's, however, little changes in the couple's sexual relationship. This is a time when the couple can make the most of their opportunities for intimacy.

How will I know when it's no longer appropriate to have sex?

There often comes a time when sex is no longer appropriate or even feasible. If you feel that you are taking advantage of your spouse with dementia, it may be time to stop having sex.

As the brain changes, a person may begin to forget how to do things such as cook and get dressed, as well as how to make love. He/she may forget the foreplay routine the couple has shared. As a result, the person may feel embarrassed and shy away from sex. As Alzheimer's progresses and affects the parietal lobe, the part of the brain responsible for processing sensory information, too much sensory input can be disturbing—making sexual contact uncomfortable.

Conversely, some people with Alzheimer's may become hypersexual—they may want or even demand far more sexual activity than the couple has even had before. The healthy spouse may or may not be comfortable with this—and may need professional advice to figure out how to handle it.

Eventually, the person with Alzheimer's disease may also forget who the spouse is or confuse the spouse with another family member, such as a sister or brother or even an adult child. When this happens, many caregiving spouses no longer feel comfortable maintaining a sexual relationship.

How can I maintain intimacy without sex?

Let me share an anecdote from my coauthor Dr. Edward Shaw. His wife, who had early-onset Alzheimer's, would become startled and upset when he came up from behind and gave her a hug and a peck on the cheek. However, she felt safer at night when snuggled under the covers and the lights were dimmed. At that time, they were able to connect as she enjoyed some gentle hugging and kissing. Surprising your spouse might have worked when you were younger, but now it may be better to be gentle, open and calm.

Other ways of maintaining intimacy with your partner without having sex are holding hands…sitting close by or holding him if he is afraid, angry or agitated…rubbing his feet or back or gently stroking his cheek…massaging his hands and arms with lotion…dancing or moving to music with him.

In later stages of the disease, will my spouse with dementia even appreciate the kind and loving things I do?

The amygdala, the emotion center of the brain that plays a key role in emotional memory, is not immediately affected by dementia or Alzheimer's. A person's deep need for love does not disappear, even after the actual actions or words are forgotten. Even in late Alzheimer's, when the amygdala is affected, one's ability to perceive emotional love endures far longer than the ability to express it. You must remind yourself daily that your loved one is capable of receiving love—even though you may not receive a thank-you, hug or kiss in acknowledgment of your expressions of love.

What if my spouse wrongfully accuses me of infidelity?

Delusions such as this may occur starting in middle-stage dementia or later. It is hard for a faithful spouse not to take an accusation of infidelity personally and lash out. First, realize that it's the disease speaking, not your spouse. Then try the three-step approach below.

Consider this hypothetical scenario in which Dan, an Alzheimer's patient, accuses his wife, Marian, of being unfaithful. *His wife should…*

- **Acknowledge.** "Dan, I hear you saying that you are worried that I am seeing someone else."
- **Affirm.** "Well, let me reassure you. We've been married for 50 years, and I've been faithful to you for 50 years—there's nothing that's going to change that."
- **Redirect.** "So let's go sit down on the couch together, turn on the TV and have some popcorn."

When Sexual Behavior Becomes Inappropriate

Elizabeth Galik, PhD, CRNP, FAAN, associate professor at University of Maryland School of Nursing in Baltimore, where she also teaches in the adult and geriatric nurse practitioner program. She specializes in the neuropsychiatric care of older adults with dementia and practices clinically as a nurse practitioner in community and long-term-care settings.

Sexual feelings don't have an expiration date. Older adults are still sexual beings, and many maintain their interest in sex into their 80s and 90s. But for people with dementia, these impulses can go awry when cognitive and personality changes lead to inappropriate sexual behavior (ISB).

Examples: Disrobing in front of others…public masturbation…uninhibited sexual talk…or the inappropriate or unwanted touching of health-care workers, other patients or even family members.

Some 5% to 20% of dementia patients exhibit some degree of ISB at some point during the course of their illness. It's more common in group-living situations (where there may be more sexual triggers/opportunities for interaction with others). It affects both men and women (though more men), and it can occur with all forms of dementia, such as those caused by Alzheimer's disease, frontotemporal dementia and vascular diseases, traumatic brain injury and others.

BROKEN BOUNDARIES

Because it's natural for adults of all ages—including those with dementia—to have and sometimes act on sexual feelings and interests, it's important to differentiate normal sexual expressions from ISB.

What can happen: Imagine that two widowed residents at a care facility spend a lot of time together. They might hold hands or kiss. This behavior may be considered normal as long as both of them have the cognitive capacity to understand who the other person is, welcome and enjoy the interactions and both are able to make informed decisions about the relationship—including the ability to say "yes" or "no."

ISB, on the other hand, is a persistent and uninhibited sexual behavior that interferes with function and is directed toward oneself or toward an unwilling partner. Patients might make aggressive and inappropriate or sexually suggestive comments to others. They might touch others in ways that are unwelcome. The behavior may occur in public or when no one else is around.

ISB is challenging to address because most people, particularly family members, are uncomfortable talking about a patient's sexuality. Health-care providers can help by initiating a conversation about sexual expression and distinguishing between sexual expression and inappropriate sexual behavior.

WHAT CAUSES ISB?

There are several causes of ISB. A loss of neurons from progressive dementia, frontal lobe injury or an acute delirium may result in ISB. Additionally, some patients with dementia have other psychiatric problems (such as bipolar disorder) that can trigger hyper-sexuality, which is a common manifestation of the mania that can characterize bipolar disorder.

Another cause: Side effects from drugs and/or alcohol. Many common medications, including the Parkinson's medication *levodopa* (Sinemet) and the sedative *diazepam* (Valium), may trigger symptoms of ISB.

When health-care providers such as physicians, nurse practitioners, neurologists and psychiatrists treat patients with ISB, they will start by looking for possible physical causes, including drug side effects. For some patients, simply changing medications can help. More often,

treatment involves nondrug approaches including education and behavioral techniques.

BEST NONDRUG STRATEGIES

There are no FDA-approved treatments specifically for ISB. Antidepressants, mood stabilizers and other drugs can help some patients, but they are used only case-by-case—and usually as a last resort due to their potential side effects, which can be quite serious. *What you can do instead…*

•**Distraction.** This can be as simple as giving someone something to do when he/she begins to exhibit unwanted sexual behaviors. The moment you hear a sexual comment, for example, try to bring the person's attention elsewhere, maybe with an activity. Alternatively, you can lead the patient away from anything that could be triggering the behavior such as a TV show.

•**Boundary reminders.** Patients with dementia might not be able to engage in lengthy conversations, but most can understand simple instructions, particularly when they're delivered in a professional, no-nonsense tone.

Example: A patient with wandering hands might be told, "No. I don't like it when you touch me. Please stop."

•**Identify sexual triggers.** Patients with dementia often misinterpret social and environmental cues. ISB is usually triggered by specific people and situations, which vary from person to person. Once you are able to identify these triggers, you can take steps to avoid uncomfortable situations and prevent misinterpretations.

Example: An elderly man who is stimulated by the presence of young women. If you have such women visiting your home, you might arrange to keep him busy with a favorite activity in a different part of the house.

Another example: Someone who gets aroused during baths or other situations that involve nudity and/or touching. You can avoid this trigger by handing the patient a washcloth and encouraging him to wash himself. And it can be helpful to have someone of the gender that the patient is not attracted to perform care duties involving nudity or touching.

•**Change the environment.** If someone is aroused by caregivers of only one sex, try to use care-givers of the other sex—even for care that doesn't involve intimacy. Change the channel on the TV when overtly sexual programs come on.

•**Hard-to-remove clothing.** You can buy "adaptive" clothing with hooks or other fasteners that make it difficult to remove—helpful for someone who disrobes, masturbates in public or tries to engage other people in unwanted sexual activity. Twenty years ago, this type of clothing tended to look institutional. Now there are more stylish options available online.

Important: The use of adaptive clothing is sometimes controversial because it prevents an individual from having access to his own body. But it can be helpful in some cases. Discuss it with your loved one's health-care provider.

Caregiving Lessons from a Dementia Coach

Kerry Mills, MPA, a dementia coach and founder of Engaging Alzheimer's, LLC, based in White Plains, New York. Mills is coauthor of *I Care: A Handbook for Care Partners of People with Dementia* and author of *Serving Residents with Dementia: Transformative Care Strategies for Assisted Living Providers*. EngagingAlzheimers.com

---

If you're one of the 15 million Americans who provides care to a family member with Alzheimer's disease or dementia, you know how tough—and emotional—it can be. You're watching someone you love be robbed of memories and independence. But you are being robbed, too—of the relationship you once had…and of your own life before you became a caregiver.

There is a way to help yourself and your spouse, parent or other relative with dementia. Compassionate, informed care techniques help improve the lifestyles of people with dementia while preserving dignity and safety…which makes your life easier, too. Mastering these "dementia coaching" tactics can help you make a positive, lasting difference in how the disease affects your entire family.

4 STRATEGIES FOR SUCCESSFUL CARE

Your goal is to provide the best care to your loved one with less stress. *I've found that these tips help…*

1. Consider yourself a care partner, not a care giver. Individuals newly diagnosed with dementia can live another 20 years—a long time to be giving your time, energy, emotions and/ or finances. The word partner recognizes that there are two of you in the relationship.

Changing how you think of your role may ease feelings of resentment and burnout—and help you feel better about taking breaks for your own physical and mental health. It also can improve the relationship.

Example: You know that hanging around the house isn't good for your spouse with dementia—or you. But your spouse isn't motivated. Saying, "Honey, you need a walk, let's go," makes you feel like you're working and makes your loved one feel bossed around. Instead, say, "Honey, I would love to go to the movies tonight, but I only want to go if you are with me. Will you join me?" The well spouse wants something and asks the person with dementia to join him/her. It's about both of them.

2. Remember they're not stubborn— they're fighting for independence. It's natural to want to control a person with dementia, much as you would an infant. But your grown-up loved one has led a rich life, full of experiences and accomplishments. When your concerns overshadow his need to maintain independence, he'll respond with resistance and frustration. Anyone would—it's a natural human tendency. Try not to get into a battle of wills.

Example: Your spouse refuses to shower. He may think he already has showered. Instead of arguing, restate the request: "This afternoon we're going out to lunch with your friend Bill. Let's make sure we're ready and look good for our visit!"

3. Dig down to the "why." Many of the behaviors of individuals who have dementia express an unfulfilled need—a craving to be active, busy, useful or safe…or simple needs such as being hungry, tired or needing to use the bathroom. If she's rambling on, don't complain…but do pay attention to clues that might let you know what's on her mind.

Example: Your wife keeps wandering in and out of the kitchen. She might be hungry—but lacks the words to let you know and may not even be aware of what she wants. Try making her a snack.

4. Stop being right. Or rather, stop insisting that you're right (even when you are). Let yourself into her world. If your loved one is recounting a story and the details are wrong, just let it be. What is gained by correcting her? If telling the story brings her joy, the facts are less important. If her mistakes are causing disturbing thoughts or behaviors, gently redirect her.

Sometimes reminding a person with great memory loss of hurtful truths can be painful—with no benefit. Telling your dad several times a day that his wife is no longer living is no favor. In these cases, not sharing the truth is more comforting than causing pain over and over. It's called therapeutic fibbing, aka comfort lies.

Example: Your mother is resisting the idea of a paid caregiver. Rather than introduce someone as an aide, you might say, "Mom, this is Carol. We met at the gym, and she loves baking. I thought the two of you could get together and swap cookie recipes."

As Carol and your mother spend time together and trust builds, Carol can make suggestions, such as, "I see your pills on the table. Can I grab them for you?" or "I'm going to use the bathroom. But do you want to go first? I can help you." Your mother will be more receptive.

SHOULD YOU HIRE A DEMENTIA COACH?

A dementia coach (or counselor) is someone with expertise in effective caregiving practices for people diagnosed with dementia—who also focuses on the needs of the caregiver. Many are health-care professionals who have worked in dementia care. Some coaches do phone and video/Skype conferencing, so geographic closeness may not be essential.

It's not an official designation, however—there is no accreditation, and services generally are not covered by insurance. Costs vary widely but range from $175 to $300 an hour. They may be deductible as a medical expense (check with your accountant). Find a dementia coach

Caregiver Alert

People caring for loved ones with a terminal illness are highly susceptible to clinical depression and anxiety, according to a new study of 395 caregivers. Details: Researchers found that 23% were moderately or severely depressed…and 33% had moderate or severe anxiety. If you're caring for a terminally ill loved one: Be sure to talk to your doctor or a therapist about your own well-being.

Debra Parker Oliver, PhD, professor of family and community medicine, University of Missouri School of Medicine, Columbia.

by searching the web and asking your local hospital or assisted-living facility for recommendations. Look for at least five years of experience working with people who have dementia.

Next, request references—and ask questions, such as…

How does your coaching work?

What are your qualifications as an Alzheimer's/dementia coach?

How long is each coaching session?

What is your fee?

How many sessions do you recommend?

You should also feel a strong connection with him/her, leaving your first in-person meeting or Skype session feeling hopeful. Your coach can work with both the person who has dementia and with the care partners. Sessions can range from a onetime consultation to weekly visits, depending on your family's needs and goals.

Get Your Elderly Mom (or Dad) to Move Closer

Barbara McVicker, author of three books on elder care including *Stuck in the Middle: Shared Stories and Tips on Caring for Mom and Dad*, which became a PBS special. McVicker was a caregiver for her parents for 10 years. BarbaraMcVicker.com

I t's stressful when your aging parents are far away. Maybe they're doing just fine, but you see signs of frailty. Perhaps you've already made a middle-of-the-night trip for a medical emergency…and you foresee more. So you want your parent or parents to move closer.

Unfortunately, Mom or Dad is likely to disagree. Even if they are becoming more fragile, the idea of packing up is daunting, and so is leaving friends, doctors and…home. Recently widowed? Change is even harder. *Here's how to get them on board…*

LAYING THE GROUNDWORK

Talk to your parents about their future, and do it sooner rather than later. Ask them how they expect to manage when they can no longer drive or fully care for themselves. They may clam up, but continue to bring it up before a health crisis—the worst time to make decisions—forces everyone's hand. Next, educate yourself—and enlist your siblings. There are many options—living with you…downsizing to a condo…finding a retirement or assisted-living community. Identify a few options that make sense. *Then…*

•**Hold a family meeting.** Your mom and dad need to have a say, no matter how right you think you are. Present the options…but it's fine to nudge them toward the one that you think is best. If at all possible, make this meeting happen in person—facial expressions and body language convey as much meaning as do words. Plus, you can give hugs.

•**Play up the positives.** Emphasize benefits that you know your parent will appreciate, such as being closer to family, including grandkids. Mom (or Dad) hates cooking and cleaning? Mention that senior housing can include housekeeping.

•**Listen to their fears.** Ask them to share their biggest worries. Be sure to show respect for these worries and emphasize how you will work with them to ease the stress.

•**Let 'em see your pain.** Few parents want to make their kids unhappy at any age. Be honest about your stresses. "I want to be able to help you. But traveling and taking time off work are not things I can regularly handle." You may feel quite emotional, and that's OK…but don't lose control!

•**Have a fallback.** Your parents still may say no, and that's their right. Be prepared with another suggestion such as moving to an assisted-living facility in their current location or hiring a geriatric care manager to oversee home care. Not ideal…but likely safer than the status quo.

Hospice Helps You and Your Loved Ones Live Better

John Mastrojohn III, RN, MSN, MBA, executive vice president and chief operating officer of the National Hospice and Palliative Care Organization (NHPCO), NHPCO. org, the largest nonprofit membership organization representing hospice and palliative care programs and professionals in the US. To learn more about hospice, consult CaringInfo.org.

Everyone's life ends. But not everyone has the same quality of life at the end of life. Many are in pain or not comforted physically, emotionally or spiritually. Others die in a hospital when they would have wanted to die at home, surrounded by loved ones in a beloved place.

Yet sadly, countless individuals who could receive hospice care don't get it. Many don't even know it's an option. And among those who do use hospice, many take advantage of it only in the last week or two of life. But research shows that hospice can provide important benefits—and for a much longer period of time than just the final few days.

Scientific evidence: In a study published in *Journal of Clinical Oncology*, researchers from Harvard Medical School and two cancer centers talked with 2,307 family members of individuals who had died.

Results: When hospice was used, patients had more appropriate relief from pain, better symptom relief and higher-quality end-of-life care…they received care that was more in accordance with their wishes…and they were more likely to have died in a preferred place (usually at home, rather than in the hospital).

What you and your loved ones need to know about hospice care…

THE FACETS OF HOSPICE CARE

Even though most people assume that they know what hospice is, few can explain exactly when it's used in the course of an illness or how it works. Medicare, the main payer of hospice care, defines hospice as a system of care for people who have approximately six months or less to live if the disease runs its normal course. In order for a patient to elect hospice care, he/she must be certified as meeting the criteria described above by an attending physician and the hospice medical director. Over 90% of people in hospice receive care at home or in the place they reside.

Hospice care is delivered by a team of doctors, nurses, home-health aides, social workers, therapists, chaplains, counselors and trained volunteers. The care plan varies according to the patient's needs, but it is not around-the-clock care (except for in the rare cases when continuous home care is needed for a brief period of crisis, such as uncontrolled pain). For that reason, family caregivers are an integral part of the care team.

Managing the patient's pain and/or controlling symptoms is a priority, and hospice provides medication and medical equipment and supplies (such as a hospital bed and/or oxygen) for these purposes. During hospice care, curative treatment for the illness itself is discontinued. *In addition, hospice care…*

•**Provides emotional support to address the myriad feelings and issues affecting hospice patients and their families.** Spiritual support is also offered for those patients who choose it and can be delivered by the hospice and/or the patient's clergy or other faith leader.

•**Offers the surviving family bereavement care and counseling,** typically for 13 months following the death of a patient. These services include written materials, phone calls, visitation and support groups.

Important: Though the Medicare hospice benefit is the predominate payer of hospice services, managed care and private insurers will often cover hospice services.

DEBUNKING MYTHS

Common myths about hospice stop many people from getting the end-of-life care they need. *For example…*

MYTH #1: **Hospice mainly serves terminal cancer patients.** Only 37% of hospice patients have cancer. Other terminal diagnoses include dementia, heart disease, lung disease, stroke, kidney disease, liver disease, HIV/AIDS and others.

MYTH #2: **The doctor must bring up hospice.** Anybody can inquire about and refer to hospice—the patient, a family member, a counselor or the doctor. But only a physician can certify that a patient is eligible for hospice care.

MYTH #3: **The hospice patient can't keep his/her own doctor.** Hospice encourages a patient to keep his primary physician. The primary physician typically knows the patient best and can consult with the hospice medical director and other hospice team members to provide the best care. Patients may still visit their primary care physician if they choose.

MYTH #4: **Hospice care hastens death.** Hospice neither hastens nor postpones dying. Just as doctors and midwives lend support and expertise during the time of childbirth, hospice provides specialized knowledge and skill for patients and families at the end of life.

MYTH #5: **Hospice means giving up.** Hospice is not about hopelessness or giving up. For example, if a patient decides to seek curative care for any disease, he can revoke the hospice benefit at any time and return to curative therapy or even try a new therapy.

FINDING HOSPICE CARE

All hospices are licensed by the state in which they operate and certified by Medicare. But not all hospices are alike. In the US, 60% are independent…20% are part of a hospital system…16% are part of a home-health agency…and 4% are part of a nursing home. Hospices are both large and small, rural and urban, and range from for-profit national chains to local nonprofits.

To find a hospice program anywhere in the US: Use the National Hospice and Palliative Care Organization's "Find a Provider Tool" at:

Moments.nhpco.org/find-a-hospice. Once you (or the certifying doctor) contact the hospice, enrollment should happen quickly.

Helpful: Look for a hospice that is accredited by an independent accrediting organization, such as the Accreditation Commission for Health Care…the Community Health Accreditation Program…or The Joint Commission.

My advice: Have the conversation about end-of-life care with your loved ones early so you understand their wishes. If you decide that you want hospice care, once you've chosen the program, you'll have an initial consultation to develop a plan of care, typically with a hospice nurse.

If the patient is comfortable with the idea, I encourage not only the family caregiver (such as a spouse) but other family members (such as adult children) to attend the initial consultation. In that way, all those involved with the patient's care will hear the same information regarding hospice care and will have the opportunity to get their questions answered. This approach also helps the hospice nurse understand the patient's needs and develop a personalized plan of care.

A Love Letter to Your Family

Stanford Medicine Letter Project, Med.Stanford.edu/letter/friendsandfamily.html, reported by Rebecca Shannonhouse, editor, *Bottom Line Health*.

When thinking about what matters most in life, things like money and career can't compare with our successes close to home—a happy marriage…love for our children…etc.

Sadly, we don't always treasure our real blessings until later in life, when so many years have passed that it can feel too late to correct mistakes or make up for lost time. You can't change the past, but you can give your loved ones (and yourself) comfort and closure. The Stanford "Dear Friends and Family" Letter Project can help.

The project, created by researchers at Stanford University, has shown that nearly everyone can benefit when he/she completes seven

Do Not Rehash

Do not rehash problems with a teenager. Talking through a child's troubles can be helpful—but excessively revisiting them and asking numerous probing questions is counterproductive. That causes teens to relive their worries and feelings instead of getting past them. Parents should become aware of any tendency they themselves have to harp on problems or to discuss them repeatedly or at length. When conversations become overly focused on negative elements and come back to those negatives repeatedly, break the cycle by suggesting a distraction, such as taking a walk together.

Roundup of experts on parent-teen relationships, reported in *The Wall Street Journal*.

life-review tasks—acknowledging who has been important in your life…remembering special moments…apologizing to those you may have hurt…forgiving those who have hurt you…expressing gratitude for the love you've received…telling those close to you how much you've loved them…and saying good-bye at the end of life.

Once you've written a letter addressing these points, you can share it with your loved ones immediately…or put it away to be read after you're gone. Letter templates are available at Med.Stanford.edu/letter/friendsandfamily.html. There's a version to use if you're healthy and another if you have a chronic illness.

The letter won't be easy to write, but it could prove to be one of the most important things you ever do.

Smartphone Addiction Changes the Brain

Hyung Suk Seo, MD, professor of neuroradiology, Korea University, Seoul, and leader of a study presented at a recent meeting of the Radiological Society of North America.

Teenagers considered to be addicted to their phones and the Internet—based on a test of their usage habits—had an imbalance of brain chemicals similar to that seen in people experiencing anxiety and depression. They tended to say that Internet and smartphone addiction interfered with their daily activities, productivity, sleep and social lives...and they had significantly higher scores on scales of depression, anxiety, insomnia and impulsivity than teens whose test scores did not indicate addiction. The addicted teens had an overabundance of the neurotransmitter gamma-aminobutyric acid (GABA) in their brains' emotional control center. Addictive substances such as alcohol are already known to alter GABA levels.

Teenage Obesity Risk

Gilad Twig, PhD, MD, physician in the Medical Corps of the Israel Defense Forces and leader of a study published in *Cancer*.

Teenage obesity is linked to high risk for colon cancer later in life. A recent study that followed nearly 1.8 million people ages 16 to 19 for an average of 23 years found that those who were overweight or obese had an increased risk for colon and rectal cancers. Overweight or obese male teenagers had a 53% higher risk for colon cancer, and females had a 54% higher risk. Being obese increased the risk for rectal cancer in males by 71% and by 100% in females.

Hugging Babies Helps Their Brains Grow

Nathalie L. Maitre, MD, PhD, neonatologist and developmental specialist at Nationwide Children's Hospital, Columbus, Ohio, and leader of a study published in *Current Biology*.

Premature babies are less responsive to affection than babies born at full term—but all babies show stronger brain response when they are given more physical affection by parents or hospital staff. Researchers believe that continuing to hug and cuddle babies after they

come home from hospital care will confer additional benefits in brain development.

Acetaminophen and ADHD

Study of data on 112,973 children born between 1999 and 2009 by researchers at Norwegian Institute of Public Health, Oslo, published in *Pediatrics*.

In a recent finding, long-term use of the pain reliever *acetaminophen* during pregnancy—for 29 days or more—led to doubling the risk for attention deficit/hyperactivity disorder in children. But use for less than seven days was associated with decreased risk for ADHD. The study did not prove cause and effect, and much more research needs to be done. Acetaminophen, the active ingredient in Tylenol and other medicines, often is prescribed during pregnancy for women who have pain or fever.

Obesity Harms Young Livers

Jennifer Woo Baidal, MD, MPH, assistant professor of pediatrics, Columbia University Medical Center, New York City, and lead author of a study published in *The Journal of Pediatrics*.

Obesity harms the livers of eight-year-olds. A bigger waist circumference at age three raises the chance that by age eight, children will have indications of nonalcoholic fatty liver disease.

Football Before 12 Raises Brain-Injury Risk

Study of 214 former football players, average age 51, by researchers at Boston University, published in *Translational Psychiatry*.

Brain problems caused by tackle football are most likely when kids start playing before

171

age 12. Children who started before that age were twice as likely to have behavioral problems in adulthood, including apathy and cognitive difficulties, and three times as likely to have clinically elevated depression scores, as kids who started playing later.

A Pill That Can Eliminate Peanut Allergies

Study by researchers at Murdoch Children's Research Institute, Melbourne, Australia, published in *The Lancet Child & Adolescent Health*.

For 18 months, children with a peanut allergy were given a daily probiotic that contained *lactobacillus rhamnosus* and a peanut protein. Four years after the treatment ended, almost 70% of the children could eat peanuts without an allergic reaction.

Fido Helps Fight Allergies and Obesity

University of Alberta, UAlberta.ca.

Children who grow up in homes with dogs have more gut bacteria that protect against allergies and obesity than those in dog-free households.

Get the Right Pet Health Insurance

Frances Wilkerson, DVM, who has practiced veterinary medicine since 1992. She founded the independent website Pet-Insurance-University.com.

If you own a cat or dog, you don't mind shelling out for food and toys—but you probably aren't spending the average $40 a month that pet health insurance costs. Fewer than 1% of pets are insured.

Dental Care for Pets

Rub dogs' and cats' teeth daily with gauze if you cannot clean them with a toothbrush. It is important to clean pets' teeth—they have plaque buildup just as people's teeth do. Rubbing the teeth with a gauze pad on which you place a small dab of pet toothpaste can help loosen and remove plaque. Or you can try Maxi/Guard Oral Cleansing Wipes or Excel Medicated Dental Wipes, which are textured to create friction to remove plaque more efficiently.

Also helpful: For cats, Purina Pro Plan Dental Crunch Cat Snacks...for dogs, C.E.T. VeggieDent Chews.

Roundup of experts on pets' dental health, reported in *Better Homes & Gardens*.

Should you? Not necessarily. If you can dip into your emergency fund to pay for expensive care, you can pass on a policy. But routine surgery can cost $3,000, and newer advances in veterinary medicine to treat cancer, heart disease and other chronic illnesses can cost much more.

Best bet: Starting insurance when a dog is a puppy or a cat is a kitten. Since your pet is unlikely to have a preexisting condition, you won't be excluded for one. It's true that premiums often rise with age, but some insurers also offer discounts for annual renewals.

If your dog or cat is older or already has a health problem, your insurance options may be more restricted.

If you shop for pet insurance...

•**Accident/illness policies,** if your pet is eligible, are better than accident-only policies. Your pet is far more likely to need medical care for an illness.

•**Think twice before paying for "wellness" coverage.** This covers routine care, including annual exams and vaccinations. Check what your vet charges—it may be cheaper to pay for these out of pocket.

•**Make sure your policy covers these four things**—cancer...chronic disease (it should be continual coverage, not for just one policy year)…hereditary and congenital diseases…and medical conditions common to your pet's breed and species.

•**Compare policies carefully.** Research the underwriters' financial strength by checking A.M. Best's rating center (AMBest.com/home/ratings.aspx). It is free, but you must register.

Your premium will vary based on what you choose for the deductible (generally $100 to $1,000 per year), copay (generally 10% to 30% of the cost of services) and the total amount that your policy will reimburse, which can vary from $2,500 up to an unlimited amount.

Safely Carry a Dog or Cat

Joseph H. Kinnarney, DVM, immediate past president of the American Veterinary Medical Association. He is a practicing vet at the Reidsville Veterinary Hospital in Reidsville, North Carolina. ReidsvilleVet.com

Pet owners often lift their dogs and cats in ways that are uncomfortable or unsafe—for the pet and/or the owner. *What to do instead…*

•**Lifting and carrying a small dog.** Kneel or stoop facing one side of the dog. Reach over the dog with the arm that is toward the dog's back end, and then arrange that hand and forearm so that they are parallel to the dog's body, on the opposite side of the dog from your body. Position that hand under the dog's chest between its front legs. The rear legs of the dog should still be between your arm and your body. While holding the dog's chest, gently move your elbow toward your body, scooping up and supporting the dog's rear legs on your arm. Position your other hand along the side of the dog that's away from your body to prevent it from falling or scrambling away and/or to provide additional support to the animal's front end if necessary. If you ever played football, picture how your coach taught you to carry the ball.

Important: Periodically confirm that the dog's rear legs still are supported by your arm, not dangling, which is bad for the dog's spine. (It's fine if the front legs dangle.)

•**Lifting and carrying a larger dog.** If your dog is too big to be comfortably supported on one forearm, instead position the dog on a dog bed, blanket or stretcher and have several people carry this. (Or put the dog in a wagon that you can pull.)

•**When you have no choice but to lift a large dog by yourself, kneel facing one side of the dog.** Wrap one arm behind the dog's rear legs, and place that hand against the far side of the dog. Wrap your other arm around the dog's chest—right in front of the top of its front legs, not up by the throat. Scoop in and up so that the arm around the front end of the dog supports the chest as much as possible without forcing the front legs backward and the arm around the back end supports both the upper rear legs and hips. Some people instead lift the rear end of a large dog by placing one arm under the abdomen, in front of the rear legs. That's acceptable for quick lifts, but it's not preferred for extended carrying—it leaves the rear legs dangling, which places stress on the dog's spine.

•**Lifting and carrying a cat.** The small-dog directions are appropriate for cats as well. But when carrying a cat that's prone to scratching, also secure one of its front legs between the thumb and forefinger of your carrying hand and the other front leg between the forefinger and middle finger of your other hand so that the cat can't scratch you.

Best Way to Bring Home a Second Pet

Roundup of experts in pet care, reported in Health.

Introduce two dogs in neutral territory, such as a park—with both dogs on leashes—so that the first dog does not see the second as an intruder and competitor. Bring a new cat home in a carrier, and keep it for a few days in its own room with its own food and litter box. Spend extra time with your older pet when the new one arrives—use play and affection, not treats, which can make pets gain weight. Walk dogs one at a time, or ask a friend to come with you on walks so that each dog has its own human walking companion. If you have two dogs, feed them in different places in the house or across the room from each other until they adjust fully. If you have a cat and a dog, separate meals carefully—it is best to feed cats in areas dogs cannot reach, since cat food is too high in protein for dogs.

Dogs Really Do Understand People

Study of MRI scans of 13 dogs led by researchers at Eötvös Loránd University, Budapest, Hungary, published in *Science*.

When listening, dogs use brain regions analogous to those that humans use to understand what other people say. Dogs' brains show that they are truly happy only if the tone of voice associated with praise is matched by actual words of praise being spoken. As with humans, the right side of dogs' brains deals with emotion and the left side of the brain with processing meaning—and it is only when both sides agree that they are hearing praise that a dog shows true happiness.

Keep Your Dog Cool When the Weather Is Hot

Your Dog magazine.

Cooling vests come with gel packs that you put in the freezer and then insert into compartments on the vest. Summer boots circulate air around a dog's paws and help protect them against hot surfaces. Cooling mats are gel-infused—cooling action starts when the dog lies on the mat and can last three hours. Pet strollers are similar to baby strollers, but they are soft all around and have high protection on all four sides. They let your pet take a break in the shade and away from the hot pavement. Bike trailers attach to bicycles to let a dog ride safely behind the bike, enjoying a cool breeze.

CHAPTER 11

Food and Diet

"Forgotten" Disease-Fighting Greens

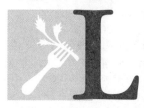

Leafy greens are the superstars of the vegetable brigade. Kale, widely considered the reigning king, is unusually high in calcium, magnesium and vitamin K…and, like other greens, is loaded with disease-fighting phytochemicals, such as lutein and vitamin C.

But let's be honest—kale's somewhat bitter taste isn't for everyone…and even if you love this veggie, you're probably not going to eat it every day. What other disease-fighting greens do you need in your diet?

TARGETED NUTRITION

Basic nutrition is just one reason that experts advise Americans to eat at least five servings of greens and other vegetables daily. But if you're concerned about specific medical conditions, research has shown that some leafy greens are particularly effective. *For example…*

•**Arugula and cancer.** Arugula is a peppery green with a sharp taste that adds a distinctive zip to otherwise bland salads. The pungent flavor has earned it the nickname "salad rocket."

The zesty flavor of arugula is largely due to its high concentration of sulfur-containing compounds. We think of arugula as a salad green, but it's actually a crucifer—in the same plant family as superfoods such as broccoli, cabbage and kale. Like other crucifers, it contains a group of anticancer compounds known as glucosinolates, which have detoxifying effects.

How arugula helps: Compounds in arugula, including sulforaphane and indole-3-carbinol, increase the body's excretion of a form of estrogen that has been linked to breast cancer. A Chinese study found that women who regularly ate a daily serving of cruciferous vegetables

Michael T. Murray, ND, a licensed naturopathic physician based in Paradise Valley, Arizona. Dr. Murray has published more than 30 books, including *Bottom Line's Encyclopedia of Healing Foods*, with coauthor Joseph Pizzorno, ND. DoctorMurray.com were 50% less likely to develop breast cancer. Another study found that just one weekly serving was enough to reduce cancer risk (including oral, colorectal and kidney malignancies).

Bonus: The sulforaphane in arugula has another benefit. It appears to help the body eliminate H. pylori, a bacterium that causes most peptic ulcers and greatly increases the risk for gastric cancer.

•Spinach and macular degeneration. As the US population ages, there's been a dramatic increase in age-related macular degeneration, a leading cause of blindness. Could a few weekly servings of spinach make a difference? There's good evidence that it might.

How spinach helps: Spinach is exceptionally high in lutein, a plant pigment that concentrates in the eyes and deflects damaging light from sunshine. Studies have found that people who consumed 6 mg of lutein daily—the amount in about one-half cup of cooked spinach—were 43% less likely to develop macular degeneration. Research published in *JAMA Ophthalmology* shows that people who consume generous amounts of lutein are also less likely to develop cataracts than those who eat less.

Important: Whether you prefer your spinach raw or cooked, be sure to have it with a little bit of oil or fat—a drizzle of olive oil is plenty—or a small amount of some other fat such as chopped nuts or avocado. Lutein is a fat-soluble nutrient, which means it is absorbed more efficiently when it's consumed with a little fat.

•Parsley and UTIs. Most people think of parsley as a colorful garnish—pretty to look at, but not much of a food. But around the world, parsley is found in tabbouleh, pesto (with or without basil) and other fragrant dishes…and it's a good green to eat if you get frequent urinary tract infections (UTIs).

About half of all women will eventually get a UTI…men get them, too, but less often. Patients with recurrent UTIs (defined as two separate infections within six months or three within one year) often depend on antibiotics—and resign themselves to the likely side effects of these drugs, such as diarrhea.

How parsley helps: It contains apigenin, a compound that acts as a diuretic and also has anti-inflammatory effects. According to a report in the journal *Case Reports in Medicine*, women who combined parsley with other herbal treatments (such as garlic) had an impressive decrease in urinary frequency and other symptoms—by 80%, in one case. Parsley's UTI-fighting effect is presumably because of apigenin's diuretic effect.

Another benefit: Reduced risk for cancer. Chlorophyll and other compounds in parsley have anticancer effects—including the ability to help inhibit the cancer-causing effects of fried foods.

Since parsley is so concentrated in nutrition and phytochemicals, just a few sprigs (or about one-quarter cup) consumed whenever possible provides exceptional health benefits. Chopped parsley can be added to salads, sauces, soups and grilled fish.

•Kale and osteoporosis. Kale's reputation as the king of veggies is based, in part, on its ability to promote bone health. People often think that milk is a great calcium source, but the absorption of calcium from kale and other leafy greens is actually higher—between 40% to 64%, compared with about 32% from milk.

And that's not all. In addition to being rich in calcium, kale also is an excellent source of vitamin K, a critical nutrient that helps anchor calcium into bone. One cup of raw kale supplies more than 600% of the recommended daily vitamin K intake. If you're concerned about bone health, you should definitely make an effort to eat more kale.

Another benefit: Improved heart health. Kale and other greens, as well as beets and celery, have been found to improve blood pressure and blood flow. While a high intake of fruit and vegetables is associated with healthy blood pressure and reduces risk for heart disease and stroke, kale and cruciferous vegetables are linked to even greater protection.

A good goal: Three to four servings of kale and other greens a week.

Important caveat: In normal amounts, kale is among the healthiest foods you can eat. But some people go overboard. Too much kale, like other cruciferous vegetables, can cause flatulence (gas) for many people. Eating too much raw kale (for example, more than three servings a week) can also interfere with the production of thyroid hormone, leading to the formation of a goiter. And because kale is such a rich source of vitamin K, anyone taking *warfarin* (Coumadin), an important anticlotting drug that interacts with this vitamin, should consult a doctor before eating kale or any leafy greens.

6 Best Foods for Your Skin

Torey Armul, MS, RD, CSSD, LD, a registered dietitian, nutritionist and national media spokesperson for the Academy of Nutrition and Dietetics. She is author of *Bun Appétit: A Simple Guide to Eating Right During Pregnancy.* Armul provides private counseling and consulting services in Columbus, Ohio. eatrightPRO.org

Want healthier skin and fewer wrinkles? Men and women can look younger and lower their risk for skin cancer, psoriasis, eczema and more by eating certain foods. *The following foods have been scientifically proven to boost the health, strength and appearance of your skin…*

YELLOW BELL PEPPERS

Yellow bell peppers are one of the most abundant sources of vitamin C. The body depends on vitamin C to form collagen, a protein that provides strength, support and elasticity to skin, hair, muscles and other tissues. Collagen also assists with cell regrowth and repair. As we age, our bodies produce less collagen, which can lead to reduced elasticity of the skin and more wrinkles.

The relationship between vitamin C and skin appearance was studied in more than 4,000 women in a report published in *The American Journal of Clinical Nutrition.* Researchers found that higher dietary intake of vitamin C was associated with lower likelihood of skin dryness and fewer wrinkles, as assessed by dermatologists. These results were independent of age, race, sun exposure, body mass index and physical activity.

Why not eat oranges, famous for their vitamin C, instead? A typical large orange contains 163% of the recommended daily value (DV) of vitamin C. That's good—but just half a yellow bell pepper contains nearly 300% of the DV of vitamin C. (Red and green peppers have less vitamin C than yellow ones but still are excellent sources.)

Eat yellow peppers raw to maximize the nutrient content. Vitamin C is sensitive to cooking and, as a water-soluble vitamin, leaches into cooking water. If you prefer to cook yellow peppers, keep the heat as low as possible for your recipe. Use the cooking juices, too (whenever possible), so that the vitamin C in the water is not wasted.

SWEET POTATOES

Sweet potatoes are an excellent source of carotenoids, the antioxidant pigments that give many foods their bright red, orange, yellow and green colors—and help keep skin cells healthy.

In a study published in *British Journal of Nutrition,* participants who ate more carotenoid-rich vegetables had significantly fewer facial wrinkles.

Eating carotenoids also can make you look healthier overall and more attractive to others. Carotenoid levels in skin contribute to healthy skin coloration. In fact, researchers from University of St. Andrews, Scotland, found that people whose faces were rated as healthy by others had consumed an average of 2.9 fruit and vegetable portions each day…and whose faces were rated separately as attractive had consumed 3.3 daily portions.

Carotenoids are fat-soluble, which means that they're better absorbed when paired with a fat-containing food—so sprinkle nuts or drizzle olive oil over your sweet potatoes for a delicious skin boost.

SALMON

Although protein in your food does not directly affect protein in your body's collagen, some research shows that amino acids (the building blocks of protein) are related to collagen synthesis in the skin.

Some amino acids are "essential," meaning that they're necessary for life but are not made in the body. They must be provided by food or supplements. Salmon contains all the essential amino acids—and essential amino acids play a unique role in skin health. In a study published in *Amino Acids*, researchers found that consuming a combination of essential amino acids significantly increased the rate of collagen synthesis in mice with UV-damaged skin.

Salmon also is a good source of monounsaturated fat, which was found to be positively associated with skin elasticity in older women in a study published in *British Journal of Nutrition*.

Don't love fish? Essential amino acids also are found in poultry, eggs, beans and whole grains.

WALNUTS

Walnuts are rich in omega-3 polyunsaturated fatty acids, which help the body make the collagen needed for healthy skin. Omega-3s help reduce inflammation and have been shown to reduce symptoms in inflammatory skin diseases such as psoriasis and acne.

The European Journal of Cancer published research comparing omega-3 fat intake to the development of malignant melanoma in more than 20,000 women. Data showed that higher intakes of omega-3s were associated with an 80% lower risk for skin cancer, leading researchers to conclude that these fats "have a substantial protective association" against melanoma.

Like essential amino acids, omega-3 fats are vitally important but are not made in the body. You must get them from your diet or supplements. Aside from walnuts (and salmon, discussed above), other excellent sources of omega-3s include flaxseed oil, ground flaxseed, chia seeds, canola oil and tofu.

RASPBERRIES AND POMEGRANATES

There is exciting research on collagen and how it is affected by ellagic acid, an antioxidant found in certain fruits and vegetables.

A study published in *Experimental Dermatology* found that mice who received ellagic acid had significantly reduced collagen breakdown from UV light, compared with mice who did not receive ellagic acid. The treatment group also developed fewer wrinkles. While most research focuses on the treatment of skin damage, this study was unique in its ability to show the role of nutrition in the prevention of collagen breakdown, wrinkles and skin damage.

Foods that are high in ellagic acid include raspberries and pomegranates (as well as blackberries, strawberries and cranberries).

CHICKPEAS

Zinc is an important ingredient for skin health because it supports the regeneration of new skin cells. The benefits are most apparent with skin repair and wound healing, but zinc also may be able to help with other skin problems such as rashes, eczema and acne.

A study published in *BioMed Research International* found a correlation between participants' zinc levels and the severity of their acne symptoms. Researchers believe that this is partly due to zinc's ability to inhibit the overgrowth of Propionibacterium acnes, a bacterium that contributes to acne.

Legumes were the focus of another study in *The Journal of the American College of Nutrition*. Researchers found that higher intakes of legumes, such as chickpeas, appeared to protect against sun-induced wrinkles in people with a variety of ethnic and geographic backgrounds.

Chickpeas are a good source of zinc, as are other beans, oysters, poultry, tofu, oatmeal and zinc-fortified cereals.

Better Than Drugs: Berries Are So Powerful Even Scientists Are Stunned

Bill Gottlieb, CHC, a health coach certified by the American Association of Drugless Practitioners and former editor in chief of Rodale Books and Prevention Magazine Health Books. He is author of 16 health books including Speed Healing, *published by Bottom Line Inc. BillGottliebHealth.com*

If you were asked to make a list of "superfoods"—nutrient-loaded foods that effectively fight disease—you'd probably include items such as kale, beans, walnuts, broccoli, green tea, wild-caught salmon...and berries.

What few people realize: As a superfood, berries—blueberries, strawberries, raspberries, blackberries, cranberries and the like—are in a class by themselves. They can be more health-giving than medications or supplements, according to experts at Harvard Medical School and Harvard T.H. Chan School of Public Health. The antioxidants in berries—anthocyanins, the compounds that give these fruits their lustrous colors—deliver a pure dose of prevention and healing to the brain, heart and every other system and cell in the body. And you don't have to eat a bushelful to get the benefits.

Here's what you need to know about the amazing power of berries…

BERRIES AND YOUR BRAIN

For more than a decade, scientists at the Jean Mayer USDA Human Nutrition Research Center on Aging at Tufts University have been studying the effect of berries on the brain—in cells and in laboratory animals. They have found that regular ingestion of blueberries, strawberries and/or blackberries can help improve "plasticity," the ability of brain cells to form new connections with one another…generate new brain cells…stop inflammation and oxidation from damaging brain cells…ease the destructive effect of stress on the brain…prevent and reverse age-related memory loss, particularly short-term, or "working," memory…and protect against amyloid-beta, the plaques in the brain that cause Alzheimer's disease. Now research has shown that blueberries can help rejuvenate the aging human brain…

Startling new findings: The researchers from Tufts studied 37 people, ages 60 to 75, dividing them into two groups—one group consumed one ounce of freeze-dried blueberries every day (the equivalent of one cup of fresh blueberries)…the other a blueberry placebo. At the beginning, middle and end of the three-month study, the participants took tests measuring learning and memory. By the end of the study, those in the blueberry group had a 20% improvement in their scores on a memory test compared with those in a placebo group.

Strawberries are good, too. The Tufts researchers gave participants either freeze-dried strawberry powder (the equivalent of two cups of fresh strawberries) or a placebo. After three months of daily intake, the strawberry group had much greater improvements in memory than the placebo group.

What to do: Eat one cup of blueberries or strawberries daily, either fresh or frozen. Choose organic. Every year, the Environmental Working Group announces its "Dirty Dozen," a list of the produce with the most pesticides. In 2017, strawberries topped the list and blueberries ranked number 17.

BERRIES AND YOUR HEART

Hundreds of studies show that anthocyanins battle oxidation and inflammation, the evil twins of chronic disease—including heart disease. *Berries can…*

• **Reduce high blood pressure**—the number-one risk factor for heart attack and stroke. Researchers from Florida State University studied 48 postmenopausal women with high blood pressure, giving them either one-third cup of freeze-dried blueberry powder daily or a placebo. After two months, the women getting the blueberry powder had a drop in systolic blood pressure (the upper number in a blood pressure reading) of 5.1% and a drop in diastolic blood pressure (the lower reading) of 6.3%—decreasing the risk for heart attack and stroke. Their arteries were also more flexible. There were no changes in the placebo group.

• **Reduce other risk factors for heart disease.** The cranberry is no slouch when it comes to guarding the heart. Scientists from the USDA's Human Nutrition Research Center studied 56 people, average age 50. Half drank two eight-ounce glasses of no-sugar-added cranberry juice daily…the other half made no changes to their diets. After two weeks, the scientists measured several risk factors for heart disease. Those drinking the juice had lower levels of C-reactive protein (CRP), a biomarker for heart-damaging inflammation…lower levels of triglycerides, a heart-hurting blood fat…and lower levels of blood sugar.

Bottom line: More berries, fewer heart attacks. In a study published in *Circulation*, researchers examined 18 years of health data from 93,600 women and found that those who ate three or more servings of blueberries and strawberries per week (one serving is one-half cup) had a 34% lower risk for heart attack, compared with women who ate them less than three times weekly.

What to do: If you have heart disease or any risk factors for heart disease (high blood pressure, high LDL cholesterol, high blood sugar, high CRP, a family history of heart disease), eat three cups of blueberries or strawberries per week.

BERRIES AND CANCER

Cellular research and animal research have shown that berries can fight just about every kind of cancer. *Example:* A scientific paper recently published by researchers from the Medical College of Wisconsin in Antioxidants shows that cranberries can help fight 17 different cancers, including bladder, blood, brain, breast, colon, esophageal, oral, prostate and stomach cancers.

But the real test of berries' anticancer power is whether berries can help people with cancer. Research published in 2016 shows that they can…

•**Oral cancer.** Researchers at The Ohio State University Comprehensive Cancer Center gave lozenges of freeze-dried black raspberry powder (which contains very high levels of anthocyanins) to people with oral cancer for two weeks. Analyzing the tumors, they found that several genetic markers of cancer severity—prosurvival genes and proinflammatory genes—were significantly reduced by up to 21%.

In an earlier study, researchers at University of North Carolina and three other universities gave a "bioadhesive" black raspberry gel or a placebo to 40 people with premalignant oral lesions (neoplasia), which often progress to oral cancer. After four months, the lesions of those using black raspberry had shrunk in size and were less likely to advance to cancer.

•**Colon cancer.** In several studies on colon cancer at the National Cancer Institute and other institutions, daily intake of 60 grams of black raspberry powder (the equivalent of 15 servings of black raspberries) reversed dozens of biomarkers of the disease. These studies showed that the powder can kill cancer cells, block the growth of new blood vessels to tumors (angio-genesis), kill cancer cells (apoptosis) and stop cancer cells from dividing and growing (proliferation).

What to do: If you are at risk for oral or colon cancer…or are being treated for one of those diseases…or are a survivor of any of them—talk with your doctor about adding black raspberry powder to a daily smoothie. (You could never eat enough black raspberries to get the cancer-reversing effect.)

Good product: Freeze-dried black raspberry powder from BerriHealth (BerriHealth.com).

For preventing cancer, eat five or more servings of fruits and vegetables every day—including berries.

Need an Energy Boost? These 5 Foods Do the Trick

Lisa Young, PhD, RD, CDN, a nutritionist in private practice and an adjunct professor of nutrition at New York University in New York City. She is author of *The Portion Teller Plan.* PortionTeller.com

Hitting a wall at 3 pm—even though you had a full night's sleep? Your first instinct may be to reach for a cup o' joe or a sugary treat just to keep you going.

Why this is a mistake: It's common for our blood sugar levels to drop in the late afternoon, making us feel tired and hungry. But the mind-buzzing, heart-racing effects of so-called quick fixes soon lead to a crash-and-burn, putting us right back where we started.

WHAT WORKS BETTER

Once you accept that quick fixes are really nothing more than "fool's gold," you can embrace the true source of sustained vitality—energy-producing real foods.

What you need to know: Often it is not a single ingredient itself that invigorates but how that powerhouse is combined with flavorful and nutritionally satisfying add-ons.

Rule of thumb: The best foods for natural all-day vibrancy typically balance a complex carbohydrate with a healthy fat and a punch of protein—a combination that takes longer to digest and stabilizes blood sugar levels for hours.

For advice on the best foods to eat for all-day energy, we spoke with leading nutritionist Lisa Young, PhD, RD, CDN, to learn about her top choices for maintaining day-long vim and vigor…

AVOCADO

Avocado contains heart-healthy monounsaturated fat and provides nearly 20 vitamins and minerals.

My favorite way to eat avocado: Sliced or smashed on whole-grain toast. In addition to being a perfect base for creamy avocado, whole-grain toast boasts its own benefits and makes for a great energy-boosting combo—it fills you up with fiber and is low in saturated fat.

CANNED SALMON

What's easier than peeling back the lid on a ready-to-serve portion of this versatile, tasty fish? Especially when two ounces of canned salmon contain just 90 calories and only 1 g of saturated fat in a convenient protein source. *Note:* To reduce possible toxins, I recommend wild salmon sold in a BPA-free can.

My favorite way to eat canned salmon: On salad greens topped with heart-smart olive oil and a side of polenta. Cornmeal-based polenta, which is loaded with complex carbs to keep blood sugar levels stable for hours, even comes in ready-made refrigerated tubes. You can cook up a slice or two in just minutes on the stove or in the oven!

FARMER'S CHEESE

Protein-packed foods such as farmer's cheese—born from farmers' efforts to use milk left over after cream is skimmed for butter—can help you stay on top of your game. Two tablespoons of farmer's cheese offer 4 g of protein with only 2.5 g of fat and 40 calories.

My favorite way to eat farmer's cheese: On Ezekiel 4:9 bread with cinnamon and/or fresh walnuts on top. You can spread farmer's cheese, with its ricotta-like texture, on Ezekiel bread—itself an efficient protein source as well as a unique blend of six grains and legumes. A dash of cinnamon not only adds the yin-yang of sweet and savory, but also helps control blood sugar levels. A few diced walnuts provide satisfying crunch and omega-3 fats that promote cardiovascular health.

QUINOA

Quinoa (pronounced "keen-wah") contains iron, B vitamins, magnesium, calcium, potassium and other nutrients, boasting zero saturated or trans fats. Even better, it takes only about 15 minutes to prepare.

My favorite way to eat quinoa: With chopped veggies and garnished with chickpeas. By topping with chickpeas, you'll boost the overall protein, vitamin and mineral content—and stay fuller longer. Or you can try a quinoa-based hot cereal.

SORGHUM

Sorghum, a substantial source of protein and dietary fiber, is a versatile, gluten-free grain that keeps your belly full and your energy levels high.

My favorite way to eat sorghum: In a tomato and red pepper slaw. *To prepare:* After simmering and draining your desired amount of sorghum, add some color by folding in a julienned slaw of tomatoes and red peppers.

Tomatoes, with their energy-boosting carbs and fiber, are also a major source of the anticancer nutrient lycopene…while red peppers aid in the absorption of iron from food, which boosts energy by promoting optimal blood oxygen levels.

How to Liven Up Your Grilling

Janet Bond Brill, PhD, RDN, FAND, is a registered dietitian nutritionist. She is the author of *Blood Pressure DOWN, Cholesterol DOWN* and *Prevent a Second Heart Attack.* DrJanet.com

You may not realize it, but that outdoor grilling you do on the weekend can be healthier than you might think. Unfor-

Vegetables: Cooked vs. Raw

All forms of cooking can destroy some nutrients (such as vitamin C and B vitamins) in vegetables. But the flip side is that some nutrients actually become more bioavailable after cooking, since cooking helps release the nutrients from the cell walls of the plant. These include lycopene (in tomatoes and red peppers) and beta-carotene (in carrots, spinach and kale). Mushrooms, asparagus and cabbage all supply more antioxidant compounds when cooked.

Vitamin B-6 and folate in broccoli and the polyphenols in onions that help protect against cancer and cardiovascular disease are better preserved in raw vegetables.

Sharon Palmer, RDN, author of *Plant-Powered for Life*, Duarte, California. SharonPalmer.com

tunately, most people douse their grilled food with sugar-spiked BBQ sauce and/or ultra-high-sodium seasonings.

My favorite grilling secret: Use vitamin C–rich fruits, such as limes and strawberries, to give your grilled food a burst of flavor. Vitamin C is a powerful antioxidant that promotes healthy skin, boosts the immune system and decreases inflammation. *Four tips for healthier grilling…*

•**Go fish!** Instead of the charred meat that scientists now believe can increase one's cancer risk, opt for an ultra-lean protein source—such as a super-low-calorie "white fish" fillet. This quick-cooking, mildly flavored fish isn't linked to the same cancer risk as charred meat and generally isn't very expensive. Popular kinds of white fish are tilapia, cod, bass, grouper, haddock, catfish and snapper.

•**Get a veggie fix.** Grilling is a great way to squeeze out mouthwatering flavor from plain vegetables. Instead of bell peppers and onions, go for something a bit more unusual such as asparagus, zucchini and brussels sprouts. Grill the veggies until tender and very lightly charred.

•**Keep it simple with seasonings.** For fish, simply squeeze on some fresh lime juice and drizzle with a touch of extra-virgin olive oil. For vegetables, slather on a mixture of extra-virgin olive oil and a good aged balsamic vinegar.

•**Add salsa.** A vitamin C–rich strawberry salsa is perfect on grilled fish.

Try the recipes below for a delicious and nutritious summer meal…

Lime-Grilled Fish with Strawberry Salsa

1 Tablespoon extra-virgin olive oil
1 Tablespoon fresh lime juice
4 firm, white-fleshed, mild fish fillets (1 pound total)
1 cup strawberry salsa (see recipe below)
1 lime, cut into 4 wedges

Directions: Coat your grill with vegetable oil spray. Then preheat on high for 10 minutes. (*Caution*: It's dangerous to coat a hot grill.) Combine the olive oil and lime juice, and brush onto the fish. Grill four to five inches from the heat source until the fish is opaque (you may want to use a fish grilling basket)—about five minutes, depending on the thickness of the fish. Avoid charring as much as possible, adjusting the heat as needed. Serve immediately, topped with salsa (see below) and fresh lime slices. Makes four servings (each serving is one fish fillet, about 3.5 ounces, with one-quarter cup of salsa).

Seasonal Strawberry Salsa

1 pint fresh strawberries, chopped
1 small red onion, chopped
1 cup tomatillos or green tomatoes, chopped (approximately four tomatillos or tomatoes)
¼ cup fresh cilantro, minced
1 jalapeño, seeded, minced
1 fresh lime (zest it, then squeeze about 2 Tablespoons of juice)

Directions: Mix all the ingredients. Spoon onto cooked fish, and serve immediately or refrigerate until ready to serve. Makes 16 one-quarter-cup servings.

Nutritional information per serving for fish with strawberry salsa (based on using tilapia): Calories, 160…fat, 5 g…cholesterol, 55 mg…carbohydrates, 6 g…dietary fiber, 1 g…protein, 23 g…sodium, 350 mg.

Healthier Grilling

Alice Bender, RDN, head of nutrition programs, American Institute for Cancer Research, Washington, DC.

Grilling meat, poultry and fish at high temperatures can lead to the formation of two types of potential carcinogens, polycyclic aromatic hydrocarbons (PAH) and heterocyclic amines (HCA).

A healthier option: Create your meal with grilled vegetables and fruit. Because they require a lot less grill time, fewer PAHs are formed. Cut veggies, such as portobello mushrooms, eggplant or zucchini, into chunks for kabobs, cook in a grill basket or grill whole. Brush with olive oil or marinade to prevent sticking. Choose fruit that is a day away from being ripe so that it will hold up on the grill. Watch closely, as fruit and veggies generally cook quickly. Try apples, pineapples or peaches.

Get the Right Dose

Michael Holick, MD, PhD, professor of medicine, physiology and biophysics, Boston University School of Medicine, and the author of *The Vitamin D Solution.*

Vitamin D dosage depends on many factors, including sun exposure, diet and body weight. Most Americans are deficient in this important vitamin, which helps the body absorb calcium and may protect against osteoporosis, cancer and hypertension. Vitamin D is found in fortified milk, oily fish and eggs, but it is difficult to get adequate amounts from diet alone. Timed, unprotected sun exposure will help your body produce vitamin D—you can calculate your needs with the free D Minder Pro app.

Supplements also are a good choice, especially for people who do not get enough natural sun exposure. I take 4,000 international units (IU) of vitamin D a day. People who are obese (with a body mass index of 30 or greater) need more vitamin D than a normal-weight person, as the vitamin is diluted by fat. A 1,000 IU dose is inadequate unless you are getting enough sun exposure and consume foods high in vitamin D.

You Say Tomato, I Say Lycopene!

Janet Bond Brill, PhD, RDN, FAND, is a registered dietitian nutritionist. She is author of *Blood Pressure DOWN, Cholesterol DOWN* and *Prevent a Second Heart Attack.* DrJanet.com

Tomatoes are the second-most popular "vegetable" (botanically speaking, they're a fruit) in the world. That's great, because there are so many wonderful health benefits to reap from tomatoes' disease-fighting plant chemicals—especially from the powerhouse nutrient lycopene, which gives tomatoes their deep red color. Lycopene also is a powerful antioxidant that protects against free radicals—the destructive molecules that disrupt cells and contribute to premature aging, tissue damage and many degenerative diseases. *Five key facts about lycopene…*

•**Cancer protection.** Research has found that lycopene helps protect against certain types of cancer, including prostate, lung and stomach cancers.

•**Cardio protection.** Lycopene is especially effective at guarding against cardiovascular disease. A meta-analysis of 25 studies found that high lycopene consumption (about two tomatoes or one-half cup of tomato sauce daily) was associated with a 26% reduction in stroke risk, a 37% reduction in death from all causes and a 14% reduction in cardiovascular disease.

•**Tomatoes = lycopene.** While many foods, including guava, watermelon, papaya, apricots and pink grapefruit, are rich in lycopene, more than 80% of the dietary lycopene consumed in the US comes from tomato products.

•**Color matters.** For the highest lycopene content, choose red, dark purple and black tomatoes over yellow ones. These deep-colored tomatoes contain much more lycopene.

•**Cook your tomatoes.** Cooking breaks down cells where the lycopene is stored so that more of it is available to be absorbed by your body. Processing and condensing tomatoes, such as for tomato paste, also concentrates the lycopene content—think pasta or pizza sauce.

Cooked cherry tomatoes are an especially easy way to get more tomatoes into your daily fare. I slice them and sauté them with garlic and fresh basil in extra-virgin olive oil for a simple pasta sauce or topping for fish. Cooked tomatoes go well with flatbread creations…and, of course, caprese salad topped with a sweet balsamic glaze is another delicious way to eat tomatoes. To get the most health benefits from lycopene, try to eat tomatoes every day.

To help you do that, try this flavorful recipe. Extra-virgin olive oil enhances lycopene absorption and adds its own antioxidant boost.

Roasted Tomatoes with Garlic

Yield: 8 servings, about one-half cup each.

2 pounds plum tomatoes (preferably organically grown)

4 garlic cloves, cut lengthwise into slivers

1 teaspoon salt

½ teaspoon freshly ground black pepper

2 Tablespoons extra-virgin olive oil

Drizzle of balsamic reduction glaze

½ cup chopped fresh basil (for garnish)

Preheat oven to 450°F, with rack in center position. Lightly oil a shallow baking pan. Cut tomatoes in half crosswise, and arrange cut side up in the pan. Stud each tomato half with slivers of garlic, then sprinkle with salt and pepper. Drizzle tomatoes evenly with olive oil and balsamic reduction glaze. Roast until soft and wilted, about 20 minutes. Remove from oven, garnish with fresh basil and serve warm. Yum!

A Green Light for Red Meat, but Skip the Franks

Study titled, "Association between Dietary Factors and Mortality from Heart Disease, Stroke, and Type 2 Diabetes in the United States," by Renata Micha, RD, PhD, Tufts Friedman School of Nutrition Science and Policy in Boston, Massachusetts, and colleagues, published in *JAMA*.

We all know that eating too many hot dogs and too few salads isn't a healthy thing. But which food choices make the most difference in whether we'll be cut down by the big killers—heart disease, stroke and diabetes?

Skipping bologna, bacon, hot dogs and other cured meats is the best move, it turns out. But eating steak occasionally? Pretty safe, according to new research.

Background: A zillion studies have looked at relationships between specific foods and nutrients and the risks for specific diseases. But there hasn't been enough research into the big picture. Which foods and nutrients play the biggest roles? Investigators created a way to figure that out.

Study: Tufts University started with major dietary guidelines to determine optimal amounts of 10 key nutrients and/or foods. Then they used high-quality diet/health studies to create a statistical risk model capable of determining the portion of deaths from cardiometabolic disease—those due to heart disease, stroke or type 2 diabetes—that could be prevented if people followed those recommendations.

Results: Overall, a suboptimal diet was related to nearly half—45%—of deaths due to heart disease, stroke and/or diabetes. Not surprisingly, if people followed dietary guidelines to eat enough fruits, vegetables, seafood rich in omega-3 fats and whole grains—while skipping sugar-sweetened beverages—death rates from those diseases would drop significantly. But the biggest contributors to increased mortality were actually consuming too much sodium, too few nuts and seeds and processed meats.

Eating unprocessed meat—beef, chicken, pork—was relatively insignificant. In fact, over the period that these studies covered, even people who had a high consumption of unprocessed red meat such as beef and pork increased their risk of dying from the three cardiometabolic diseases by only 0.4%. While the lowest risk was associated with a daily maximum of no more than one-half ounce a day—one 3½-ounce portion a week—eating more than this, even a lot more, didn't substantially increase risk in this study.

Processed meats were much bigger dangers. People who ate a diet high in processed meats—defined as meats preserved by smoking, curing, salting or adding chemicals, including bacon, salami, sausages, hot dogs and deli/luncheon meats—faced an 8% increased risk for death. While those who ate the most processed meat were at higher risk than those who ate less, the researchers note that the ideal amount of processed meats for longevity is…none.

The same goes for sugar-sweetened beverages—less is better, but none is best.

Here are all the numbers showing which eating habits—either eating too much or too little of certain foods—seemed to lead to cardiometabolic death…

WHAT FOODS AND BEVERAGES RAISE YOUR RISK

You'll increase your risk of dying from cardiometabolic disease by…

5%…if you consume too much sodium. (*Goal*: Less than 2,000 mg a day).

5%…if you eat too few nuts and seeds. (*Goal*: At least two ounces of nuts/seeds a day).

2%…if you eat too much processed meat. (*Goal*: None.)

6%…if you eat too few vegetables. (*Goal*: At least four servings a day.)

5%…if you eat too little fruit. (*Goal*: At least three servings a day.)

4%…if you consume too little omega-3-rich seafood. (*Goal*: Enough to supply an average of 250 mg of omega-3 fatty acids a day. That's about one 3½-ounce serving of salmon a week.)

4%…if you drink a lot of sugar-sweetened beverages. (*Goal*: Drink none.)

9%…if you eat too few whole grains. (*Goal*: At least 4½ ounces a day).

4%…if you eat too much unprocessed red meat. (*Goal*: No more than 3½ ounces a week.)

Red Meat's Link to Disease

Red meat is linked to more than just heart disease. People who ate the most red meat had the highest risk of dying from cancer, heart disease, stroke, respiratory disease, diabetes, infections, chronic kidney disease and chronic liver disease. People who consumed more than five ounces per day of red meat had a 26% increased risk of dying during the study, versus those who ate less than five ounces per week.

Study of nearly 537,000 adults led by researchers at the US National Institutes of Health, Bethesda, Maryland, published in *The BMJ*.

Surprising finding: Over the 10 years of the study (2002 to 2012), Americans have been eating better—more nuts and seeds, whole grains, fruits and polyunsaturated fats and fewer sugar-sweetened beverages.

Bottom line: A study such as this cannot prove cause and effect, but it most likely helps us figure out which diet changes are most likely to improve our health. One key take-away is the importance of eating healthful foods more frequently—not just eating unhealthful foods less frequently. To be sure, watching sodium and skipping processed meats is a good idea, but eating more "good" stuff is at least as powerful a way to protect your health.

Soy: Superfood or Scapegoat?

Janet Bond Brill, PhD, RDN, FAND, is a registered dietitian nutritionist, a fellow of the Academy of Nutrition and Dietetics and a nationally recognized nutrition, health and fitness expert who specializes in cardiovascular disease prevention. Based in Allentown, Pennsylvania, Dr. Brill is author of Blood Pressure DOWN, Cholesterol DOWN *and* Prevent a Second Heart Attack. *DrJanet.com*

O ver the last decade or so, soy has gone from superfood to scapegoat as health pros debate its potential health benefits, including heart disease prevention. Given all this back and forth, you may wonder if this food is still worth eating.

The short answer: Yes, as long as you stick to largely unprocessed whole foods, such as tofu, edamame, tempeh, soy nuts and soy milk, and skip the more highly processed ones—think soy hot dogs, burgers and protein bars. The problem with highly processed soy foods is that they contain additives such as sodium, fillers and preservatives used to extend shelf life. Others contain only isolated soy protein, so you lose the benefits of whole soy. *Here's why soy should still be part of your diet…*

•**It's a healthy alternative to red meat.** All beans provide protein, but soybeans are exceptional. One-half cup of cooked soybeans provides 15 g of high-quality protein—double the amount found in other legumes. Like animal protein, soy contains all the essential amino acids in just the right proportion. It's also packed with fiber, phytochemicals, good fats such as omega-3s and lots of vitamins and minerals—ingredients that are often lacking in some animal proteins. You can toss soybeans in a salad to add crunch, use them instead of chickpeas for hummus or add them to quinoa as a tasty side dish.

•**It contributes to heart health.** While no single food can reduce your risk, eating a mostly plant-based diet that includes healthy fat and is rich in fiber and phytochemicals (this could include soy, copious amounts of fresh fruits and vegetables, nuts and extra-virgin olive oil)… working out at least 30 minutes a day…and not smoking can improve your cardiovascular health.

•**It is widely consumed in countries with lower rates of chronic disease.** No matter what the studies say, many scientists believe that high soy consumption explains why many Asian countries, where soy has long been a major staple, have lower rates of heart disease, cancer, stroke, osteoporosis and diabetes compared with the US.

So do your heart a favor and keep eating soy—starting with this recipe…

Curried Roasted Cauliflower and Tofu over Brown Rice

This quick and easy recipe is a perfect way to incorporate soy into a delicious heart-healthy dish…

- 1 container extra-firm tofu (14 ounces), drained and cut into one-inch cubes
- 1 fresh head cauliflower, cut into small pieces
- 3 Tablespoons extra-virgin olive oil
- 3 Tablespoons curry powder
- 1 teaspoon ground ginger
- 1 teaspoon ground cumin
- 1 teaspoon salt
- 1 large Vidalia onion, halved and sliced
- 2 Tablespoons currants
- 2 cups cooked brown rice (or quinoa)

What to do: Preheat the oven to 400°F. In a large bowl, combine the tofu with the cauliflower and one tablespoon of olive oil. Heat two tablespoons of olive oil in a skillet over medi-

um-high heat. Add the curry, ginger, cumin and salt and stir until blended. Add the onion and stir until light brown. Add the currants and onion mixture to the large bowl and toss with the tofu and cauliflower until they are well coated. Spread the mixture on a baking sheet. Bake, stirring occasionally, for 40 minutes. Serve over brown rice or quinoa. *Yield*: 4 servings.

Get Pesticides Off Apples

To remove pesticide residue from conventionally grown apples, mix one teaspoon of baking soda in two cups of water, submerge the apples in a bowl with a cover for two minutes, then rinse.

Even better: Buy organic.

Study by researchers at University of Massachusetts and Massachusetts Pesticide Analysis Laboratory, both in Amherst, published in *Journal of Agriculture and Food Chemistry.*

---

8 "Forever" Foods Every Healthy Kitchen Needs

Torey Armul, MS, RD, CSSD, a spokesperson for the Academy of Nutrition and Dietetics, counsels clients on sports nutrition, weight management and family/prenatal nutrition through her private practice in Columbus, Ohio.

When are you most likely to order take-out food? If you're like many people, it's when you're low on groceries at home. Keep your cabinets and your freezer stocked with these eight staples, and you'll never be without a fast but healthy meal.

FROZEN SHRIMP

If you're out of fresh meat, you'll get a convenient protein-rich alternative with frozen shrimp. They're a good source of B vitamins and iron, which can help boost your metabolism and keep you feeling your best. Because of their smaller size, frozen shrimp also can be easier to cook and prepare than frozen beef, pork or chicken.

In fact, you can save yourself a step by buying precooked shrimp. That way you just need to reheat them and season as desired. Thaw the shrimp in a bowl of hot water for three to five minutes and remove the tails. Next, season with olive oil and dried herbs and spices, such as chipotle chili pepper, garlic powder or basil. Reheat for just a few minutes on the stovetop, in the oven or on the grill. Shrimp can be served by itself or added to rice, pasta, tortillas, tacos or salad.

FROZEN BROCCOLI

Vegetables are one of the first foods to spoil in every grocery haul. Don't let that be a reason to skip your veggies! Fruits and vegetables should make up half of what we eat, although few Americans are meeting this recommended daily intake. Once your stash of fresh veggies runs out, frozen makes an excellent substitute. They are packaged at the peak of freshness, which means that they retain their nutritional content. Some frozen veggies taste more like fresh than others—that includes broccoli, which also is especially nutritious. Not a fan of broccoli? Always keep on hand frozen cauliflower, peas, green beans, asparagus, brussels sprouts or a frozen vegetable "medley" that you like.

Easy one-pot dinner: Add your favorite frozen vegetables to a pasta pot a few minutes before the pasta is finished cooking. (Don't worry, the vegetables won't make the pasta too cold.) Then drain the pasta and vegetables together and serve. Easy!

TUNA PACKETS

Tuna packets are another convenient source of protein, with the addition of heart-healthy omega-3 fats. They're ready in an instant, but unlike cans, they don't require draining (the nutritional content is similar to that of canned tuna, however). Packaged tuna has a long shelf life, making it a pantry prerequisite when your other options are limited.

Branch out from plain tuna with flavored tuna packets, such as lemon pepper, hot buffalo style, sweet and spicy (my favorite!) and sun-dried tomato and basil. They add taste and variety to your meal without adding too much additional sodium or calories. I use flavored tuna packets to spice up my usual sandwiches, salads and pasta dishes.

CANNED SOUP

Canned soup gets a bad rap for containing too much salt, fat, sugar, preservatives…or all of the above. I still recommend it because it can be a full, balanced meal. The trick is to buy only soups that aren't loaded with unhealthy ingredients. The best soups are broth- or vegetable-based (such as butternut squash, tomato, minestrone or chicken noodle) rather than cream-based. Look for soups labeled "low sodium," which means that they contain 140 mg or less of sodium per serving. "Reduced sodium" indicates only that the soup has less sodium than the original version, so it may not be low in salt after all. While you're comparing labels, choose the soup with less saturated fat (2 grams or less) and more fiber (2 grams or more) per serving.

You also can bulk up a can of soup by adding frozen vegetables, canned beans, leftover rice, packaged tuna or really any healthy food you have around.

Here's another kitchen hack: Canned soup makes a ready-made sauce. Some of my favorite soups to use as sauce are butternut squash, chunky tomato, Italian-style wedding and lentil vegetable. Just add the soup to cooked rice, pasta, quinoa, poultry or fish for a delicious sauce that's ready in seconds. Low-sodium varieties will help to moderate your daily sodium intake.

CANNED CHICKPEAS

Beans are one of the most underrated foods at the store. They are cheap yet remarkably nutritious, loaded with plant-based protein and fiber. Chickpeas, also known as garbanzo beans, are an excellent source of iron, folate, phosphorus and manganese. They are exceptionally convenient and versatile. Eat them plain, with a dash of salt and pepper or mixed into your meal. Enjoy them warm or cold. Mash them to create a creamy hummuslike appetizer or to complement a main dish.

While you're stocking up on chickpeas, grab some canned lentils, black beans and kidney beans, too. They share a similar nutritional profile and can be seamlessly added to soups, salads, rice bowls, tacos and omelets.

MICROWAVABLE RICE

There is no faster meal-starter than a packet of microwavable rice. It's ready in just 90 seconds, and the brown and wild rice varieties are major sources of fiber. Rice is a healthy base for a variety of Asian and Mexican dishes, or it can add flavor and nutrition to traditional soups and salads. Should you worry about arsenic levels in rice? Not if you eat a variety of whole grains and practice good portion control.

You do pay for the convenience of microwavable rice, however. I wait for sales to stock up on the microwavable packages.

WHOLE-WHEAT PASTA

Dried pasta will last for a year or more in your pantry, making it a healthy choice when you're out of fresher foods. It's ready in minutes and can be a delicious way to add nutrients to your meal. Most people think of pasta as a carbohydrate-rich indulgence rather than a nutritious meal choice. However, it all comes down to choosing the right kind and watching your portion size.

Buy 100% whole-wheat pasta—meaning that whole wheat is the only ingredient. It typically has a shelf life of one to two years. Whole-wheat pasta is an excellent source of fiber, which keeps your digestive tract healthy and running smoothly. It also contains a moderate amount of protein.

Typical pasta portions are way too large. Limit yourself to a healthy one-cup serving of cooked pasta, and add vegetables and beans to help fill you up.

FROZEN STRAWBERRIES

Few foods are more perishable than fresh fruit. Luckily, frozen berries are a great alternative. One cup of frozen strawberries is low in calories but delivers 18% of your recommended daily fiber intake and 150% of your daily vitamin C. Like vegetables, fruit is frozen at its peak ripeness, preserving nutritional value.

Nosh on berries straight from the bag for a sweet and satisfying dessert (just give them a few minutes to thaw slightly). Want to sweeten up your breakfast with healthy antioxidants?

Sauté frozen fruit in a saucepan for a berry sauce to drizzle over pancakes, yogurt and oatmeal. Strawberries also are great in smoothies and stirred into yogurt.

Save money when buying frozen fruit by waiting for sales, which usually happen when the fruit is in season. Diversify your choices with frozen mango, cherries, peaches and blueberries, all of which make a low-calorie dessert.

Coffee: The Ultimate Health Drink

Bob Arnot, MD, an internist and former chief medical and foreign correspondent for NBC and CBS. He is the author of 12 books on nutrition and health, and the host of the Dr. Danger reality TV series. His current book is *The Coffee Lover's Diet: Change Your Coffee, Change Your Life.* DrBobArnot.com

When it comes to good-for-you beverages, popular drinks such as red wine and green tea tend to get the most press. But the real heavyweight among health drinks in America is coffee.

Hundreds of scientific studies show that daily coffee drinking can lower one's risk for serious conditions such as heart attack and stroke…diabetes…obesity…cancer…Alzheimer's disease…Parkinson's disease…and perhaps even depression.

New scientific evidence: In a 16-year study of more than 500,000 people, published in *Annals of Internal Medicine*, those who drank three or more cups of coffee daily had up to 12% (men) and 7% (women) lower risk of dying from any cause over the study period, compared with people who didn't drink coffee.

My story: With so much remarkable scientific evidence about coffee, I recently traveled the globe to find the healthiest and most delicious coffees. *What I discovered…*

THE BEST BEANS

What makes coffee so healthy? There's no question that it's rich in antioxidants known as polyphenols. But coffee's real health-promoting muscle comes from a particular type of polyphenol called chlorogenic acid (CGA), which is uniquely effective in dousing the fires of inflammation and stopping oxidation.

The key fact is that some coffee beans contain far more CGAs than others. For example, the beans with the highest content of CGAs are typically grown at high altitudes and close to the equator in countries such as Kenya, Ethiopia, Colombia and parts of Brazil, where environmental conditions trigger the production of polyphenols (including CGAs) that can protect their cells—and yours.

My advice: Always drink high-CGA coffees. Among the commercial coffees we tested, one of the highest in CGAs you can buy at the grocery store was Dunkin' Donuts Original Blend...with McCafé Premium Roast Decaf, Medium Roast, not far behind. However, artisanal hand-roasted coffees have 50% more CGAs than what you'll find at the grocery store.

Note: Even though caffeinated coffees can have about 25% more CGAs than decaffeinated versions, decaf is also a rich source of these powerhouse polyphenols. Most flavored coffees don't use high-quality CGA-rich beans because the flavoring overwhelms the taste.

THE BEST ROASTS

Coffee lovers often gravitate to the bold flavor of dark roast brews, but this could be a mistake when it comes to health benefits. That's because the very high temperatures that are required for dark roasts destroy polyphenols (including CGAs) and can generate toxic products such as acrylamide, the carcinogenic chemical found in french fries and potato chips.

Bonus: Light and medium roasts that preserve CGAs and other polyphenols are also naturally delicious enough to forgo fattening additives such as cream and sugar, which blunt the health benefits.

My advice: For the biggest health boost, forgo dark-roasted beans and opt instead for a light roast. Medium roast is the next best option.

THE BEST GRIND

If you are looking for the most healthful coffee, fresh ground is the way to go. With pre-ground coffee, the most delicate flavors are almost instantly lost...and it usually falls short on CGAs.

There's a plethora of choices when it comes to coffee grinders. I recommend a conical burr grinder, which includes two cone-shaped, revolving cutting surfaces. This type of grinder is better than a metal blade grinder because you get a much more uniform size, which improves flavor.

Best product: Mahlkönig.

Good product: A Cuisinart has conical burrs—and a range of grind settings.

My advice: To achieve the most flavor when trying a new coffee, start with a very fine grind and move incrementally to a coarse one. If the coffee is too finely ground, it can taste bitter. Medium-coarse grind produces a lovely cup of coffee and still delivers lots of polyphenols.

THE BEST BREW

Brewing techniques fall into two categories—pour-over and immersion. In pour-overs, you place coffee grounds in a filter and pour a stream of water over them, and coffee drains into a container below. With immersion, the water completely envelops the coffee grounds.

My favorite pour-over device is the Kalita. Another good choice is the Chemex, which is one of the most popular pour-over devices in the US.

Other good choices: Keurig devices complete an automatic pour-over extraction cycle with minimal mess and time. Some excellent organic K-cups from Kenya, Colombia and Ethiopia test high for polyphenols and score very high for taste.

Among immersion devices, I favor the Aeropress—it's relatively inexpensive and makes a great cup of coffee.

FOR BEST RESULTS

Research shows that three to five cups of coffee daily is the optimal amount for better health.

However: Many people are genetically slow to metabolize caffeine. You're likely a slow caffeine metabolizer if more than two cups of caffeinated coffee make your heart race, trigger irritability or disturb your sleep. In that case, drink high-polyphenol decaffeinated coffees.

Coffee Might Be Bad for You

Marilyn C. Cornelis, PhD, assistant professor, Northwestern University Feinberg School of Medicine, Chicago.

C offee is the ultimate health drink, right? After all, a regular java habit is linked with protection against heart disease and more. But that doesn't mean it's healthy for you. It even might be dangerous.

The caffeine gene: When it comes to caffeine, about 15% of people are slow metabolizers due to a variant of the gene CYP1A2. They're more sensitive to the effects of caffeine, and it lingers much longer in their bodies.

Result: A much higher risk of developing high blood pressure and heart disease. In research published in *JAMA*, coffee was linked to heart attacks—but only in people with this gene variant. Another study found that moderate coffee drinkers who were slow caffeine metabolizers were 72% more likely to develop high blood pressure.

Insomnia and anxiety: Caffeine affects people differently when it comes to sleep and anxiety, too. Consider sleep. The average person clears half the caffeine from his/her body in about four to six hours—but it can take up to 24 hours for slow metabolizers! As for anxiety, people with panic disorder and social phobia are more sensitive to caffeine than people without these disorders.

Commonsense test: Want to know if you have the slow-metabolizing CYP1A2 variant? If you sign up for the gene-typing service 23andMe (about $200), you get this information in the "wellness report." Or you could simply monitor your systolic blood pressure to see if it goes up five points or more after drinking a cup. If so, cut back.

Coffee Ups the Crave

Coffee can make you crave something sweet. Coffee suppresses adenosine receptors, which help generate feelings of sleepiness. By suppressing those receptors, coffee makes people feel more alert, but it also dampens the ability to taste sweetness. Being unable to taste sweetness makes the brain crave it more.

Study of 107 people by researchers at Cornell University, Ithaca, New York, published in *Journal of Food Science*.

How to Still Eat Sugar and Stay Healthy

Sharon Palmer, RDN, a Duarte, California–based registered dietitian nutritionist and author of *The Plant-Powered Diet* and *Plant-Powered for Life*. She is also editor of the newsletter *Environmental Nutrition* and nutrition editor for *Today's Dietitian*. SharonPalmer.com

"O nly the dose makes the poison"—Paracelsus (1493-1541), Swiss physician and alchemist.

Lots of us are trying to skim a little more sugar from our diets these days. And rightly so. Eating too much sugar—even a single daily can of sugary soda—is linked with an increased risk for obesity, heart disease, diabetes and other unhealthy results.

Chances are you would be healthier if you eliminated almost all sugar from your diet. But is that practical for you? The good news is, you don't need to do that to reach the peak of your health potential. You don't need to stop eating sweet things! You do, however, need to know what to avoid, and it's not all obvious stuff like sugary soda.

Here's how to still eat sugar—and stay healthy.

WHAT TO LIMIT: ADDED SUGAR

A peach has natural sugar. So does a sweet potato—and milk. But these "natural" sugars in fruits, vegetables and dairy foods aren't the real concern. That's because the sugars found naturally in foods often come packed with fiber, which slows the absorption of these sugars, as well as important nutrients that contribute to health.

The sugar that's added to processed foods and recipes is another matter. It's no surprise that there are plenty of added sugars in sugary beverages, cakes, candies, ice cream and other "sweets." But many recipes used by restaurants and home cooks, and many processed foods you buy at the market, are jammed with hidden added sugar—even ones that don't taste sweet! It's this hidden sugar that could—quite literally—kill you, and that you owe it to yourself to minimize.

HOW MUCH ADDED SUGAR IS OK TO EAT?

The *2015-2020 Dietary Guidelines for Americans* set an upper limit on added sugar—10% of total calories per day. Based on a typical 2,000-calorie-a-day diet, that limit allows you 200 calories from added sugar, which works out to 50 grams, or 12½ teaspoons, of added sugar each day.

Does 12½ teaspoons of pure sugar deliberately put into your food each day sound like too little to you? The fact is, we're eating more than that. The average American woman consumes about 240 calories, and the average man 335 calories, from added sugar, each day. Some people are eating less, of course, but that means others are eating even more. Sometimes, a lot more.

It's easy to go over the limit. After all, a can of soda can have 10 teaspoons (40 grams) of sugar. Since one gram of sugar has 4 calories, that's 160 calories from added sugar right there. On top of that, many foods that aren't "sweets" have added sugar, including yogurt, breakfast cereals, salad dressings, breads, soups, pasta sauces, condiments…even basic vegetables. Consider the popular Le Sueur brand of canned peas. The manufacturer promotes them as "harvested when they're at their sweetest"—and then just to be sure, we suppose, adds pure sugar to every can. And that's not unusual.

HOW TO CUT BACK ON SUGAR BUT STILL ENJOY SUGAR

The first step if you want to stop flooding your body with sugar, of course, is to cut back on obviously high-sugar foods such as cookies, ice cream and soda and other sugary drinks. But then, you must start checking nutrition labels for sugar content—not just on some kinds of prepared foods but on every kind. Remember, you are not necessarily looking for no sugar—most food has some sugar naturally. To get a grip on hidden sugar, compare grams of sugar on food labels within categories of products—one pasta sauce to another, one breakfast cereal to another, etc.—and buy those with little sugar. Unfortunately, it can be difficult to ferret out which sugars are "added" and which are "naturally occurring" in a product via the food label, which lists only "sugars" by amount in grams per serving. Help is coming, though—the FDA will require new food labels by 2020 that specify the amount of "added sugars."

Until then, look for sources of added sugar in the ingredients list. The closer an ingredient is to the top of the list, the greater amount by weight is in the product. It's easy to spot ingredients listed specifically as sugar, white granulated sugar, raw sugar, honey, maple syrup, molasses, etc. *But the following ingredients also mean "added sugar"…*

Agave syrup
Anhydrous dextrose
Corn syrup
Corn syrup solids
Dextrose
Evaporated cane juice
Fructose
High-fructose corn syrup (HFCS)
Invert sugar
Lactose
Malt syrup
Maltose
Nectars (e.g., peach nectar, pear nectar)
Sucrose

Pay attention to prepared ready-to-eat foods that you take home and restaurant meals, too. Most supermarkets and chain restaurants have nutritional information available—all you have to do is ask. What you find may help you make smarter choices, with less added sugar, from the menu. The same is true for home-cooked meals. If your family recipe for meatloaf calls for lots of sugar, why not try making it with less—or none?

Final tip: You don't have to eliminate sugary treats to have a healthy diet. But save your added sugar grams for where they really give you the most pleasure—a scoop of high-quality ice cream, a really good cookie, a square of gourmet dark chocolate.

New Natural Sweeteners Can Help You Cut Back on Sugar

Janet Bond Brill, PhD, RDN, FAND, is a registered dietitian nutritionist and the author of *Blood Pressure DOWN, Cholesterol DOWN* and *Prevent a Second Heart Attack*. DrJanet.com

It's not news that consumption of refined sugar in the US has skyrocketed—the average American now consumes an incredible 23.5 teaspoons a day, almost double what the average American consumed 100 years ago! But why are we doing this to ourselves? Refined sugar not only contributes to weight gain but also has been linked to increased risk for diabetes, heart disease, anxiety, depression and other health conditions. What's more, the desire for sugar can be addictive, making it extremely difficult to cut back.

Luckily, there's an ever-growing number of natural sugar alternatives that can be a big help if you'd rather not use an artificial sweetener or go cold turkey, which is very difficult to do. All can satisfy the craving for sugar and provide lower calories than table sugar. *Some of the newest and best natural sweeteners on the market…*

•**Lite & Sweet** is a blend of xylitol and erythritol, sugar alcohols derived from berries and other fruits. It comes in bulk and packet form—one teaspoon has four calories (there's 16 calories in a teaspoon of table sugar). Lite & Sweet looks like regular sugar—and when using it for baking and cooking, it can be substituted for regular sugar teaspoon for teaspoon.

Both xylitol and erythritol are considered safe for human consumption if consumed in small doses. However, if you have too much of them, they can have a laxative effect.

•**Nature Sweet** is a combination erythritol, fructose, chicory root fiber and two plant-derived sweeteners. The first is stevia, which comes from the leaves of the stevia plant and has up to 200 times the sweetness of table sugar. The second plant-derived sweetener comes from monk fruit, a subtropical melonlike gourd, and is about 150 to 200 times sweeter than regular sugar. The new kid on the block at Starbucks, one packet of Nature Sweet (it comes in a green packet) has zero calories. In addition to using it in beverages, Nature Sweet can be used in recipes where the primary role of sugar is to sweeten, not to add bulk or tenderness, such as in sauces, salad dressings, fruit pies and cheesecake.

All sweeteners in Nature Sweet have been approved by the FDA for use in the US and do not appear to pose any health risks when used in moderation.

•**Just Like Sugar** is made primarily from chicory root fiber. Chicory root offers a high concentration of the prebiotic inulin, which supports the growth of "friendly" bacteria that are associated with improved bowel function and better general health. Sold in bulk form, it has zero calories per serving. It can be used like table sugar to sweeten beverages, etc. Plus, there is a version that can be used specifically for baking.

Caution: Some people experience bloating, gas, stomach cramping and/or diarrhea when consuming excess fiber, and individuals sensitive to pollen and other related plants may have an allergic reaction to the chicory in this product.

Substituting a natural sweetener in your favorite daily beverage, instead of using refined sugar or drinking a presweetened beverage, can be a great first step in cutting back on sugar and put you on the road to better health!

9 New Ways to Lose the Last 10 Pounds

Torey Armul, MS, RD, CSSD, LD, is a spokesperson for the Academy of Nutrition and Dietetics. She counsels clients on weight management, sports nutrition, pregnancy and family nutrition through her private practice in Columbus, Ohio.

You've changed your diet. You've exercised. And it worked—you lost weight. But not that last 10 pounds. Sound familiar?

Those last few pounds really are more difficult to lose. One reason, ironically, is that you weigh less now—so you need fewer calories to maintain your weight. Your body also fights back, resisting further weight loss through hormonal and metabolic means. Your resting metabolic rate falls, so you burn fewer calories at rest. Hormones kick in to increase your appetite. The result may be a weight plateau—or even weight regain.

What to do? If you can't bear the thought of cutting more calories or spending more time exercising, here are some unconventional methods to get you over the finish line…

DRINK GREEN TEA

A green tea habit may help you lose weight.

One reason: Gut bacteria. A recent study showed that mice that received green and black tea extracts had fewer gut microbes linked to obesity and more linked to lean body mass. Green tea is particularly rich in gut-friendly polyphenols. In a study published in *Clinical Nutrition,* women who consumed green tea extract every day for 12 weeks lost an average of 2.5 pounds—without following a reduced-calorie diet.

GET OUTSIDE—AND GO HIGH

Do you exercise mostly indoors? Head out! Exercising outside burns more calories, due to harder terrain and wind resistance, and can improve your mood and increase your enjoyment of the workout.

Fun fact: Gardeners weigh less than nongardeners, according to research—11 pounds less for women, 16 for men.

To really jump-start your weight loss, though, book your next vacation in the mountains. Research published in *Obesity* found that spending one week at a high altitude (8,700 feet) led study participants to eat less than those at sea level and to lose an average of three pounds. Both metabolic rate and levels of leptin (the "satiety" hormone) were higher.

GO BEYOND CALORIES

Counting calories still is the primary way most people approach weight loss—but different foods with the same calorie counts can have very different effects on satiety levels and weight.

Case in point: Plant-based proteins—beans, legumes, nuts, seeds, soy and grains such as quinoa—help you feel more full than animal-based proteins. Fiber is one reason. In one study, participants who ate a plant-based rather than an animal-based breakfast spontaneously ate about 100 fewer calories at lunch.

SHARE A SELFIE

If you've kept your weight goals to yourself, it's time to share them aloud. Make a public commitment. It will increase accountability and help build a community of support. That comes in handy when you need motivation or experience a setback.

One study from Northwestern University found that people in an online weight-loss group who "friended" others in the group and posted photos of their progress lost more weight than those who were less active online. In another study, those who shared goals with friends were more likely than those who didn't to meet them (62% versus 43%). Social-media outlets such as Twitter and Facebook can help, too, studies show—just be sure to unfollow people who don't support you or who make fun of your goals.

ADD SOME WEIGHT ON PURPOSE— MUSCLE WEIGHT

Building strength may not have been your focus in the initial stages of your weight loss, but it's crucial now. As you lost weight, your metabolic rate decreased. Strength training helps bring it back up. In one study, for example, a 26-week strength-training program increased resting metabolic rate by 7%.

Muscles are not miracle calorie burners, though. Their ability to radically change metabolism often is hyped in the media. The average actually is about 50 calories a day, according to a research review—not much if you're seeking a big weight loss. But adding muscle is great if you want a little edge to lose those last few pounds, since 50 calories per day translates to losing five extra pounds a year.

DON'T LET ANOTHER NIGHT GO BY

You know that sleep is essential for health, but you might not realize how even a little sleep deprivation can drive cravings and slow metabolism.

Amazing statistic: After a single night of poor sleep, study subjects ate an average of 385 extra calories the next day, according to statistical analysis of multiple studies. In fact, just two consecutive sleep-deprived nights (four hours each night) may be enough to alter your metabolism, according to research published in *Endocrine Development*. It increases the body's level of the hunger-stimulating hormone ghrelin and decreased hunger-reducing leptin. To lose those last 10 pounds, commit to healthier sleep habits.

TIME-RESTRICTED DAYTIME EATING

"Time-restricted eating," in which you consume all of your calories each day within a 10- or 12-hour window, is a new fad with potential weight-loss benefits. But to make it work best, eat your calories relatively early in the day. One two-month study from the University of Pennsylvania's Perelman School of Medicine found that participants who ate all their calories between 8 am and 7 pm weighed less than those who did so between noon and 11 pm—and they all consumed the same number of calories. For the daytime eaters, ghrelin peaked earlier and leptin peaked later. That helps deter late-night cravings.

If you're truly hungry late in the evening, don't be a martyr! Instead, choose a snack with fiber and protein, such as a handful of nuts…or fruit with Greek yogurt.

REDEFINE YOURSELF

One of the greatest predictors of weight-loss success is in your own head. A study published in *International Journal of Obesity* found that regardless of actual weight status, people who perceived themselves as overweight were significantly more likely to gain weight. It may not be easy, but give yourself credit for the weight you have lost (even if you haven't hit your goal), and try to think positively about yourself and your weight. Love and respect yourself just as you are.

TAKE A BREAK

Dieting all the time is exhausting—and can be self-defeating. Research published in *International Journal for Obesity* found that men who took a two-week break from dieting lost more weight than those who dieted continuously. During their dieting break, the men ate simply to maintain their weight. So take a break when you feel you need it, be kind to yourself and envision yourself meeting your goals.

Send Your Diet on Vacation

Nuala Byrne, PhD, head, School of Health Sciences, University of Tasmania, Launceston, Australia.

Fifty-one obese men on diets were placed in two groups—one dieted continuously for 16 weeks…the second group took a two-week break every two weeks (eating just to maintain their weight).

Result: Intermittent dieters lost more weight than continuous dieters (an average of 31 pounds and 20 pounds, respectively) and maintained a greater weight loss (24 pounds versus six-and-a-half pounds) six months later.

Theory: Restricting calories slows down the metabolism. Taking a diet break resets the metabolism.

Treat the Treat as a Meal

Jane Ogden, PhD, professor of health psychology, University of Surrey, UK, and leader of a study of 80 people, published in *Appetite*.

Treating food as a meal, not a snack, may help you eat less.

Recent study: A pasta dish was presented two ways. One way was as a snack, eaten standing up from a plastic bowl with a plastic fork. The other way was as a meal, eaten while seated at a table from a ceramic plate with a metal fork. Volunteers were then given additional foods to taste-test. Those who had eaten the pasta "snack" ate more of the new food than those who had eaten the pasta "meal."

Painless Weight-Loss Trick

Study of nearly 600,000 people with type 2 diabetes by researchers at Kyushu University, Fukuoko, Japan, published in *BMJ Open*.

Easy weight-control approach:* Eat slowly. Slow eaters were 42% less likely to be overweight than fast eaters…and normal-speed eaters were 29% less likely to be overweight than fast eaters. Study participants who reduced their eating speed during the six-year study were more likely to lose weight.

Possible reason: It takes 20 minutes after eating for the brain to receive signals of satiety. In that time, faster eaters consume more calories.

Mediterranean Diet Mistakes You're Probably Making

Kelly Toups, MLA, RD, LDN, director of nutrition at Oldways, a nonprofit dedicated to improving public health through healthy cultural food traditions, Boston. Oldwayspt.org

In some ways, the famously good-for-you Mediterranean diet is a victim of its own success. It's got such a healthy glow that promoters selling diets that are radically different—even diametrically opposed—try to bask in it. But even people who are doing their level best to eat the real thing often misunderstand the diet and make mistakes that can substantially undermine its enormous potential.

That matters because there is more scientific evidence for the health benefits of the real Mediterranean diet than for any other diet in the world. Eating the Mediterranean way—the real Mediterranean way—has been shown to protect people from heart disease and stroke, as well as obesity, diabetes, dementia and colon cancer.

People who eat this way also have healthier DNA and live longer, on average, than people who don't.

Latest finding: Adults age 60 and older who most closely followed the diet over an average of four years were 38% less likely to experience frailty such as muscle weakness and fatigue, compared with those who followed it less closely.

One reason: The diet is rich in antioxidants and anti-inflammatory nutrients that help keep muscles strong as we age.

So let's get introduced to the Mediterranean diet right—as if it were for the first time—and get all the benefits…

WHAT IS THE REAL MEDITERRANEAN DIET?

The diet evolved in olive oil–producing regions near the Mediterranean Sea. At its most basic, it's mostly vegetables, legumes, fruit, nuts and seeds ("plant" foods), olive oil and seafood…some poultry and dairy…and very little red meat, sweets or processed foods. The Mediterranean Diet Pyramid, developed 25 years ago by researchers at Harvard School of Public Health and Oldways, a nonprofit that promotes healthy food traditions and lifestyles, remains an excellent guide today…

•**Eat every day.** Fruits, vegetables, grains (mostly whole grains), olive oil, legumes (such as beans and lentils), nuts and peanuts, seeds, herbs and spices.

•**Eat often—at least twice a week.** Fish and other seafood.

•**Eat often—daily or a few times a week, in moderate portions.** Fermented dairy (yogurt, cheese) and eggs.

•**Eat less often, such as weekly.** Poultry.

•**Eat infrequently—once or twice a month.** Red meats and sweets.

•**Drink.** Water, and if you drink alcohol, only wine in moderation.

•***Get plenty of physical activity.***

•***Make meals relaxed and enjoyable.*** A less stressful eating experience is part of the healthy Mediterranean way, too.

THAT'S NOT MEDITERRANEAN!

Easy-peasy, right? You'd think so. But it's surprisingly easy to deceive yourself. *Here are some things that the true Mediterranean diet is not…*

•**It's not low-fat.** It's easy to find low-fat "Mediterranean" cookbooks. But the real Mediterranean diet includes plenty of fat. The truth is, all that delicious olive oil is one reason why it's so easy to eat all those vegetables. And yet studies show that sticking to the real thing—fat and all—helps people lose weight and keep it off. One reason is that the vegetables are so rich in fiber that they're very filling.

•**It's not low-carb.** The book *The Pioppi Diet: A 21-Day Lifestyle Plan* is promoted as a "take on the Mediterranean diet," yet it is essentially a very-low-carb diet that also calls for periodic fasting days and recommends coconut oil. None of these attributes are part of the traditional Mediterranean diet, which includes plenty of grains, including moderate portions of refined pasta mixed with olive oil and veggies, fish or beans—and whole grains including bulgur wheat, farro (an ancient form of wheat) and barley.

•**Pizza? Think again.** Despite its Italian name, American-style pizza is fast food and generally not good for you. It's one of the biggest sources of calories, sodium and saturated fat in the American diet. To make it healthier, make the crust whole-grain and top it with vegetables (not meat) and only a little cheese.

•**It's not vegetarian and certainly not vegan.** Beef, pork and lamb traditionally were considered luxuries and were reserved for special occasions, maybe a few times a month. But the Mediterranean diet is not a vegetarian diet and certainly not a vegan one. Seafood is key, but it's fine to eat moderate amounts of poultry, eggs and dairy—especially fermented dairy foods such as yogurt and cheese.

•**It's not about superfoods.** No single food—not even olive oil—explains this diet's power. It's an eating pattern. Just adding one or two components—washing down your rib roast with a Barolo—won't do much. It's about

shifting your overall approach and maintaining it for many years.

•**It's not a license to drink.** Alcohol plays a part in the Mediterranean diet, but again, it's the pattern that counts—moderate drinking (up to one drink a day for women, two for men), mostly wine, almost always with meals. Beer isn't unhealthy—it's just not a big part of this dietary pattern. And drinking heavily, especially without eating—such as the cocktail hour—is the opposite of the Mediterranean way.

Now that you can spot Mediterranean-diet mistakes, you can get closer to the real thing—with its enormous health benefits, not to mention sheer deliciousness. Nobody's perfect, and your diet doesn't need to be either. But you can get close to this way of eating by taking a series of small steps—replace chips with nuts or fruit for snacks…choose beans or seafood over beef…replace soda and juice with water…drink wine at meals rather than booze on an empty stomach…switch to fresh fruit for dessert and save baked sweets and ice cream for special occasions.

BEST MEDITERRANEAN DIET COOKBOOKS

We asked Kelly Toups for her favorite Mediterranean cookbooks. *Her choices include a classic, a newer book and one from the Oldways collection…*

Mediterranean Cookery by Claudia Roden. Well before Greek yogurt and olive oil were kitchen staples in the US, there was Claudia Roden, one of the foremost authorities on Mediterranean cuisine. Her simple-yet-elegant recipes have stood the test of time.

The Complete Mediterranean Cookbook by America's Test Kitchen. This colorful collection of more than 500 recipes is a wonderful way to immerse yourself in the bold flavors of the diet.

The Oldways 4-Week Mediterranean Diet Menu Plan. The menu plan takes you on a 28-day journey through many of the delicious and satisfying tastes of the Mediterranean diet. It includes plans for each day.

CHAPTER 12

Infectious Diseases

A Pandemic Could Be Looming—Why We Are Vulnerable

The 100th anniversary of the flu pandemic of 1918–1919—which killed approximately 50 million people, both young and old, over a period of about nine months—looms ominously over the world.

Even with all the medical advances that have been made in the last century, it's possible that a similar deadly pandemic could occur again, according to many infectious disease experts. To learn more about the possible risks of a modern-day pandemic and the best ways to protect ourselves, we spoke with Miryam Z. Wahrman, PhD, a leading authority on communicable diseases.

We seem to hear the term "epidemic" more than "pandemic." What's the difference? An epidemic occurs when an infectious disease spreads rapidly to many people, exceeds what is expected based on recent experience and is typically concentrated in a particular geographic region. One example is the 2014–2016 outbreak of the Ebola virus, which was centered in West Africa and killed more than 11,000.

A pandemic is an epidemic that spreads across a large region (potentially globally), is spread from person-to-person and affects a high proportion of the population. Besides the flu pandemic of 1918, another example is the 2009–2010 H1N1 influenza pandemic that killed an estimated 200,000 people worldwide.

Do you think a new pandemic is coming? Based on the prevalence of infectious diseases in every corner of the globe, the history of past epidemics and the frequency of worldwide travel, there's a high likelihood that new (or old) pathogens will emerge in the near future.

Miryam Z. Wahrman, PhD, a professor of biology at William Paterson University in Wayne, New Jersey, where she specializes in microbiology, hand hygiene and the interactions between bacteria and environmental surfaces. Dr. Wahrman is also the author of *The Hand Book: Surviving in a Germ-Filled World*.

There are constantly outbreaks of infectious diseases all over the world, including in developed countries. Some diseases originate in animals and are passed to humans, where they become serious threats to large populations. Other disease outbreaks occur as a result of a deliberate choice of people not to vaccinate or occur when viruses, bacteria or other microbes genetically change and evolve into new forms that evade our immune systems, or resist antibiotic treatments. It is critically important to track diseases all over the world in order to document outbreaks that could lead to epidemics or pandemics.

Can anyone predict which disease may cause a pandemic? While it's impossible to definitively predict which viruses or bacteria will spread widely, many scientists believe that the flu strain H7N9, known as the avian flu, has the greatest potential to become an epidemic—and eventually spread globally into a pandemic.

H7N9, a subtype of influenza A, has been circulating in poultry for years. In 2013, China reported the first known cases of a new strain of H7N9 in humans. The World Health Organization (WHO) reports that since 2013, 1,554 humans have been infected with H7N9 in China and roughly 40% of patients have died from the disease.

In the latest wave of H7N9, October 2016 to July 2017, the highest number of cases was reported, suggesting that according to the WHO, "the virus is spreading, and…further intensive surveillance and control measures…are crucial." There have been no reports of H7N9 in the US yet, and it appears that the virus is transmitted from poultry to humans and seldom from human to human. However, if that transmission pattern changes, it would herald the potential for H7N9 to become an epidemic/pandemic.

Some diseases in bats are also candidates for eventual transmission to humans.

Why are we at risk for another pandemic? Our world population has more than doubled in the last 50 years, which means there are more people to infect—and to infect others. Also, more people than ever are traveling the globe. An infected person can travel to the other side of the world in as little as a day.

Global climate change is another concern. As parts of our environment become warmer, disease-carrying insects move to new areas and expose more people.

Also, while antibiotics have increased life expectancy, use and abuse of these medications lead to the development of antibiotic-resistant bacteria, or "superbugs," that are difficult or impossible to treat. Two such superbugs, found mainly in health-care facilities, are *Clostridium difficile* and methicillin-resistant *Staphylococcus aureus* (MRSA). They kill thousands in the US each year, although infections have declined due to improved medical procedures.

Can pandemics be prevented? With the development of the Internet and advances in telecommunications and air travel, scientists are better able to collaborate and share data. By sharing resources and scientific research between countries, diseases can be contained.

Also, the development of vaccines and new antibiotics against these contagious diseases is critical. Pharmaceutical companies are reluctant to spend resources developing and producing vaccines and antibiotics because it is not as profitable as selling drugs used for chronic diseases.

What can we do to protect ourselves? One of the very best ways to keep germs at bay is to practice proper handwashing. Don't wait for a pandemic to comply.

My advice: Wash your hands with plain liquid soap and warm water, scrubbing for at least 20 seconds. Antibacterial soaps have become popular, but some studies have shown that they promote the development of drug-resistant bacteria.

Also, studies have shown that using a single-use paper towel in public restrooms is more effective at ridding bacteria from the hands than warm-air dryers or jet dryers, which have been found to spew harmful microbes into the air. When soap and water are not available, hand sanitizers, such as Purell, are a good choice, but they do not get rid of superbugs such as C. difficile.

It's critical to wash your hands before touching your eyes, nose or mouth—the most common routes for germs to enter the body. Also, be sure to wash your hands before eating. And insist that health-care workers wash their hands before touching you or your loved ones.

Are there any other precautions that people should be taking? Phones, smartphones, keyboards and tablets have been shown to harbor bacteria and other harmful germs. It's a good idea to clean these devices by wiping the surface down, as needed, with a microfiber cloth or tissue lightly moistened with 70% rubbing alcohol.

When "Dementia" Is Really Lyme Disease

Richard I. Horowitz, MD, an internist and medical director of the Hudson Valley Healing Arts Center in Hyde Park, New York. He has treated more than 12,000 patients with chronic Lyme disease over the past 30 years. He is a past president of the International Lyme and Associated Diseases Educational Foundation, and the author of *How Can I Get Better: An Action Plan for Treating Resistant Lyme & Chronic Disease.* CanGetBetter.com

People who have been told that they have Alzheimer's disease or another form of dementia owe it to themselves to ask their doctors one important question—"Could it be Lyme disease?"

Case in point: Singer Kris Kristofferson struggled for years with memory problems. His doctors suspected Alzheimer's disease or brain damage from sports-related head injuries.

Surprising news: He was recently told that he really had Lyme disease, which often causes cognitive problems that can be misdiagnosed as Alzheimer's disease.

What most people don't realize: While doctors routinely look for the physical symptoms of Lyme disease, such as a rash, fatigue, joint and muscle pain and unexplained fevers, many don't realize that psychological and cognitive impairments, including depression, anxiety, short- and long-term memory loss and other symptoms often confused with Alzheimer's disease, are also important clues.

THE BRAIN AT RISK

Lyme disease is a bacterial infection transmitted by tick bites. The organisms that can cause human infection readily travel from the place where a tick bite occurred into the brain, the sac surrounding the brain (the meninges) or the spinal cord as well as to the muscles, joints, heart and other parts of the body.

What happens next: Infection and inflammation of brain tissue can lead to memory and concentration problems and may also cause psychiatric problems, such as visual and auditory hallucinations that resemble schizophrenia. Infection of nerves in the spinal cord can cause numbness, tingling, burning or stabbing sensations in the arms and legs and/or across the trunk, which can come and go and even migrate to other parts of the body.

Shocking fact: About a quarter of all people diagnosed and treated early for Lyme disease go on to develop a chronic and hard-to-treat infection that often leads to some of the neurological symptoms described earlier, as well as headaches, neck stiffness, light and sound sensitivity and sleep disorders. The percentage is much higher among Lyme patients who aren't given early antibiotic treatment, who are undertreated or who remain undiagnosed.

WHY IT'S MISSED

Doctors should suspect Lyme disease when patients complain about problems with memory, concentration or other cognitive functions—particularly in parts of the country where Lyme and other tick-borne diseases are rampant (mainly the Northeast and upper Midwest). But Lyme is spreading. Doctors should consider it in dementia work-ups.

Experts advise Americans who live in tick-infested areas to be alert for the earliest sign of Lyme infection—a bull's-eye–shaped rash surrounding the site of the tick bite. However, only about 50% of Lyme patients ever develop a rash...or they confuse the rash with a spider bite, skin infection or bruise. Unless they know for a fact that they were bitten by a tick—and most don't—they don't even consider that Lyme might be the culprit.

More worrisome are the cognitive/psychological symptoms that affect more than 90% of the Lyme patients I've treated. These include memory loss and concentration problems, depression and psychiatric disorders...as well as symptoms easily mistaken for those caused by

Alzheimer's disease and other neurodegenerative disorders.

Diagnostic complication: Even when Lyme is suspected, it's often difficult to diagnose. That's why doctors should start with a clinical diagnosis that is supported by lab testing. Hallmarks of Lyme include pain that migrates around the body and symptoms that come and go. When used together, the two main blood tests for Lyme disease—the Western blot and the ELISA test—miss about half of all infected patients. To improve accuracy, newer tests such as the C6 ELISA and EliSpot, which show higher sensitivity in detecting evidence of Lyme disease, can also be done. Other options (such as DNA and RNA tests, Nanotrap, etc.) are available, and spinal taps and PET scans may also be helpful.

Best advice: When outdoors, wear protective clothing treated with permethrin (an insect repellent), use tick sprays (those containing IR3535 and picaridin are safer) and do frequent tick checks. Remove any ticks immediately using fine-tipped tweezers and grasping the tick as close to the skin as possible, pulling upward without squeezing. Save the tick so it can be tested and examined by your health-care provider.

Suspect Lyme disease if you experience sudden concentration or memory problems, anxiety and mood swings, headaches, migratory joint or muscle pain, dizziness or other symptoms—especially if you have no history of these problems. Such symptoms can occur within days to months of the bite.

TREATMENT CHALLENGES

People who aren't treated quickly for Lyme (or those who have Lyme disease along with another tick-borne disease, such as *babesiosis* or *bartonellosis*) might not improve when they're given the standard antibiotic therapy—usually oral *doxycycline* (Oracea), *amoxicillin* (Moxatag) or *cefuroxime* (Zinacef). Because Lyme is more curable when treated early, your doctor might begin medication if you have symptoms (such as migratory joint pain) even before test results are confirmed or if you've had a tick bite but are not displaying symptoms of illness. About three-quarters of Lyme patients who take antibiotics within a month of the infection won't develop long-term symptoms and can be cured.

Important: If you've had antibiotic treatment for Lyme but continue to have neurological symptoms, the infection has likely spread to the nervous system. This may require different combinations of antibiotics for a longer treatment period. There are many treatment options, depending on specific symptoms, your medical history, the type of infection(s) and other considerations, such as allergies and the state of your immune and gastrointestinal systems.

How I have treated Lyme patients with persistent neurological symptoms: During the first month of treatment, I might prescribe doxycycline with *hydroxychloroquine* (Plaquenil), an antimalarial drug that helps to increase effectiveness, with or without the antibiotics *metronidazole* (Flagyl) or *tinidazole* (Tindamax) to kill cystic (dormant) forms of bacteria. I find that two or three drug regimens work best for chronically ill patients.

Important: Treatment must be tailored to the individual.

ANTI-INFLAMMATORY SUPPORT

The presence of cognitive/psychological symptoms with Lyme disease always means that inflammation is affecting the brain and/or surrounding tissue. When you're infected, microglial cells in the brain secrete inflammatory substances that cause fatigue, mood changes and problems with memory and concentration. It's critical to shut down the infection and accompanying inflammation. *What helps…**

•**Anti-inflammatory supplements,** such as curcumin, broccoli seed extract, resveratrol and green tea extract. Take them one at a time or all together. Also consider an antioxidant such as glutathione.

•**Stevia,** available in supplement form (the Nutramedix brand is effective), has been shown to kill the Lyme bacterium, and it reduces and breaks up Lyme biofilms, "sheets" of bacteria that resist the effects of antibiotics. Gradually work up to 15 drops, twice a day. (*Note:* This is not the same stevia found in the sweetener section of the grocery store.)

*If you use prescription medication, have a chronic medical condition or are pregnant or nursing, consult your doctor before taking any supplements.

•**A good night's sleep is critical during Lyme treatments.** Sleep deprivation increases inflammation…impairs immunity…and increases cognitive/psychological symptoms.

•**An anti-inflammatory diet,** including lots of healthy, low-carbohydrate fruits and vegetables…no sugar…and little or no red meat. I often recommend a mercury-free fish oil supplement as well.

Deadly Tick Disease on the Rise (It's Not Lyme)

Jennifer L. Lyons, MD, chief, division of neurological infections and inflammatory diseases in Brigham and Women's Hospital's department of neurology, and assistant professor of neurology at Harvard Medical School, both in Boston.

The ticks that carry Lyme disease may be even more dangerous than you thought. They also can carry a virus that can cause a potentially fatal disease called *Powassan virus encephalitis*. And warmer winters may lead to rising tick populations, increasing the risk. It also is possible that other ticks may carry the virus.

It can take a tick as little as 15 minutes to transmit Powassan encephalitis to a person. Most people who contract it have no symptoms. But infections that do cause symptoms are extremely serious—10% to 15% of people who develop symptoms do not survive.

Symptoms usually start with fever and a sense of generally feeling unwell, with a series of nonspecific flulike muscle aches and pains and sometimes a rash or headache. This is followed a few days to a few weeks later by severe headache, weakness, possible seizures, inability to think clearly and possibly inability to breathe on one's own.

Everyone with symptomatic Powassan encephalitis should be hospitalized. Treatment includes mechanical ventilation, blood pressure support and management of electrolytes. There is no vaccine to prevent Powassan encephalitis, and there are no medicines to cure it. With prompt care, patients typically recover after a few days to a few weeks, but at least half of those who survive will have permanent neurological damage. Per-

manent effects may include seizures, cognitive disability, weakness or loss of sensation in limbs or coordination difficulties.

Powassan encephalitis can strike anyone—many cases are in otherwise perfectly healthy individuals. For now, the disease, thankfully, is rare. The Centers for Disease Control and Prevention estimate only about 75 cases nationwide over the past decade, mostly in the Great Lakes region and the Northeast. There is no evidence that pets can get encephalitis due to the Powassan virus, but they can carry ticks into the house.

Self-defense: If you are likely to be in areas with ticks, use an insect repellent that contains DEET. Also wear permethrin-embedded clothing—and choose light-colored garments to see ticks.

---

6 Surprising Foods That Can Give You Food Poisoning

Robert B. Gravani, PhD, CFS, professor emeritus of food science at Cornell University, Ithaca, New York. He is past president of the Institute of Food Technologists.

Perfected by nature. That's the motto for Live Spring Water. It is "raw" water—unfiltered, untreated spring water—the latest trend in health-conscious circles. Cost: $36.99 for a two-and-a-half-gallon jug…$14.99 for a refill.

Save your money…and you might be saving yourself something even more valuable—your health. According to the Centers for Disease Control and Prevention, the nation's top health protection agency, drinking "raw" water could increase the risk for serious food-borne illnesses including, potentially, cholera and typhoid. You also could swallow disease-causing parasites including *Giardia*, *Cryptosporidium* and *Cyclospora*. While no outbreaks have been reported from the bottled variety—and Live Spring, for one, says that it tests its water sources once a year for contamination—public health authorities believe that it's only a matter of time before someone gets sick from bottled raw water.

Unless you like to chase the latest trends, you probably don't have a cooler filled with raw water in your kitchen. *But chances are you do have one or more of the following five other surprising sources of food-borne illnesses…*

•**Melon and other fruits with thick skin.** You might assume that a fruit with a thick, inedible skin—such as cantaloupe, mango, papaya and even avocado—would be perfectly safe. After all, you're not eating the skin. But there have been several food-poisoning outbreaks associated with such fruits.

Risky moment: When you cut into the fruit, you can transfer bacteria from the skin to the flesh.

Protect yourself: Thoroughly wash fruits that have a thick skin before you cut through them, using water and a produce brush to get at nooks and crannies—soap isn't necessary.

•**Raw flour.** You're probably thinking, Who eats raw flour? But if you ever nibble raw cookie dough or lick cake batter off your finger—you do! Recently, dozens of people across the country got sick from eating raw dough made from flour contaminated with the E. coli bacterium. A whopping 10 million pounds of flour were recalled because of the outbreak.

Protect yourself: Don't eat raw cookie dough or anything that contains raw flour. And that's a doubly good idea because many recipes containing flour also include another food that is dangerous raw—eggs.

•**Homemade soups and stews.** If you have made a big pot of soup or stew and then left it on the stovetop for hours to cool, you are putting yourself at risk for a lesser known, yet pervasive, bacterium called *Clostridium perfringens*—estimated to cause a million cases of food-borne illness each year in the US. Even though the soup was boiled, the organism forms spores that can survive the cooking process—and then germinate as the food slowly cools.

Protect yourself: Cool soups and stews as quickly as possibly—only briefly on a countertop, then in the refrigerator.

Tip: Transfer hot liquids into large, shallow containers to let the liquid cool down quickly. As soon as it stops steaming, pop it in the fridge.

Alternative: Buy a nifty gadget called an ice paddle that you fill with water and then freeze—it cools hot liquids quickly with just a little stirring. Then put the now-cool soup or stew into the fridge. Eat within four days, and be sure to reheat to a simmer before serving.

•**Cooked meats—even ones that have been stored properly.** Everyone knows that raw meat can possibly harbor *salmonella* and other bacteria. But even foods that are cooked when you buy them, such as deli meats… smoked seafood…store-made deli salads…and precooked hot dogs can harbor *Listeria*. It's a bacterium that grows in moist, cool temperatures—such as a refrigerator or cooler.

Protect yourself: Eat meats that you buy cooked soon after purchasing them, and toss anything that remains five days after you opened the package. With unopened packages, use the "best by" date as a rule of thumb for when to toss. In this way, you won't be eating these foods after the bacterium has had a great deal of time to multiply.

Note: If you buy frozen hot dogs or freeze the hot dogs when you get them home, you're safer—Listeria won't multiply in the freezer.

•**If there are any spills from deli salads in your refrigerator, clean them up promptly.** Once a week, wipe the walls and shelves of the fridge with warm, soapy water, then rinse…and keep the temperature at 40°F or lower.

Listeria is especially dangerous to pregnant women and people with compromised immune systems (from diabetes or cancer, for example). They should be especially cautious and heat not only hot dogs but also lunch meat and smoked seafood until they're steaming.

•**Raw pet food.** This one is a risk both for you and your cat or dog. Raw pet food (meat, bones, organs) is a popular "natural" trend. It's supposed to be closer to the kind of food that a feral dog or cat would eat in the wild. But it's very easy for these foods to get contaminated with salmonella, Listeria and other pathogens that can make pets and humans sick—the FDA has recalled several brands due to contamination.

As with humans, in pets these food-borne illnesses can lead to vomiting, diarrhea and sometimes fever. Even if your pet doesn't get sick, you can become ill if you contract these bacterial infections after handling pet food.

Protect yourself: It's best to avoid raw food entirely and serve your pet only food that has been cooked, either store-bought or home-made. If you do handle raw pet food, be sure to wash your hands in hot, soapy water for at least 20 seconds.

STAYING SAFE

Now that you know about these often-ignored dangers, you can protect yourself. But don't ignore the better-known food-safety risks, either. *These include…*

•**Rare or even medium-rare hamburgers.** Make sure burgers reach an internal temperature of 160°F.

•**Raw milk.** It's dangerous. Avoid it.

•**Bagged salad greens.** These have been the cause of many recalls. Better to buy bunches of spinach or heads of lettuce…rinse thoroughly in cold water (no need for soap)…dry thoroughly and refrigerate until use.

•**Sprouts.** Never eat any kind of sprout raw.

SIGNS OF FOOD POISONING

Think you've got food poisoning? Many cases are mild and go away on their own with a little home TLC including rest, staying close to the bathroom and restoring lost fluids.

But be certain to call your doctor if you have…

•**High fever (over 101.5°F)**

•**Blood in your stool**

•**Frequent vomiting** that prevents you from keeping liquids down

•**Signs of dehydration,** including decreased urination, a dry mouth and throat and/or feeling dizzy when you stand up

•**Diarrhea** that lasts more than three days

Update on Shingles: A New Vaccine and Better Self-Care

Lindsay C. Strowd, MD, assistant professor of dermatology at Wake Forest Baptist Health in Winston-Salem, North Carolina. Her research has appeared in *Journal of the American Academy of Dermatology, The American Journal of Dermatopathology* and other professional journals.

Shingles is one of those dreaded conditions that you may not think too much about—until it's your turn to endure the ravages of this painful viral infection.

Recent development: There's a new vaccine that provides better protection than the previous one. But despite all the attention it's getting, many people are still unaware of some key details.

Reality check: Because some people—vaccinated or not—still do develop shingles, you also need to know how to best treat the condition and use self-care measures to curb the suffering.

THE SHINGLES VACCINE

The first vaccine for adult shingles, Zostavax, was FDA approved in 2006. It was found to prevent shingles in about half of people who received the single shot.

What you may not realize: Shingles is much more than a skin rash. It's a viral infection that starts with a rash but usually doesn't stop there. The rash can be intensely painful and can lead to severe nerve pain that's potentially permanent. And in some cases, shingles can increase stroke risk.

Shingrix, the shingles vaccine that was FDA approved in late 2017, is about 97% effective against shingles during the first year. Its effectiveness wanes over time, but experts predict that it will continue to reduce infections by about 85% over four years. Research has shown that it's particularly effective in older adults, who face the highest risk for shingles.

What you may not realize: The new vaccine is also recommended for those who were previously vaccinated with Zostavax. Even if you've already received the older vaccine, the CDC recommends getting the new one.

Also important: Just because you've already had shingles, it doesn't mean you're off the hook—you can get shingles more than once. *Other key facts to know about the new vaccine…*

• **It requires two doses instead of one.** While the original shingles vaccine was given in a single dose, Shingrix requires two doses—given about two to six months apart.

• **It's pricey.** Shingrix is about $280 for both shots total, roughly the same cost as the single-shot original vaccine. Most insurance, including Medicare, is expected to cover the new vaccine, but you'll want to check before getting the shots.

• **There's some discomfort from the shot,** which involves mainly arm swelling and localized pain—this is typical with most injections. But about half of patients age 70 and older report more bothersome side effects, including widespread muscle pain, fatigue and/or headaches. Most side effects are temporary and last about 24 to 48 hours.

• **The vaccine's duration is uncertain.** Most vaccines lose their protection over time. The older shingles vaccine seems to lose some of its protection after about five or six years. Shingrix has not been used long enough to determine exactly how many years of protection it will give. And patients may need revaccination at some point after the original vaccination series.

• **Shingrix uses killed viruses,** while Zostavax uses live viruses. Those with impaired immune systems cannot receive live vaccines. If you have been told in the past that you cannot get the shingles vaccine due to an impaired immune system, ask your doctor about Shingrix.

• **Shingrix can be given starting at age 50,** while Zostavax was given to those age 60 and older.

My advice: Everyone age 50 or older and any adult with an impaired immune system should ask a doctor about getting the new vaccine.

IF YOU DO GET SHINGLES

If you get vaccinated but develop shingles anyway, the rash will typically be milder with less severe pain, and the illness will be shorter in duration. Plus, there will be less risk for serious complications such as permanent nerve damage.

Shingles typically starts with one to five days of shooting or burning pain, numbness, tingling, itching and/or skin sensitivity. Some people also have flulike symptoms—headache, chills and fever. The affected skin will then develop redness and small blisters filled with fluid. If you get these symptoms, see your doctor right away—early diagnosis and treatment can help shorten the course of the attack and improve symptoms. Antiviral medication may shorten the duration of the illness and help with pain relief. It also can reduce risk for nerve pain complications but must be given soon after the rash appears, ideally within 72 hours.

If the pain is severe: Ask your doctor about *gabapentin* (Neurontin), an antiseizure drug that also relieves nerve pain. Topical lidocaine, available over-the-counter, can help with pain as well.

Complications: The shingles rash sometimes occurs on the face or near the eyes. In these cases, the virus can enter the optic nerve and cause vision loss. And in very rare cases, the shingles virus can infect the brain and cause inflammation of the brain (encephalitis). Important: Seek immediate medical care if the rash is near your eye or on your nose or it continues spreading to other parts of your body.

Best self-care options…

• **Try a cool-water compress…**or oatmeal/baking soda baths, which can reduce itching and discomfort. For a compress, soak and wring out a soft washcloth with cool water and apply it to the rash for five to 10 minutes, several times per day. For baths, add colloidal oatmeal/baking soda to cool bathwater. Soak for 10 minutes once a day.

• **Coat the rash with a thick ointment such as petroleum jelly,** Aquaphor or unscented A&D Ointment, then cover the area with a bandage. Ointments are soothing, and the bandage will protect the area from the friction caused by clothing.

• **Wear loose, natural-fiber clothes (such as cotton).** They're more comfortable than polyester or other synthetic fabrics.

THE SHINGLES TRAP

About 90% of adults had chicken pox (varicella-zoster virus) early in life. Once you've been exposed to this virus, it retreats to the nervous system and lies dormant. The virus can reactivate later in life, usually after age 50, and cause shingles.

Sometimes shingles will be reactivated during periods of extreme stress on the body—for example, during a bad illness. People with weakened immune systems—the elderly…those with chronic diseases…and/or patients taking immune-suppressing medications for conditions such as rheumatoid arthritis or lupus or using chemotherapy drugs—are at greater risk of developing shingles.

Don't Let the Flu Turn into Pneumonia

William Schaffner, MD, an infectious disease specialist at Vanderbilt University Medical Center in Nashville and medical director of the National Foundation for Infectious Diseases. NFID.org

MyFluVaccine.com

The flu lands hundreds of thousands of people in the hospital each year and kills tens of thousands. But flu that leads to pneumonia is even deadlier.

Startling statistic: Flu-plus-pneumonia ranks eighth in leading causes of death in the US.

THE FLU/PNEUMONIA COMBO

Every year, pneumonia affects more than one million Americans—and about 50,000 die. People most susceptible to pneumonia include the elderly, especially nursing home residents and individuals who have chronic health conditions such as heart or lung disease. The flu-to-pneumonia progression isn't the only cause of pneumonia, of course, but since the combo is so deadly—and often so preventable—it's worth special attention.

Here's what happens: You get the flu, a contagious respiratory illness caused by an influenza virus. You get the typical symptoms—sore throat, cough, body aches, fever, headaches and chills. But the flu also makes your lungs more susceptible to a bacterial infection caused by *Streptococcus pneumoniae* (S. pneumoniae), the most common cause of pneumonia in adults.

When that happens, air sacs fill with pus and other liquid, making it harder for oxygen to reach the bloodstream and making it difficult to breathe. Death can come from organs that are starved of oxygen—or from a blood infection (sepsis).

Here's how to protect yourself…

STEP ONE: GET A FLU SHOT

If you don't get the flu, you won't be at risk for that combination of flu virus/S. pneumoniae that is so dangerous to susceptible people. Getting a flu shot is the best way to protect yourself. It is recommended for everyone over the age of six months. While not 100% effective, it does offer substantial protection.

Why a flu shot is so important: A bad flu year means that pneumonia cases could potentially soar. The 2019 flu shot should be a good match for the kinds of flu viruses coming our way, which, according to the World Health Organization (WHO), includes two new strains.

STEP TWO: MAKE SURE YOU'RE UP-TO-DATE ON PNEUMONIA VACCINATION

Effective vaccines exist against S. pneumoniae, which, as described earlier, causes the vast majority of pneumonia cases in adults. Everyone age 65 and older should be vaccinated—yet only about 50% of healthy adults in this age group are. Some adults need protection before they turn 65—smokers and anyone with a chronic health condition (heart or lung disease, diabetes, asthma, etc.). For the best protection, you'll need two different vaccines, spaced out over a year or more…

•**Start with a onetime-only dose of the pneumococcal conjugate vaccine called PCV13 (Prevnar 13),** which protects against 13 types of pneumococcal bacteria.

•**One year later,** get a dose of pneumococcal polysaccharide vaccine PPSV23 (Pneumovax), which protects against 23 strains of pneumococcal bacteria. Prevnar 13 primes your immune system so that Pneumovax works better than it would if you took it by itself.

•**Based on your age and health,** your doctor may advise another dose of Pneumovax five years later.

STEP THREE: WATCH YOUR MEDS

Certain health conditions and medications can affect your susceptibility to pneumonia…

•**Steroids and other immunosuppressive drugs** can make you more susceptible to pneumonia. These drugs interfere with the immune response, so your body can't fight off infection as easily.

Low-dose steroids, even taken long-term, may not increase pneumonia risk, but higher doses (such as 20 mg a day) can do so in as little as two weeks. If you need a high-dose steroid to control your condition, be especially vigilant during flu season—get vaccinated, wash your hands frequently, stay away from crowds, and call your doctor at the first sign of illness such as a sore throat.

•**Acid-suppressive medications,** such as proton pump inhibitors including *omeprazole* (Prilosec), as well as histamine-2 receptor antagonists including *ranitidine* (Zantac), inhibit the production of stomach acids. But these acids help keep harmful gut bacteria in check.

Less acid means more potential for harmful bacteria to colonize and eventually enter the lungs. Unless your doctor prescribes these on a long-term basis (a rare occurrence), use them only for short periods of time—no more than four weeks for heartburn/gastroesophageal reflux disease (GERD), for example.

•**Pneumonia occurs less often in adults who get routine dental checkups.** Routine dental visits can help decrease the overall amount of bacteria in your mouth, including those that can cause pneumonia in susceptible people.

Bonus: A healthy mouth reduces heart disease risk, too.

IF YOU DO GET THE FLU…

Since the flu shot doesn't always prevent infection, be on the lookout for symptoms including feeling feverish, chills, body aches, sore throat and fatigue. If you suspect that you have the flu, call your doctor. You may be a candidate for prescription antiviral medication such as *oseltamivir* (Tamiflu), which can shorten your illness duration and possibly decrease the odds of it progressing to pneumonia. But you need to take it within a day or two of the first symptoms for it to be effective.

More from William Schaffner, MD…

Pneumonia and Your Heart

Adults hospitalized with pneumonia have a heightened risk for cardiovascular problems including sudden heart attack, often with no warning signs.

What happens: Oxygen deprivation from a bout of pneumonia can starve cardiac muscle cells so that they function less well or even die off. One study found that within the first month of pneumonia diagnosis, the risk for stroke, heart attack or death due to heart disease grew by as much as fourfold…and remained elevated for years. Patients recovering from pneumonia also are predisposed to developing it again—another good reason to prevent it in the first place.

Animal Infections That Can Make You Sick

Kevin R. Kazacos, DVM, PhD, professor emeritus of veterinary parasitology at Purdue University College of Veterinary Medicine in West Lafayette, Indiana. One HealthInitiative.com

---

When we think of protecting ourselves against infectious diseases, our beloved pets (and even those wild critters that live in our backyards) usually don't come to mind. But they should.

What most people don't realize: Every year, tens of thousands of Americans get sick from diseases spread from animals to people. In fact, current estimates are that about 60% of all human pathogens and 75% of newly recognized infectious diseases affecting humans originate in animals.

TWO TO WATCH OUT FOR

Examples of infections spread by animals (zoonotic diseases) that don't get the attention they deserve…

•**Cat scratch fever.** About 12,000 Americans are infected each year with cat scratch fever due to a scratch or bite from an infected cat. Caused by the bacterium *Bartonella henselae*, it is spread to cats by infected fleas, which excrete the organism in their feces ("flea dirt"), thus contaminating the cat's fur and claws.

How do humans contract it? People can become infected if an infected cat breaks the skin by scratching or biting them, or if a cat licks an open wound or abrasion on a person's skin.

What are the red flags? Typically, the bite or scratch site becomes infected, with swelling, redness and the development of a bump or blister at the site, occurring three to 10 days after being bitten or scratched.

Other symptoms include tender and swollen lymph nodes near the site, fatigue or overall discomfort, headache and low-grade fever. The disease usually goes away on its own, with no treatment, in four to eight weeks. The infection is not transmitted from person to person.

While rare, serious complications may develop, including blood infection, high fever and inflammation of the brain, heart, eyes or other internal organs. People with a weakened or compromised immune system (those with cancer or taking immunosuppressant medications, for example) and young children are more susceptible to complications.

How is it prevented? Avoid "rough play" with cats, particularly kittens, which could lead to scratches and bites. Any scratches and bites you might get should be washed immediately with soap and running water. Cats should not be allowed to lick any cuts or open wounds on a person's skin.

To protect cats from contracting the infection from fleas, use oral or topical flea products and treat the animals promptly if they become infested. Keep your cats indoors as much as possible to avoid other infected cats (and their fleas) and to prevent them from picking up fleas from the outside environment.

•**Raccoon roundworm (baylisascariasis).** This disease is caused by the larvae of a parasitic roundworm, Baylisascaris procyonis, commonly found in the intestine of raccoons and occasionally in dogs. The worms lay hundreds of thousands of eggs daily, which are shed in the animal's feces. The eggs in the feces or soil usually take two to four weeks to become infective.

A wide variety of animals, including rabbits, rodents, birds, dogs and primates, can become infected if they ingest infective eggs from areas of raccoon fecal contamination. Typically, infected animals show signs of progressive brain disease (encephalitis), such as incoordination, circling, head tilts and tremors, often ending in death.

How do humans contract it? People become infected by accidentally ingesting infective eggs from areas or articles contaminated by raccoons (or infected dogs in rare cases). Raccoons typically establish localized defecation sites—a kind of communal toilet—called latrines. These latrines, which can have a very high concentration of the eggs of the *B. procyonis* roundworm, can be found in backyards, on logs in woods, in attics, on rooftops and anywhere the animals have access to.

Young children are at greatest risk of infection because they sometimes place soil and other materials (including feces and contaminated objects or their fingers) into their mouths. Adults can also become infected if they accidentally ingest eggs following contact with contaminated areas or when cleaning up raccoon feces in their garage, backyard or other area without gloves, and if they do not wash their hands well.

What are the red flags? Infection can manifest as subtle to severe brain disease that appears two to three weeks after exposure. In heavy infections, symptoms may include sudden lethargy and unresponsiveness, incoordination, loss of speech and fine motor skills, decreased head control, vision problems and seizures that may progress rapidly to stupor, coma and death.

In addition to encephalitis, the worms may cause vision problems and blindness, either as a result of ongoing brain damage or from separate migration to the eye, which often occurs in cases without brain involvement.

How is it prevented? Home owners should consult a reputable pest control company for advice on the best ways to prevent raccoons from entering their properties.

Young children should be taught to recognize and avoid raccoon latrines and to wash their hands after being outdoors—especially after playing in wooded areas or the soil. Sandboxes should be covered when not in use because raccoons may establish latrines there.

Adults should wear gloves when dealing with areas that could possibly be contaminated and should wash their hands thoroughly. Latrines can be cleaned up and decontaminated by careful removal of feces and the use of heat (such as scalding water or steam) to kill any residual eggs. Very hot water (greater than 145°F) will kill eggs on clothing and other articles.

Important. If a child or adult who has been exposed to a raccoon latrine is suspected of ingesting any of the infected material, a course of *albendazole* (Albenza), a strong antiparasite medication, should be started while the person is being monitored to stop any larvae from entering the nervous system or eyes.

For a listing of zoonotic diseases and more details on avoiding them: Consult the Iowa State University Center for Food Security & Public Health (CFSPH.iastate.edu) and the Centers for Disease Control and Prevention (CDC.gov).

HOW ANIMALS SPREAD DISEASES

With the ongoing threat of Lyme disease and Zika virus, ticks and mosquitoes tend to get the most attention these days. But illnesses caused by the pets we live with…animals we may come in contact with at petting zoos…and those that take up residence in our backyards can also make us sick. Infections that are spread from animals to humans (known as zoonotic diseases) can be caused by viruses, bacteria, fungi and parasites.

Common ways people become infected with a zoonotic disease…

•**Direct contact with the feces,** urine, saliva, blood, nasal secretions or other body fluids (or hair or skin) of an infected animal. Example: Salmonellosis and cat scratch fever (see page 207).

•**Indirect contact with areas where animals live and roam,** or objects or surfaces that have been contaminated with infectious agents that animals left behind, such as animal pens or cages, aquarium tanks, food and water dishes, the soil or water where animals live, etc. Example: Raccoon roundworm (see below).

•**Vectorborne** when the disease is transmitted via an intermediate species (the vector, usually a blood-sucking insect), which carries and spreads disease-producing microorganisms.

Examples: Diseases transmitted by mosquitoes, ticks and fleas, including West Nile virus, Lyme disease and plague.

•***Salmonellosis.*** This is a diarrheal illness caused by Salmonella bacteria, which are present in the gastrointestinal tract of many animals, including domestic and wild birds, mammals, reptiles and amphibians.

How do humans contract it? People become infected by accidentally ingesting the feces of infected animals, directly or indirectly, after handling or petting animals or working with them. Common sources include baby chicks and ducklings, turtles, lizards and calves. It is also a common food-borne illness following ingestion of undercooked meat or eggs or unpasteurized dairy products.

What are the red flags? Symptoms of diarrhea, abdominal cramping and fever usually occur one to three days after exposure and typically resolve within a week. In some cases, especially in the very young or elderly or people with weak immune systems, more serious complications may occur requiring hospitalization and treatment.

How is it prevented? The best defense is hand-washing following contact with animals or their feces—whether it's a pet, wildlife, livestock or an animal in a petting zoo. Certain animals, such as turtles and lizards like iguanas, should not be kept as pets in households with very young children.

Also important: Safe food preparation methods, thorough cooking of animal products (meat and eggs), and consumption of pasteurized dairy products.

•**Ringworm (dermatophytosis).** This common skin infection is caused not caused by worms but by a variety of fungi. The condition gets its name from the ring-like rash it causes on the skin.

How do humans contract it? The fungi produce infective spores that are present on an animal's hair or in the environment. People and animals, including dogs, cats, large animals, rabbits, rodents and wildlife, get infected by touching an infected animal's (or person's) skin or hair or by touching things that can harbor the fungi—such as blankets, brushes and towels.

What are the red flags? It usually takes from one to four weeks after exposure to show signs. Animals often develop hairless patches of reddened, itchy scaly skin that are circular and become ringlike over time as the infection spreads out from the center. The fungus is more common in young puppies or kittens, due to their immature immune system and in older ones with weakened immune systems. People develop similar lesions that are itchy, inflamed and red on the outer edges with scaling and a ring-like appearance.

How is it prevented? Wash your hands after handling pets or other animals. Be especially careful around animals with obvious or suspect skin lesions. Clean and disinfect areas where your animal spends time, including crates and bedding. Vacuum to remove infected hair or flakes or skin, and wash with a strong detergent and a diluted bleach (1:10) to kill the spores of the fungus.

If your pet is found to have ringworm (your veterinarian can perform a microscopic exam and culture on samples of your pet's hair and skin)…wear disposable gloves and long sleeves when handling the animal…and wash your hands immediately afterward. Pets and people are typically treated with topical antifungal creams, medicated shampoos or prescribed baths/rinses, although oral antifungal drugs are also used.

Important: If your pet is found to have ringworm, it may be necessary to treat all pets in your household. People with weakened immune systems should not handle animals with ringworm.

Is Your Arthritis Really an Infection?

David Lans, DO, FACP, a clinical assistant professor of medicine at New York Medical College in Valhalla, New York, chief of rheumatology at NewYork-Presbyterian/Lawrence Hospital in Bronxville, New York, and an internist and a rheumatologist in private practice at Integrative Rheumatology of Westchester in New Rochelle, New York.

When you think of arthritis, what probably comes to mind is osteoarthritis, the wear-and-tear disease that affects more than 30 million Americans.

What you may not realize: Other types of arthritis can ravage joints, including arthritis caused by infection. For example, a recent study published in *Arthritis Care & Research* found that more than 16,000 people go to the emergency room every year with septic arthritis, an infection that can cause irreversible damage and deformity to joints.

Infections play a role in many cases of arthritis, both acute and chronic. Because these types of arthritis are less common than osteoarthritis, they are often misdiagnosed or overlooked. *What you need to know about…*

•**Septic arthritis.** Triggered by bacteria in the bloodstream that settle in a joint, this is the most serious form of infectious arthritis. Without prompt treatment, deep bone infections may occur and take months to resolve. One-third of people with septic arthritis suffer joint damage—and 10% die.

About half the time, the infection is in the knee, and pain and swelling are so severe that walking is difficult. The joint will also be red and hot. And you'll have a fever and chills and feel very sick. The knee is a common site for septic arthritis because of its large size and location.

People who have weakened immune systems, including adults over age 65 and children, are the most common victims of septic arthritis.

Contact Lenses and Bacteria

Bacteria can form biofilms (layers of microorganisms) that adhere to lenses, making them more resistant against antimicrobial solutions such as lens cleaners. Biofilm formation is a major factor in eye infections related to contact lenses. *To reduce chances of infection...*

•**Wash your hands with soap and water before inserting lenses.** Use the cleaning solution recommended by your doctor or labeled for your type of lenses. Follow the cleaning and storage instructions.

•**Avoid sleeping in contact lenses,** even if you have the "continuous wear" type, since overnight wear is a big risk factor for infection. If you are not careful about cleaning, consider a daily disposable lens. Smokers and those who have diabetes or a weakened immune system are at a greater risk for infection.

Lindsay Ciocco, OD, FAAO, instructor of ophthalmology, The Johns Hopkins Wilmer Eye Institute, Baltimore.

You're also at higher risk if you already have a joint problem, such as osteoarthritis, gout or rheumatoid arthritis, which is an autoimmune disease...if you're taking medications for rheumatoid arthritis, which suppress the immune system...if you have an immune-weakening disease, such as diabetes or cancer...or if you have fragile skin that is easily injured and heals poorly (a fairly common problem among older adults and those with diabetes), allowing bacteria ready access into your bloodstream.

Many types of bacteria can cause septic arthritis. The most common bacterial culprits are Staph and Streptococcal species. If the infection isn't stopped, bacteria can destroy cartilage, causing permanent damage.

What to watch out for: Sudden, severe pain in a knee or other joint, and flulike symptoms, including fever and chills.

Treatment: Go to the emergency room or see a doctor—immediately. The joint will be drained with a needle or tube (arthroscopy), and the fluid will be cultured to identify the bacteria. It's likely you'll also get blood tests to help pinpoint the infection and X-rays to see if the joint has been damaged.

If you're diagnosed with septic arthritis, you'll receive IV antibiotics, followed by oral antibiotics. The usual antibiotic treatment duration is about six weeks. If antibiotics aren't effective, you may need surgery to drain the infection.

•**Reactive arthritis.** This type of arthritis can plague joints for weeks to years. Doctors aren't certain if reactive arthritis is an infection of the joint...or a joint-centered inflammation triggered by an infection elsewhere in the body. Either way, the arthritis is typically caused by either a sexually transmitted bacterial infection, such as chlamydia or gonorrhea, or a gastrointestinal infection, such as C. difficile or salmonella. Food poisoning is a common trigger.

What to watch out for: Joint pain that develops a few weeks or months after a sexually transmitted or gastrointestinal infection.

Treatment: A blood test will be given to detect the bacteria. If it's positive, you'll take antibiotics that target the organism. Nonsteroidal anti-inflammatory drugs (NSAIDs), such as ibuprofen (Motrin)...corticosteroids...or antirheumatic drugs, such as *methotrexate* (Trexall), may also be prescribed.

•**Lyme arthritis.** Lyme disease, a bacterial infection from a tick bite, is found throughout the US, but mainly in the Northeast, from Maine to Virginia, and in Minnesota, Wisconsin, Michigan and northern California. Some people never overcome the infection and develop chronic Lyme disease. Among those, more than half develop Lyme arthritis—one or more swollen joints (usually a knee), with pain (typically mild) that is intermittent or constant.

What to watch out for: Lyme arthritis usually develops several months after the tick bite. As with all types of arthritis, joint swelling and pain can occur.

Treatment: Lyme arthritis often resembles reactive arthritis. To make a definitive diagnosis, your doctor will order a blood test to detect antibodies to *B. burgdorferi,* the bacterium transmitted from the tick bite. The doctor may also remove fluid from your joint for a polymerase chain reaction (PCR) test, which detects the presence of DNA from B. burgdorferi.

If one or both of these tests are positive, your doctor will probably prescribe oral or intravenous antibiotics for one to three months. In most cases, this treatment cures Lyme arthritis, especially if it's initiated early on.

However, in some patients, the treatment fails, and chronic arthritis, as well as other symptoms (such as fatigue, headache and difficulty concentrating), may persist. If the disease isn't controlled, a drug used for rheumatoid arthritis—a disease modifying antirheumatic drug, or DMARD—often helps control the Lyme arthritis. Some patients require long-term treatment, while others improve over a period of months.

•**Viral joint infections.** Many viruses can trigger acute arthritis, but the joint pain that results is usually mild and goes away on its own after a few weeks. Viral infections that can cause arthritis include…

•Zika virus, from mosquitoes that carry it.

•Epstein-Barr, the virus that causes mononucleosis.

•Hepatitis A and B, the liver-infecting viruses that cause about one-third of virus-triggered arthritis.

•Parvovirus, a respiratory infection common in adults who are routinely exposed to children, the primary carriers of this infection, which causes a distinctive face rash.

What to watch out for: Sudden, mild joint pain (viral arthritis can affect almost any joint).

Treatment: Your physician will order a blood test for antibodies to specific viruses that can cause acute arthritis. Pain control is the goal, typically with an over-the-counter NSAID, such as ibuprofen or *naproxen* (Aleve).

Syphilis Rates High

Philip A. Chan, MD, is an internal medicine and infectious disease specialist and assistant professor of medicine at Brown University, Providence.

Syphilis rates are the highest in 20 years. From 2014 to 2015, the number of cases in the US rose 17.7%, from 63,453 to 74,702. Social media likely plays a role because dating apps such as Tinder and Grindr make it easy to have sex with people that users don't know well.

Self-defense: Get tested annually or, if you have multiple partners, get tested every three months. The disease is easily treated when found early. Late-stage syphilis can cause dementia and cardiovascular problems.

Swimmer Warning: Even Chlorine Doesn't Kill This Dangerous Parasite

Michele Hlavsa, RN, MPH, an epidemiologist with the Centers for Disease Control and Prevention's National Center for Emerging and Zoonotic Infectious Diseases, Atlanta. She is chief of the CDC's Healthy Swimming Program. CDC.gov

That crystal-clear pool water could be harboring *Cryptosporidium*, a parasite that can cause up to three weeks of diarrhea, stomach cramps, nausea and vomiting. Reports of widespread outbreaks of infection by the parasite, known as crypto for short, have doubled in just two years in the US, from 16 outbreaks in 2014 to 32 in 2016, and thousands of Americans are infected annually. Nearly 2,000 people were infected last year in Ohio alone. Crypto is now the most common cause of diarrhea outbreaks linked to pools and water playgrounds in the US, and it can be life-threatening for people with weakened immune systems.

This parasite usually is spread through swallowing contaminated water at swimming pools and water playgrounds. Unlike most pathogens, it can survive up to 10 days in properly chlorinated water. Advanced water-treatment systems such as those using ultraviolet light or ozone do a better job of killing crypto. Public swimming pools and water playgrounds are especially vulnerable to causing large-scale outbreaks because of the large numbers of people who use them, but crypto also can be contracted in private pools and hot tubs and in natural bodies of water.

What to do: Don't swallow any water when you go swimming—especially when swimming in a public pool or visiting a water playground. If you do not swallow any water, you are unlikely to become infected even if crypto is present. One way to reduce the odds of ingestion is to keep your face out of the water as much as possible.

The parasite is transmitted into pool water from infected individuals via contaminated feces. To avoid being the source of contamination in a pool, don't go swimming if you have been experiencing diarrhea, and don't allow children to do so either. (This includes very young children in diapers—if a child has diarrhea, even the "swim diapers" designed for use in pools will not provide adequate protection for the water.) If your doctor tells you that your diarrhea is a result of crypto, do not go swimming until you have been diarrhea-free for two weeks.

Hidden Infection Risk

Juan-Jesus Carrero, PharmD, associate professor of renal epidemiology, Karolinska Institutet, Stockholm, Sweden.

As kidney function declined, the risk for infections, such as urinary tract infections and sepsis, grew almost sixfold, a study of 1.1 million people found. Because kidney disease often goes undiagnosed, many people are at high risk for such infections without knowing it.

What to do: Be sure your doctor monitors your kidney function with a serum creatinine blood test or an albuminuria urine test—especially if you've had more infections than usual.

Your Cash Could Make You Sick

Philip M. Tierno, Jr., PhD, a microbiologist and director of clinical microbiology and diagnostic immunology at New York University Langone Medical Center, New York City. He is author of *The Secret Life of Germs*.

Your cold hard cash could give you a cold—or worse. Recent research conducted by New York University's Center for Genomics & System Biology identified roughly 3,000 types of bacteria on paper money, including germs that cause food poisoning, staph infections and pneumonia.

Cut Risk for UTIs by 50%

Cut your risk for urinary tract infections (UTIs) in half by drinking an extra six cups of water a day. Young women who had frequent UTIs and drank six more cups of water daily were 48% less likely to have another UTI (the women had been drinking about four cups of fluid a day before the study). And the water drinkers were able to reduce their use of antibiotics by 47%. Fluid intake may reduce UTI risk by preventing bacteria from adhering to the bladder and reducing overall bacterial concentration.

Thomas Hooton, MD, clinical director, division of infectious diseases, University of Miami School of Medicine, and coauthor of a study of 140 healthy premenopausal women who had at least three UTIs in the previous year, presented at the recent IDWeek 2017 conference in San Diego.

Touching a germy bill will not necessarily make you sick. Typically, a relatively large number of germs must enter the body to cause infection, and that usually does not occur when you handle money in normal ways—but there are exceptions.

Example: A single norovirus virion (the infectious form of a virus) can cause infection.

The health risks from germ-covered money increase greatly when money is handled by someone who also handles food, such as a sandwich-shop worker or street-food vendor. This opens the door for germs to be transferred from money to the food we eat, allowing many more of the germs to enter the body.

Coins tend to harbor fewer germs than paper money because certain metals used in coins, including copper, nickel and zinc, naturally inhibit germ growth. Crisp, new bills tend to harbor fewer germs than old, worn ones because US paper money has antimicrobial properties that seem to diminish with time and usage.

What to do: Wash your hands or use a hand sanitizer as soon as possible after handling money. Choose a hand sanitizer with an alcohol percentage of 85% or higher—unlike most germs, the norovirus can survive 60% to 65% alcohol hand sanitizers.

CHAPTER 13

Medication Alerts

Medications That Increase Your Risk of Falling

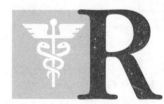**R**ead the package insert for any medication and you'll likely see dizziness listed as a possible side effect. Still, few of us take dizziness seriously. But we should. Dizziness can lead to a fall...and that could lead to a serious injury.

MORE MEDS, MORE RISK

More than half of all Americans are taking two prescription medications—20% are taking five or more, according to Mayo Clinic research. So it's important to recognize that side effects, including dizziness, are more pronounced with every drug you take. The increased effects are not additive—they are exponential. After a while, the question is not if you will fall, but when. Falls are one of the leading causes of long-term disability in older adults.

Here are widely used medications that commonly cause dizziness and falls. Chances are you use at least one of the following medications.

PAIN MEDICATIONS

The risks of opioid pain medications (including disorientation and dizziness) are well-known, but there is an increased fall risk even with over-the-counter (OTC) pain relievers. These seemingly benign medications influence many body systems, including the central nervous system (CNS), and can cause dizziness, even at normal doses.

Examples: Nonsteroidal anti-inflammatory drugs (NSAIDs), such as aspirin, *ibuprofen* (Advil) and *naproxen* (Aleve).

Surprisingly, aspirin may be the worst offender. In addition to its effects on the CNS, aspirin bombards the vestibular nerve that feeds balance information from the inner ear to the brain. Many people can't take aspirin (even the baby aspirin dose of 81 mg) without expe-

Jack Fincham, PhD, RPh, professor of pharmaceutical and administrative sciences at Presbyterian College School of Pharmacy in Clinton, South Carolina.

213

riencing severe dizziness or even vertigo—the nauseating perception that the room is spinning or tilting.

Note: Muscle relaxers are also sometimes prescribed for pain. These drugs cause significant drowsiness.

Examples: *Carisoprodol* (Soma), *cyclobenzaprine* and *orphenadrine*. When paired with a pain reliever, the combination of dizziness and drowsiness is a perfect recipe for a fall.

SLEEP AIDS AND ALLERGY DRUGS

Diphenhydramine is an antihistamine recommended to clear a stuffy nose and induce drowsiness at bedtime.

Examples: Benadryl, Tylenol PM, Advil PM and Aleve PM.

Like aspirin, *diphenhydramine* affects the CNS and the vestibular system, causing dizziness. It also slows down mental abilities such as thinking and processing information, so you may be less able to recognize side effects.

Because this drug is included in medications as a sleep aid, many people assume that they can sleep away the side effects. But diphenhydramine has a long half-life—in older adults, it can stay in their systems for up to 18 hours. The medication-induced dizziness can cause a fall if you get up during the night, for example, to use the bathroom.

ANTIDEPRESSANTS

All antidepressants work at the level of neurotransmitters—the chemical messengers, such as serotonin, norepinephrine and dopamine, that allow us to think, act and experience emotion.

The most widely used antidepressants are selective serotonin reuptake inhibitors (SSRIs), which work by making serotonin more available to the brain, elevating mood and decreasing anxiety.

Examples: *Fluoxetine* (Prozac), *paroxetine* (Paxil) and *sertraline* (Zoloft).

Migraine drugs also work by affecting serotonin availability.

Examples: *Sumatriptan* (Imitrex) and *zolmitriptan* (Zomig).

Serotonin and norepinephrine reuptake inhibitors (SNRIs) are a newer type of antidepressant that makes both serotonin and norepinephrine more available to the brain.

Examples: *Duloxetine* (Cymbalta), *venlafaxine* (Effexor) and *desvenlafaxine* (Pristiq).

Bupropion (Wellbutrin) affects the availability of both norepinephrine and dopamine.

Note: The smoking-cessation medication Zyban also contains bupropion.

Besides affecting mood, these antidepressants carry messages to the brain from the balance centers of the inner ear, so they can affect your equilibrium. In addition, a faulty message can make the communication between brain and body less responsive. When you stand up or move, you may be less able to control your body position, increasing the risk of toppling over.

BLOOD PRESSURE DRUGS

There are many types of blood pressure medications, including…

- **Diuretics** ("water pills"), such as *furosemide* (Lasix).

- **Beta-blockers,** such as *propranolol* (Inderal) and *atenolol* (Tenormin).

- **Angiotensin-converting enzyme (ACE) inhibitors,** such as *enalapril* (Vasotec) and *lisinopril* (Zestril).

- **Angiotensin II receptor blockers (ARBs),** such as *losartan* (Cozaar) and *olmesartan* (Benicar).

- **Calcium channel blockers,** such as *amlodipine* (Norvasc).

All medications that lower your blood pressure can also diminish your ability to quickly adapt to changing blood pressure needs, such as when you change your body position. Therefore, a common side effect of these drugs is orthostatic hypotension—a sudden spell of light-headed dizziness that happens when you quickly stand up after sitting or lying down.

ANTICONVULSANTS AND NEUROPATHY DRUGS

Drugs for epilepsy, fibromyalgia and neuropathy can alleviate pain by putting the brakes on nerve impulse transmission. But this may limit the brain's ability to respond normally and quickly, significantly reducing alertness and increasing dizziness.

Examples: Gabapentin (Neurontin), *pregabalin* (Lyrica) and *carbamazepine* (Tegretol), all commonly used to treat diabetic nerve pain and fibromyalgia…and *clonazepam* (Klonopin) and *phenytoin* (Dilantin), both used as antiepileptic drugs.

WHAT TO DO

Literally every drug has the potential to cause dizziness and increase your risk of falling. *What to do…*

•**For occasional-use medications**—assess your level of discomfort. If you don't really need a drug, don't take it. If you must take a medication, develop an alternate plan that may include a medication change that is approved after consultation with your health-care provider.

•**For long-term medications**—never stop taking them without advice from your health-care provider. Many medications need to be tapered and will create rebound side effects if stopped abruptly.

•**For all new medications**—be alert for signs of dizziness or drowsiness. Are your body and mind as quick and responsive as usual? Do you feel alert? These side effects may be subtle or pronounced, but they should not be ignored. If they occur, avoid any activity that could result in a fall, including using stairs or ladders. If you must use stairs, steady yourself with handrails and move slowly up or down the stairs.

As your body adjusts to a medication, you may be prescribed a higher dosage to get the appropriate therapeutic effect.

Important: Watch for new side effects with each dosage change. They can appear even after the drug has been taken for an extended period.

•**If you experience orthostatic hypotension**—be sure to take your time standing up… and don't immediately start walking. Take a moment to steady yourself. If you become lightheaded, sit down immediately. This practice is useful for anyone taking medication.

•**If you feel dizzy or have other troubling side effects while using any medication**—call your doctor…or talk to your pharmacist, who may be more accessible. Ask if there is another treatment that might have fewer side effects and less dizziness.

•**Before driving or exercising**—observe how you are reacting to the medication. Does an effect diminish in intensity after a while? If so, try to drive small distances and exercise carefully with companions to see how you are doing.

Don't Let Your Doctor Become Your "Drug Dealer"

Anna Lembke, MD, a psychiatrist, assistant professor and chief of addiction medicine at Stanford University School of Medicine in California. She is the author of *Drug Dealer, MD: How Doctors Were Duped, Patients Got Hooked, and Why It's So Hard to Stop.*

With all the alarming headlines warning us against the full-blown opioid epidemic that is gripping the US, you'd think that patients and doctors would be on high alert for possible misuse of these drugs. Yet the problem continues…

Shocking statistics: More than 91 Americans die every day from an opioid overdose, according to the Centers for Disease Control and Prevention (CDC).

Surprisingly, only 7% of people who misuse or are addicted to these powerful painkillers get them from strangers or dealers—the vast majority are obtained with legitimate prescriptions or from friends or relatives who presumably obtained them from their doctors.

Why do doctors continue to prescribe drugs that are known to cause addiction—and why do so many patients demand drugs that are not effective for long-term pain?

To learn more, we spoke with Anna Lembke, MD, a psychiatrist and addiction specialist who has extensively studied the misuse of prescription drugs.

Which drugs are most likely to cause addiction?

The opioid painkillers—morphine, *hydrocodone*, *oxycodone* (OxyContin, Percocet), *fentanyl* (Sublimaze, Duragesic), etc.—are the main offenders. They're classified by the FDA as Schedule II drugs, meaning they carry a high risk for addiction.

Some stimulant drugs, including *methylphenidate* (Ritalin) and other medications used to treat attention deficit hyperactivity disorder, can also be addictive, particularly when they're used by patients who are also taking opioid painkillers or other mood-altering drugs.

Are prescription medications more addictive than street drugs?

They may not be inherently more addictive (this would depend on the different chemical properties), but they're more readily available—and that's a big part of addiction. In the 1960s, 80% of heroin (an illicit opioid) users started out with heroin. Today, most heroin users begin with prescription opioid painkillers before moving on to heroin.

Opioids are routinely prescribed by pain specialists, surgeons and family doctors. Patients acquire the drugs from emergency rooms, walk-in clinics and online pharmacies. They're everywhere.

Who is most likely to get addicted?

Patients with a previous history of addiction—to alcohol and/or drugs—have the highest risk. Addiction is also common in those with a family history of addiction or a personal history of depression or other psychiatric disorders. Before prescribing opioids, doctors should ask if a patient has any history of addiction or mental illness as well as if there is any family history of addiction. If a doctor does not ask about this (many don't), a patient should be sure to alert his/her doctor regarding these issues.

However, we've also found that patients with no history of addiction/drug use are also at risk. Studies have shown that about 25% of patients who use these drugs for legitimate medical reasons for three months or more will begin to misuse these medications—meaning they take more than prescribed or don't take the medica-

tion as prescribed (for example, they binge or hoard medication). This is a first step on the road to addiction.

Why do doctors keep prescribing opioids?

Many believe, mistakenly, that patients who take these drugs for pain—as opposed to using them recreationally—are unlikely to become addicted. There's an old (and flawed) statistic that pain patients have less than a 1% chance of becoming addicted. We now know that this is not true.

Other factors: Doctors want to ease pain… pleasing patients is part of their DNA. Prescribing a powerful painkiller can feel like a better alternative than possibly letting someone suffer.

How do patients get more medication than they need?

Many of them "doctor shop"—they exaggerate their symptoms while collecting prescriptions from many different doctors. Some patients claim to have lost or misplaced their prescriptions before the refill date. Others create so much disruption in doctors' offices—begging for drugs, threatening lawsuits, intimidating the staff, etc.—that they're given prescriptions just to be rid of them.

Note: Some insurance companies are now closely monitoring claims and alerting prescribers about suspicious activity, so some patients pay out of pocket to avoid getting caught.

Don't patients know that they're becoming addicted?

Surprisingly, they don't. Addictive drugs work on the brain's reward pathways. Patients feel so good when they take the drugs that they lose insight into all the negative consequences—lost jobs, damaged relationships, etc.

Who should take these drugs?

Opioids are very effective painkillers. Anyone who's suffered a severe, acute injury—a broken leg, for example—will clearly benefit in the short term. Those who have had major surgery almost always need them. They're also a good choice for those with acute pain related to cancer, such as metastatic cancer lesions on the bone. And opioids are an essential tool in the last few hours of life to help ease the passage to death.

But for chronic pain, opioids should be the very last choice. Nonmedication alternatives, such as psychotherapy, physical therapy, acupuncture, massage, meditation, etc., should be tried first, followed by nonopioid medications, such as *ibuprofen* (Motrin) or *acetaminophen* (Tylenol). These approaches can also be tried in combination.

For people who don't respond to the approaches above, opioids may be required, but doctors need to proceed with caution. I advise intermittent dosing—say, using the drugs three days a week, without using them in between. This will still reduce pain but with less risk for addiction. Patients don't take the drug regularly enough to build up a tolerance and dependence, so they shouldn't have withdrawal symptoms.

Can anything else be done to help? Doctors who prescribe these drugs should take advantage of prescription drug monitoring programs. These state-by-state databases (available in every state except Missouri) allow doctors to see every prescription (for opioids and other scheduled drugs) that a patient has received within a certain time. They'll know how many prescriptions a patient has received…how many doctors they're getting them from…the doses they're taking, etc. This information goes into the database when a patient picks up the prescription at the pharmacy.

Drugs That Can Turn Deadly: Is Your Med Making You Suicidal?

Jack E. Fincham, PhD, RPh, professor of pharmaceutical and administrative sciences, Presbyterian College School of Pharmacy, Clinton, South Carolina.

Americans use a lot of medications, filling prescriptions and buying over-the-counter (OTC) drugs several billion times each year. All these medications come with potential benefits and risks. But in the ubiquitous TV and print ads targeted to consumers, the benefits get much more attention than the risks.

Surprising danger you should know about: The use of certain medications is linked to suicidal thinking. That's right—a medication that you take to feel better might twist your thoughts, suddenly and powerfully, so that you feel bad enough to consider ending your life.

My analysis: When I recently completed a search of Clinical Pharmacology powered by ClinicalKey, a trusted database of drug information, this potential side effect is listed for 188 different drugs, including both prescription and OTC medications that are taken by several million Americans. Use of certain drugs with this possible side effect has also been linked to increased risk for suicide attempts and completed suicides.

To be fair, just because this possible side effect is listed does not mean that a drug always causes suicidal thinking…nor that the drug is to blame if this frightening problem does occur. But it does mean that cases have shown up—either in clinical trials conducted before the drug was approved or in reports sent to FDA regulators after it hit the market.

Unfortunately, it is impossible to say with any certainty how often people experience this (or any other) side effect in real-world use. That's because not everyone having a problem reports it, nor do regulators hear from people who have no problems with the drug.

Still, if suicidal thinking is a possible side effect of a drug you're taking for, say, depression, asthma, allergies or acne, it's something you want to know so that you, your doctor and the people close to you can be on the alert—and fully consider all the risks and benefits of that medication or alternatives.

Important: Do not stop taking a medication your doctor has prescribed without checking with the doctor or pharmacist. Some drugs may have additional side effects if stopped abruptly.

DRUGS ON THE DANGER LIST

Among the medications that have been linked to suicidal thinking…

•***Montelukast*** **(Singulair).** Singulair is the best known of a group of medicines known as

217

leukotriene inhibitors. Usually taken in pill form, it is used to treat asthma and, in some cases, nasal allergies. Other drugs in this class include *zafirlukast* (Accolate) and *zileuton* (Zyflo).

Since 2009, the FDA has required these drugs to carry labels saying that suicidal thinking and actions (and mental health problems such as anxiety and depression) have been reported in some patients.

My advice: Assuming you've talked with your doctor about the risks and potential benefits and have decided to use a leukotriene inhibitor, stay alert for any changes in your typical feelings and thoughts. If any occur, it may be that you could safely use another drug, such as a beta-agonist, or switch to something else entirely, such as an inhaled corticosteroid. These medications have not been linked to suicidal thinking.

•**Antidepressants.** While studies in older adults have not found a definitive link between antidepressant use and suicidal thinking, studies in children, teens and adults under age 25 have been concerning enough to lead the FDA to put so-called black-box warnings (the strongest kind) about the possible risks for young people on all antidepressants.

It's unclear why young people might be especially vulnerable to such a drug side effect. Perhaps medical providers and parents are more vigilant and more likely to report known suicidal thoughts or attempts when the patient is young. Or perhaps young brains react differently to the drugs. Whatever the reason, the FDA says the risk appears greatest in the early weeks of treatment or right after a dose is increased or decreased.

My advice: When anyone you know—but particularly a young person—is taking an antidepressant, be alert for warning signs, including worsening depression…talk of suicide…sleeplessness…agitation…and social withdrawal.

•*Varenicline* (**Chantix**). This prescription pill can help some people quit smoking. But for years, the FDA has required this medication to be labeled with a black-box warning alerting users that the drug has been linked with serious mental health problems, including suicidal thinking and behavior.

In 2016, citing new data, the FDA removed the strong warning, saying that the benefits of using Chantix to quit smoking outweighed the possible mental health risks and that those risks appear to be lower than previously suspected.

However, the risk for suicidal thinking continues to be mentioned on the manufacturer's website.

What may not be brought to your attention: Some of the best smoking-cessation tools, including nicotine-replacement products such as gums and patches, are available without a prescription and have not been linked to suicidal thinking. In-person and telephone counseling (call 800-QUIT-NOW) also can help some smokers.

My advice: If you're uneasy about taking Chantix, try one of the other approaches mentioned above. But do stay resolved to quit smoking!

OTHER DRUGS

The list of widely used medications linked to suicidal thoughts or actions also includes the OTC allergy drugs *cetirizine* (Zyrtec) and *levocetirizine* (Xyzal)…the acne drug *isotretinoin*…the nerve pain drug *pregabalin* (Lyrica)…and a variety of medications, including *carbamazepine* (Tegretol) and *divalproex sodium* (Depakote), that are used to treat seizures. Studies differ on which seizure medications are associated with the risk, so the FDA requires warnings on all of them.

Good rule of thumb: If you don't feel "right" when starting any new medication or a new dose of a medication, talk to your pharmacist, physician or other health-care provider. You also can read about the possible side effects of any medication at FDA.gov—search "Index to Drug-Specific Information."

Critically important: If you or someone you know is having suicidal thoughts, immediately call your doctor…go to a hospital emergency room…or call the confidential and toll-free National Suicide Prevention Lifeline at 800-273-TALK (8255). Help is available!

Medical "Marijuana" Without the High

David Bearman, MD, vice president of the American Academy of Cannabinoid Medicine and author of the forthcoming book *Abridged Guide to Cannabinoid Medicine Practice*. He is in private practice in Goleta, California.

Now legal in 30 states, medical cannabis (aka marijuana) can treat a wide variety of ailments from cancer pain to seizures. But what if you don't want to get high to get relief?

That's where cannabidiol (CBD), a compound derived from marijuana, comes in. Unlike its more famous cousin, tetrahydrocannabinol (THC), CBD doesn't cause even mild euphoria…or give you the munchies.

Yet CBD is the subject of some of the most exciting medical research in the field today—it has numerous potential therapeutic applications that may turn it into the next wonder drug for treating epilepsy, anxiety, Alzheimer's and a host of other diseases and ailments.

Case in point: Epidiolex, a newly developed drug (key ingredient: CBD), reduces seizures by 39% in children with a rare form of epilepsy, Dravet syndrome. It was approved by the FDA in April 2018.

CBD is widely available in many states and online, even though the Federal Drug Enforcement Agency classifies it as an illegal narcotic.

To learn more about its medical uses, we spoke with David Bearman, MD, a leading authority on cannabinoid medicine. He emphasized that people with medical conditions who are interested in CBD should first discuss it with their doctors. *His answers to our questions…*

Isn't CBD actually psychoactive—the reason medical marijuana is so controversial?

It is—but not the way people might think. Like THC, it crosses the blood-brain barrier and binds to receptors in the brain—that's how it can reduce pain. It also affects the immune system to reduce inflammation. But unlike THC, CBD doesn't cause euphoria or dysphoria—feeling uneasy, anxious or too out of touch with reality.

What forms does CBD come in?

It's available in a wide variety of forms including a liquid tincture, capsules, an oil for use in a vaporizer (aka vaping) and in sprays that can be inhaled or sprayed under the tongue. There also are topical CBD creams to help with muscle pain. Some companies also produce synthetic forms of CBD.

Is CBD addictive?

No. There is no addictive aspect to CBD whatsoever—or, for that matter, to THC.

What do we know currently about what kinds of patients CBD can help?

The list of diseases and conditions that CBD can improve and the symptoms that it can relieve actually is quite long. *I'll discuss a few…*

•**Epilepsy.** Research shows that CBD helps prevent seizures. Many doctors now are not waiting for an FDA-approved drug—they already are recommending it in tincture or capsules.

•**Anxiety.** A New York University School of Medicine review found that CBD can treat anxiety disorder, obsessive-compulsive disorder (OCD) and post-traumatic stress disorder (PTSD). Other research has found that it has effects similar to some antipsychotic drugs—it may be effective in treating patients with schizophrenia.

•**Alzheimer's and Parkinson's.** CBD's neuroprotective properties may help stem the progression of Alzheimer's disease and Parkinson's disease, among other brain diseases. While more research is needed, I believe that people at high risk for either disease—and certainly those in the early stages—should use CBD.

•**Other conditions.** CBD is being studied for its possible therapeutic effect on diabetes, stroke, rheumatoid arthritis, psoriasis, multiple sclerosis, fibromyalgia and osteoarthritis. It also contributes to the inhibition of cancer cell growth. But more research is needed in all these areas.

There always are drawbacks with any drug— what are CBD's?

CBD may cause fatigue, nausea and changes in appetite. A more serious concern is that CBD reduces the speed at which the body metabolizes the blood thinner *warfarin* (Coumadin)—if you're taking the two together, let your doctor know. He/she will want to monitor your blood-clotting factors closely and may need to reduce your warfarin dosage.

Are there conditions for which using CBD in combination with THC is more beneficial than CBD alone?

Absolutely. In my experience, CBD paired with THC works better for treating epilepsy and for reducing chronic pain. CBD's principal contribution to treating chronic pain is its anti-inflammatory properties. Often the THC dose can be low enough (5 mg or less) that there's no sense of being high. Plus, CBD partially reduces the euphoric effect of THC. A patient may want to start with CBD and then, if needed, add a little THC to see whether it makes a beneficial difference.

How can doctors and patients tell the right amount of CBD to take?

There's not enough research to make any definitive statements about dosing. Every individual is different—your size, age and the illness you're treating will affect how much you require for treatment.

My advice: Work with a knowledgeable health professional who can help you adjust the dose, the THC/CBD ratio, discuss whether to include other cannabinoids, explore the best way for you to take CBD, address possible side effects—and follow your medical progress. My advice to my patients is to start at a low dose and increase it slowly if needed.

What's the best form to take?

I generally advise taking CBD orally, not by inhalation or topically. You'll get the fastest effects with inhaling/vaping, but those effects last only about three hours. Taking CBD orally means that the effects can last up to seven hours.

The route of CBD administration depends on how rapidly you need it to start working…and how long you want the therapeutic effects to last. Different patients prefer different routes of administration—respiratory (vaping)…oral (tinctures, edibles, pills)…topical or suppository. But with so many routes of administration, it is best to discuss your preference with your physician.

Hallucinogens Go Mainstream?

Stephen Ross, MD, director of addiction psychiatry at New York University (NYU) Langone Medical Center, associate professor of psychiatry and child and adolescent psychiatry at NYU School of Medicine.

Hallucinogenic drugs may bring to mind the '60s. But new studies show that there actually might be mental health benefits for a number of hallucinogens, including psilocybin (the active ingredient in "magic mushrooms")…ketamine (a "rave" drug known as Special K)…MDMA (known as Ecstasy or Molly)…and LSD. Hallucinogens, also known as psychedelics, have so far been studied in small doses taken in carefully supervised environments and rigorously coupled with psychotherapy—so you're not about to get a prescription for one this weekend. But the research is real… and promising.

HOW HALLUCINOGENS WORK

Psychedelic drugs are thought to activate serotonin 2A receptors in the brain, which profoundly alters consciousness. When this happens, stimuli that the brain might have ignored suddenly become heightened, and the mind is opened to new experiences. From the user's perspective, there also can be a mystical or spiritual component. MDMA, according to a leading hypothesis, promotes attachment and bonding, so recounting a traumatic event to a psychotherapist in a safe environment while under its influence may remove the fear and anxiety associated with the memory and replace it with a more positive memory.

One thing these drugs don't do is trigger addiction. Psilocybin and LSD do not possess addictive properties in any ways that we measure addiction in animal and human models. In fact, they may have anti-addictive properties (see next page).

Hallucinogens can exacerbate psychosis, however, and should never be given to psychotic patients such as schizophrenics. As the experiences in the '60s and '70s demonstrated, there are well-known adverse psychological effects from uncontrolled recreational use of psychedelics. The most serious are psychosis in people with a known psychotic illness or who are at risk for psychotic illness…dangerous behavior such as violence and suicide…and severe anxiety and panic.

But once that susceptible population is screened out, psychedelics are very safe when used in controlled environments and administered by skilled clinicians. In the modern era of research with psychedelics over the last 20 years, there have been more than 2,000 doses of psilocybin administered—and zero serious adverse events.

AN ADDICTION FIGHTER

Preliminary results of an ongoing NYU study focusing on alcohol dependence suggest a very positive outcome from psilocybin. Following the first psilocybin session, the number of drinking days, as well as heavy drinking days, dropped significantly among participants. At Johns Hopkins Medical Center, another early-stage study has reported that psilocybin is effective against tobacco addiction. Other researchers are studying its use for treating cocaine addiction.

INVESTIGATIONS TO TREAT DEPRESSION, PTSD AND MORE

Here are a few more ways that psychedelic drugs are being studied for therapeutic purposes…

•**Cancer patients.** In a phase 2 study at NYU Langone Medical Center and Johns Hopkins University, a majority of people suffering cancer-related anxiety or depression experienced rapid, substantial and sustained relief for as long as eight months from a single dose of psilocybin administered in conjunction with psychotherapy.

•**Depression.** In a small British study, patients who had been clinically depressed for an average of 18 years and who had not responded to standard medications showed an improvement in symptoms one week after two doses of psilocybin. Several other small studies have found that ketamine provides rapid antidepressant effects for severe and even suicidal depression, and larger trials are now under way.

•**PTSD.** MDMA-assisted psychotherapy has shown promising results in treating post-traumatic stress disorder (PTSD). Prior medications and psychotherapy had not worked for the patients in the study, yet one year after treatment with MDMA-assisted psychotherapy, 68% of them demonstrated long-term improvement, and some no longer met the criteria for having PTSD.

•**Cognition.** The Beckley/Imperial Research Programme in the UK is undertaking the first controlled scientific investigation into whether LSD microdosing—taking such a small dose that you don't even know you're on it—enhances cognition, increases productivity, improves mood and/or boosts creativity. Their findings could result in therapeutic use for people with depression, among other conditions.

THE FUTURE

Early clinical trials have moved into the second and third phases, so it's possible we will see these treatments become available to patients in three to five years. If it happens, it will be under restrictive conditions—drugs administered by certain doctors in certain hospitals and clinics with appropriate supervision. We'll keep you posted.

A SPIRITUAL AWAKENING?

How psychedelics work against addictions isn't understood exactly. There are certainly biological explanations, in terms of rewiring the brain and changes at the gene level. But a leading hypothesis in the NYU psilocybin trial to treat alcoholism is that a spiritual transformation—the result of a drug-induced, personally meaningful mystical experience—is key. In that trial, 70% of participants reported that being on the drug was one of the top-five most significant experiences of their lives. As far back as the early 1800s, William James, the father of American psychology, suggested that spiritual/mystical experiences could help addicts, and a spiritual awakening is one of the guiding principles of Alcoholics Anonymous.

Medications That Don't Mix with Alcohol

Kevin T. Strang, PhD, distinguished faculty associate in neuroscience and physiology in the department of neuroscience at University of Wisconsin-Madison School of Medicine and Public Health. He is also coauthor of *Vander's Human Physiology*.

Many of us have become so accustomed to seeing the "avoid alcohol" warning on every new prescription we get that we've begun to tune out this advice…and few of us even consider that alcohol might react with over-the-counter (OTC) medications.

That's a huge mistake! Alcohol is a powerful drug that has widespread and sometimes unpredictable effects in the body. It makes some medications less effective…amplifies the effects of others…and can cause a toxic—or even fatal—reaction with some medications.

Below, some medications that are adversely affected by alcohol…*

ACETAMINOPHEN

Acetaminophen (Tylenol) by itself can be harmful to the liver—in fact, acetaminophen overdose is the number-one cause of acute liver failure. But the likelihood of liver failure is much greater if you also drink alcohol.

Why acetaminophen and alcohol don't mix: Alcohol is a toxin, but there's a reaction in the body that breaks apart alcohol molecules so they are less dangerous. This reaction requires a coenzyme called NAD (*nicotinamide adenine dinucleotide*) that's found in all living cells. However, we also need NAD to deal with the toxic effects of acetaminophen. The breakdown of acetaminophen in the liver creates a highly toxic by-product.

Main danger: If stores of NAD are depleted by drinking alcohol and taking acetaminophen, liver problems or even permanent liver damage can result. Acetaminophen is particularly dangerous when taken during or within a couple hours of alcohol consumption.

*It's best to abstain from alcohol when taking any of these medications. However, if you do drink alcohol while taking these meds, be sure to accurately report the amount to your doctor so that you can be appropriately monitored.

IBUPROFEN

Ibuprofen (Advil, Motrin) blocks the production of prostaglandins. These hormones, which the body releases in response to illness and injury, can cause pain, swelling and fever. But prostaglandins also play a critical role in blood clotting and blood vessel control, which impacts kidney function.

When blood flow to the kidneys is reduced for any reason—for example, during exercise or dehydration—prostaglandins are released to prompt blood vessels in the kidneys to dilate, which helps protect them from oxygen deprivation.

Why ibuprofen and alcohol don't mix: Drinking alcohol causes excess urination that can lead to dehydration. Alcohol also inhibits prostaglandins. If you take ibuprofen to help relieve a hangover or use it on an ongoing basis while drinking excess alcohol, it could block the prostaglandins that are released to protect the kidneys.

Main danger: Every episode of alcohol plus ibuprofen potentially kills a few more kidney cells, which makes kidney failure more likely over time. But acute renal failure can occur with just one episode of excess alcohol and ibuprofen.

Note: Ibuprofen combined with dehydration from diarrhea, vomiting or exercise, for example, can adversely affect the kidneys as well.

BLOOD THINNERS

Aspirin and other blood thinners, such as *warfarin* (Coumadin) and *clopidogrel* (Plavix), are often used by people who have heart disease. They work by inhibiting prostaglandins, which, as mentioned above, are involved in blood clotting.

Why blood thinners and alcohol don't mix: Because alcohol also inhibits prostaglandins, this combination results in an exaggerated anticlotting effect.

Main dangers: A higher, unpredictable anticoagulant effect in the system, which could cause dangerous bleeding anywhere in the body, such as a stroke or bleeding ulcer. Additionally, both aspirin and alcohol are known stomach irritants. Over time, the combination can increase the risk for stomach problems including gastritis and ulcers.

ANXIETY MEDS OR NARCOTICS

Benzodiazepines (such as Valium and Xanax) and the narcotic pain relievers *oxycodone* (OxyContin) or *hydrocodone* target specific neurotransmitter receptors in the brain. When triggered, these receptors depress brain activity, which helps ease anxiety and pain.

Why anxiety medications OR narcotics and alcohol don't mix: Alcohol is also a central nervous system depressant. If it's consumed when either drug is still in a person's system, the drug effect is amplified.

Main danger: The circuit in the brain that's responsible for regulating breathing contains gamma-aminobutyric acid (GABA) neurons. When there's excessive activation of GABA—which can happen when mixing these drugs and alcohol—the breathing circuits can shut down.

If you are unconscious—passed out or sleeping—you could stop breathing if you've had anxiety or pain medications and alcohol. These combinations are a major cause of alcohol-related deaths.

BLOOD PRESSURE DRUGS OR VIAGRA

There are two main types of drugs prescribed for high blood pressure—diuretics, such as *chlorothiazide* (Diuril), and vasodilators, such as nitroglycerin. Diuretics work by reducing blood volume, namely by ridding the body of excess water via urination. Vasodilators work by widening the blood vessels to lower blood pressure. Viagra, a drug used to treat erectile dysfunction, is a vasodilator as well.

Why blood pressure drugs or Viagra and alcohol don't mix: Since alcohol is a diuretic and a potential vasodilator, it intensifies the actions of blood pressure medications and Viagra. In other words, combining alcohol and any of these drugs is like taking multiple doses of the medications.

Main danger: You can have a dangerous drop in blood pressure that may cause dizziness, fainting, seizures or cardiac arrhythmias.

ALCOHOL AND OTHER MEDS

The effects of alcohol aren't limited to the drugs listed above. The cytochrome P450 system in the liver helps the body to eliminate all foreign substances—alcohol, prescription and OTC drugs and pesticides. The more foreign substances you're exposed to, the more robust this system becomes. Heavy drinkers have a very hearty cytochrome P450 system—this helps them detoxify large amounts of alcohol but also clears desirable drugs. This means a heavy drinker may not get the full benefit of any medication!

A Better Way to Take a Tablet

Jamison Starbuck, ND, is a naturopathic physician in family practice and producer of *Dr. Starbuck's Health Tips for Kids*, a weekly program on Montana Public Radio, MTPR.org, both in Missoula. She is a past president of the American Association of Naturopathic Physicians and a contributing editor to *The Alternative Advisor: The Complete Guide to Natural Therapies and Alternative Treatments.* DrJamisonStarbuck.com

---

In medical speak, sublingual means "under the tongue." What's so special about this area of the body? For starters, it's rich in tiny blood vessels. That's why a thermometer that is placed under the tongue does a good job of measuring your body temperature. But sublingual refers to more than the placement of your thermometer. Certain natural and prescription medicines can be taken sublingually, too. This allows a tablet to be absorbed directly into the bloodstream. That way, it doesn't enter the digestive system and get processed by the liver before entering the bloodstream. Doctors often recommend sublingual medicines for patients with digestive problems or liver disease because they don't bother the stomach, and the liver gets a rest from managing or breaking down medication. Sublingual medicines also are helpful for patients who have difficulty swallowing. Some heart and pain medications and vitamins are available in sublingual form, and a compounding pharmacy can convert some other oral medications and supplements into a sublingual version.

In the world of natural medicine, vitamin B-12 is one of our most common sublingual supplements. Unlike other B vitamins, B-12 requires intrinsic factor, a glycoprotein that is produced in cells lining the stomach and allows this vitamin to be absorbed into your bloodstream through your intestine. As we age, we can make less intrinsic factor. People of any age who have stomach problems such as gastritis or an ulcer also may be deficient in this vitamin protein. If you have low intrinsic factor, odds are that you're B-12 deficient.

A B-12 deficiency is significant because this vitamin is crucial for healthy brain and nerve function. B-12 works with folic acid (another B vitamin) to make a compound known as SAMe (short for S-adenosylmethionine), which boosts our moods and immunity. A B-12 deficiency can cause poor cognition, depression and fatigue. For people who are deficient in this powerful vitamin, doctors have long given B-12 shots (usually monthly). However, research has shown that daily sublingual B-12 also can be effective in getting this vitamin into your bloodstream. And a daily cherry-flavored B-12 sublingual tablet is much more pleasant than a shot!

The hormone progesterone is most readily absorbed into the bloodstream when it is given in a sublingual form or through a skin lotion. Sublingual administration is the tried-and-true method for delivering homeopathic remedies as well. That's because these remedies need to be directly absorbed into the bloodstream. So placing two little homeopathic tablets or two drops of a liquid preparation under the tongue (before or after eating) is the most effective way of delivering a homeopathic treatment.

Caution: Sublingual medications can irritate mouth sores.

My advice: Ask your doctor if there are any sublingual medications you could take instead of the oral form. Because of how efficiently sublingual medicines are absorbed, they are more potent than oral doses. For this reason, discuss the dose of any sublingual medicine with your doctor—you may be able to take a lower dose and perhaps lower your risk for side effects.

Also, because eating and drinking can interfere with absorption of the drug, ask how long you need to wait to eat or drink after taking a sublingual tablet.

Avoid the Hospital Opioid Trap

Jane C. Ballantyne, MD, FRCA, professor, anesthesiology and pain medicine, University of Washington, Seattle. She is coauthor of *Expert Decision Making on Opioid Treatments.*

The surgery went well. But now, a year later, the patient is still in trouble.

The problem is neither the surgery nor some mysterious postsurgical complication. It's those pills in his pocket—the opioid painkillers first prescribed in the hospital. When he was discharged, he took home a renewable prescription…and still is taking the pills. He feels like he needs them. And he's not alone. Medical or dental surgery often is the trigger for a long-term opioid dependency.

The truth is, it's not primarily the post-op pain that leads to dependency—it's the drugs themselves. And that's a tragedy, because there is growing evidence that long-term use of opioids actually can increase the body's sensitivity to pain.

But there is a way out—a growing movement within medicine to handle pain without opioids whenever possible. Without opioids, patients have fewer complications after surgery and recover faster—and they are able to go home sooner.

It's still important to tackle pain, of course. Indeed, it's critical. Acute postsurgical pain that isn't managed effectively can trigger pain sensitivity throughout the nervous system, which can be difficult to reverse and can lead to a chronic pain condition.

To learn the best ways to manage pain after surgery without opioids, we interviewed integrative pain-management expert Jane C. Ballantyne, MD. *Her recommendations…*

WHAT YOUR DOCTOR CAN DO

If you're planning to have an operation or dental procedure that typically results in the use of opioids, speak with your health-care provider to find out what nonopioid drug approaches are best for you. These include gabapentinoids, a class of drugs originally developed to treat seizures that has been shown to reduce post-surgical pain and opioid use.

Caution: While gabapentinoids are considered nonaddictive, some people can develop a dependence on them.

If you are having surgery in your lower abdomen, pelvis, rectum or to a leg (such as knee replacement), regional anesthesia—nerve blocks—are a good option. They work quickly with fewer side effects than general anesthesia. They can be effective for postoperative pain, too—research finds that nerve blocks provide better pain relief than opioids.

WHAT YOU CAN DO
BEFORE AN OPERATION

While there is plenty that your medical team can (and should) do, there is even more that you can do yourself to minimize postoperative pain so that you need less opioid pain relief—or even none at all.

Start by preparing your mind: When you need an operation, it's easy to catastrophize—imagine all the bad things that can happen. That fearful, anxious response actually increases your risk for postoperative pain and complications and delays recovery. One approach that can help with pain management is cognitive behavioral therapy (CBT), which helps you learn how to reframe thoughts so that they are more realistic—which often means less negative—usually in just a few sessions. To find a CBT therapist, click on "Find a CBT therapist" on the website of the Association for Behavioral and Cognitive Therapies (ABCT.org).

Any of these self-help approaches also can help…

•**Mindfulness-based stress reduction (MBSR),** a form of meditation, is as effective as CBT at managing pain. Follow free guided meditation online from the UCLA Mindful Awareness Research Center (MARC.ucla.edu/mindful-meditations). Mindfulness-related apps also can help—including Headspace (Apple and Android, $12.99 a month, Headspace.com) and Simple Habit (Apple and Android, $11.99 a month, SimpleHabit.com).

•**Guided imagery.** Listening to an instructor who helps you imagine relaxing scenes has been shown to reduce postoperative pain. You can purchase audio for a "guided meditation for successful surgery" at HealthJourneys.com (starting at $11.98 for an MP3 download, $17.98 for a CD). Start listening in the days beforehand—and continue while you're in the hospital.

•**Self-hypnosis for pain self-management.** One source for self-hypnosis CDs is the HypnosisNetwork.com. Self-hypnosis is useful both before and after your operation.

Finally, make sure that you have your favorite music to listen to before and after your procedure. That, too, can ease pain.

PREPARE YOUR BODY, TOO…

Nutrition plays a big role in how well your body can recover from surgery. If you are obese and/or have diabetes, losing 5% of your body weight and improving blood sugar control can reduce your risk for post-op infection and pain.

Short-term fixes also make a difference. Many older patients, for example, don't take in adequate protein, which can slow healing. And vitamin D levels below 30 ng/mL, endemic in the US, can increase the risk for infections as well as worsen pain. As soon as you are scheduled for surgery, ask your doctor to test your vitamin D levels and, if they're low, to recommend supplementation.

Some dietary supplements also may help. The best studied is turmeric, which is anti-inflammatory and has painkilling properties. (Curcumin is a derivative, but the whole root—turmeric—has additional benefits.) There are several published studies by surgeons on turmeric, both pre- and post-op, that show that it eases pain in recovery and reduces the need for other painkillers. It does increase bleeding time a little, though, so discuss with your surgeon whether it's appropriate for you.

AFTER THE OPERATION

Continue with whichever practices you started before the operation. In one study, young adults who used guided imagery after spinal-fusion surgery had less pain both in the next 24 hours and over the next two weeks, compared with those who didn't practice it.

These additional nondrug approaches may reduce pain considerably...

•**Electrostimulation.** Devices that deliver very low levels of electrical stimulation can stimulate pain-related nerve fibers in a non-painful way...and block painful stimuli from reaching the brain. Two readily available technologies include transcutaneous electric nerve stimulation (TENS) and pulsed electromagnetic fields. TENS machines are widely available in hospitals, and treatment usually can be obtained on request. Most insurance companies cover TENS for chronic pain, but you may need approval.

•**Acupuncture also reduces postsurgical pain and the need for pain medications,** especially if used within 48 hours after the operation. Unfortunately, few hospitals offer this option, so you'll have to make your own arrangements—and it may not be covered by insurance.

MANAGING YOUR PAIN EXPECTATIONS

It's important to discuss pain management with your medical team and to make sure that appropriate nonopioid methods are used if possible. After an operation, be assertive with the medical staff to make sure that your pain-relief needs are met. But it's also important to realize that you likely will experience some pain—it's unrealistic to expect no pain after surgery. Accepting that also is part of the process.

The Dangers of "Feel Good" Sedatives

Cara Tannenbaum, MD, professor in the faculties of medicine and pharmacy at Université de Montréal and the Michel Saucier Endowed Chair in Geriatric Pharmacology, Health and Aging at Centre de Recherche de l'Institut Universitaire de Gériatrie de Montréal, both in Canada.

Imagine that you've had a particularly bad year. Maybe you've lost a close friend...suffered from financial problems...or struggled with frequent insomnia.

A doctor—maybe a psychiatrist, but more likely an internist or a family physician—might suggest that a sedative will help you get through the rough patch. The drug will probably be a benzodiazepine, a class of "sedative hypnotics" that includes popular medications like *alprazolam* (Xanax), *lorazepam* (Ativan) and many others. Or it could be a related "Z" drug, such as *zolpidem* (Ambien) and *zaleplon* (Sonata).

You'll immediately start to sleep better and worry less. But every day that you take it, the risk for side effects—including addiction—increases. Experts now believe that the risks are so high that "benzos" should never be the first choice for insomnia and/or anxiety...and that their use should be limited to four weeks or less.

DANGEROUS DRUGS

Benzodiazepines are among the most popular drugs ever developed. A recent study found that more than 5% of American adults took at least one of these drugs during a one-year period. Shockingly, the majority of these prescriptions were written for patients age 65 and older.

The same study found that about one-third of the older patients who took a benzodiazepine did so for months, years or even decades—even though these drugs are intended for short-term use.

Why it's a problem: Benzodiazepines and the related "Z" drugs bind to brain receptors that cause sedation. They're highly addictive in patients of all ages...but the risk for side effects is much higher in older adults because of an age-related decline in kidney function and an increase in fat mass, both of which cause the drugs to accumulate in the body. A dose that would quickly be metabolized and excreted in a younger adult might stay active for days in older adults.

Older patients who take these drugs are at increased risk for a number of health issues. For example, they are five times more likely to suffer from memory/concentration problems… four times more likely to experience daytime fatigue…and twice as likely to fall, suffer hip or wrist fractures or have car accidents. There's even some evidence that benzodiazepines may increase the risk of developing Alzheimer's or other forms of dementia.

Important: When benzodiazepines are taken with opioid painkillers, the risk for opioid overdose increases significantly.

TOO MANY PRESCRIPTIONS

Doctors know that benzodiazepines are inherently risky but continue to prescribe them freely. It's estimated that 20% to 25% of all inappropriate prescriptions (that is, medications for which harms outweigh the benefits and safer alternatives exist) in older adults involve one or more of these drugs…and about half of doctors will continue to renew prescriptions (citing patient resistance to tapering, among other factors) despite the risks.

It's common in medicine to prescribe potentially risky drugs when the benefits clearly outweigh the risks. But for most patients, benzodiazepines do not pass this simple test. It's estimated that 13 patients would have to take one of these drugs for one patient to benefit (the "number needed to treat").

Put another way, for every 13 patients taking these drugs, 12 are not gaining benefit. Conversely, about one in five patients who takes benzodiazepines suffers from serious impairments (the "number needed to harm"), such as memory problems, lack of concentration and daytime drowsiness, that interfere with function.

Why do doctors continue to prescribe them? It's partly because patients demand these drugs. They believe that benzodiazepines help them, and doctors don't want to deprive their patients of well-being. There's also a financial aspect—insurance companies and HMOs that routinely pay for drug prescriptions often don't cover long-term, nondrug treatments for insomnia and/or anxiety.

For about 10% of patients, benzodiazepines are essential treatments. They're used, in some cases long-term, for seizures and some mental disorders, including disabling anxiety. They can be lifesavers when used short-term for patients who are withdrawing from alcohol or other drugs. But the vast majority of prescriptions are written for patients who would do just as well—or better—with nondrug treatments.

GOING DRUG-FREE

When I meet with patients who take these drugs, many say that they would like to stop because of side effects, such as fatigue, memory loss, incontinence, etc. But the drugs are addictive. People who try to quit often experience intense insomnia, anxiety and other symptoms during the withdrawal period, which typically lasts one to four weeks.

Good news: We conducted a study that looked at 261 patients who were taking these drugs for at least three months. After six months, 62% of those in an intervention group (who were given a patient-education brochure that discussed drug risks, nondrug treatments and advice on discontinuing drugs) had asked their doctors/pharmacists for advice about stopping…and 27% did stop, compared with 5% in a control group.

Some of these patients had been taking benzodiazepines for 40 years and then stopped within six months because of the brochure! A few of the patients started using cognitive behavioral techniques to help them sleep, and eight patients began taking an antidepressant because underlying depression was unmasked.

Caution: If you've taken a benzodiazepine for months or years and have developed a physical dependence, don't quit "cold turkey." (After two to four weeks, everyone develops a physical dependence.) Abruptly stopping the drug can cause confusion, heart palpitations, nausea and sometimes mental disturbances, including hallucinations. (See previous article, "The Dangers of 'Feel Good' Sedatives," for more information.)

About half of patients who quit a benzodiazepine will experience at least some side effects. To make the process easier (and safer), experts recommend gradually decreasing the dose—under the supervision of a doctor—over several months. Some patients might go four to five months before they're completely drug-free. *How it works…*

•**During the first two weeks,** a patient might be advised to take a half dose on Monday and Friday. The other days, he/she will take the same dose as before.

•**For the next two weeks,** the "half-dose" days might expand to include Wednesday, Saturday and Sunday. During subsequent weeks, patients will reduce their doses still more. The exact amounts will depend on the patient, the degree of side effects, etc.

•**Anticipate discomfort.** When you start reducing doses, you will experience withdrawal. I warn patients that they'll feel like they have jet lag for a week or two. Stick it out! If you absolutely can't function while you're tapering, it's OK to take the same dose for a while longer—but never go back to a higher dose.

•**To deal with daytime sleepiness,** I advise patients to avoid taking a nap and to keep active. Expose yourself to bright light (either outside or with bright indoor lamps). The goal is to get back on a natural energy and day–night wake cycle. This includes not going to bed until you're ready to sleep.

•**If you're taking one of these drugs to deal with anxiety,** talk to a health-care professional or a therapist to identify the root cause of your discomfort and to help you get through stressful situations.

Support groups for anxiety-related disorders can help you learn to manage stress more effectively.

Relaxation techniques, such as stretching, yoga, massage or tai chi, can be worthwhile, too.

•**To deal with insomnia,** consider cognitive behavioral therapy for insomnia (CBT-I) and the use of a sleep diary. These are the most effective nondrug therapies for insomnia.

For more information on tapering off a benzodiazepine, go to DeprescribingNetwork.ca

You May Be Using the Wrong Painkiller

Jianguo Cheng, MD, PhD, professor of anesthesiology and director of the Cleveland Clinic Multidisciplinary Pain Medicine Fellowship Program, and president-elect of the American Academy of Pain Medicine. Recognized by Becker's Review as one of the 70 Best Pain Management Physicians in America, he has published more than 200 research papers, articles and book chapters.

Millions of Americans fight their pain and inflammation with an over-the-counter (OTC) nonsteroidal anti-inflammatory drug (NSAID), such as *ibuprofen* (Motrin, Advil) or *naproxen* (Aleve, Naprosyn)—or a prescription anti-inflammatory, such as *celecoxib* (Celebrex). But if you've got heart disease and/or kidney disease, finding a pain reliever that won't worsen your other condition is tricky.

What most people don't realize: Even in healthy people, NSAIDs—especially when taken for longer or at higher doses than directed by a doctor—increase risk for heart attack and stroke and can potentially harm the kidneys. For those who already have heart disease and/or kidney disease, these risks are even greater.

It's widely known that NSAIDs can cause stomach bleeding as a side effect, but the potential risks to the user's heart and kidneys are not nearly as well recognized.

Important: Short-term use of any NSAID (no longer than 10 days) is always preferable to long-term use. In fact, you may not need drugs at all (see next page). *Pain relief options if you have…*

HEART DISEASE

Background: NSAIDs raise one's risk for heart attack and stroke by increasing blood clot formation. These medications can also interfere with certain high blood pressure drugs, such as diuretics…angiotensin-converting enzyme (ACE) inhibitors…and beta-blockers, and cause the body to retain fluid—a problem that often plagues people with heart failure.

If you have known risks for heart disease: For people with risk factors such as high blood pressure, diabetes, an enlarged heart or an abnormal EKG reading with no clinical symptoms, NSAIDs may be used, under a doctor's supervision. Celecoxib is generally safer for pain than naproxen or ibuprofen because it is associated with fewer gastrointestinal and/or renal complications.

People treating high blood pressure with an ACE inhibitor drug, such as *captopril* or *benazepril* (Lotensin), should aim for lower doses of celecoxib than typically prescribed (for example, less than 150 mg per day) and use it for no more than 10 days.

If you have known heart disease: NSAIDs increase the risk for new cardiovascular events in people with established heart disease and may lead to heart failure in those with severe heart disease. NSAIDs should be avoided in those with recent heart attack, unstable angina or poorly controlled heart failure. For these individuals, non-NSAID medications, such as *acetaminophen* (Tylenol), may be considered.*

Note: Aspirin is also an NSAID but does not carry the same cardiovascular risks. Low-dose aspirin is widely used for its blood-thinning effects to reduce risk for heart attack or stroke in those who have cardiovascular disease or are at increased risk for it. A doctor should prescribe and monitor such daily aspirin therapy.

KIDNEY DISEASE

Background: NSAIDs can reduce blood flow to the kidneys and/or cause the body to retain fluid, taxing the kidneys.

If kidney disease is mild: It may go unnoticed, except you may have slightly higher blood levels of creatinine (a waste product normally removed by kidneys). Short-term and low-dose NSAIDs, including aspirin, may be used if creatinine levels are not substantially elevated (less than 1.5 mg/dL). Creatinine levels should be monitored if NSAIDs are used in these cases.

If kidney disease is severe: If you have kidney disease and routinely retain extra fluid, it's a severe case. You should avoid all NSAIDs—including daily low-dose aspirin for heart attack prevention. A person with severe kidney disease may use acetaminophen if his/her liver function is normal.

---

*With some cases of heart disease (and/or kidney disease), a topical NSAID, which is absorbed differently from a pill, may also be an option.

Avoid Beta-Blocker Side Effects

Beta-blockers lower blood pressure by preventing adrenaline from stimulating beta-receptors in the kidneys, heart and arteries. The most common side effect is fatigue. Others include cold hands and feet, thinning hair and less commonly shortness of breath and weight gain.

In most hypertensive patients, a beta-blocker is not necessary since other drugs (ACE inhibitors, angiotensin receptor blockers, diuretics or calcium channel blockers) work as well and have fewer side effects. If a beta-blocker is necessary, use the lowest dose possible.

Also, many doctors are unaware that some beta-blockers are less likely to have side effects than others, depending on whether they dilate arteries, how much drug circulates into the brain and how the drug is metabolized. In comparison with the current best-selling beta-blocker, *metoprolol* (Toprol), some older beta-blockers, such as *bisoprolol* and *betaxolol*, may be better tolerated, and newer beta-blockers, including *carvedilol* (Coreg) and *nebivolol* (Bystolic), offer the advantage of dilating (relaxing) arteries.

Samuel J. Mann, MD, hypertension specialist, New York-Presbyterian Hospital, New York City, and the author of *Hypertension and You*.

Important: When used as directed, acetaminophen is generally safe but can interfere with liver function when taken in excessive doses (more than 3 g per day) and/or when combined with alcohol.

HEART AND KIDNEY DISEASE

What if you have both heart and kidney problems? If your blood work indicates that your liver function is normal, acetaminophen (see above) can often be used for pain, under a doctor's direction.

NONDRUG PAIN RELIEF

Drugs are not the only option—nor should they even be your first choice—especially if you have heart disease and/or kidney disease. *Non-drug therapies that can reduce or replace your use of pain medication...*

•**Noninvasive.** Physical therapy, aqua therapy, exercise, tai chi and yoga are powerful pain-fighters. Acupuncture and massage have also been shown to help, as have behavioral approaches such as cognitive therapy. Most people see results within days to weeks.

•**Minimally invasive.** Nerve blocks—injected anesthetics or nerve ablations (using heat) that are designed to turn off pain signals—are generally given once every few weeks or months and can produce lasting pain relief without resorting to long-term drug use.

Another option: Neuromodulation, in which a small device (electrodes and a pulse genera-tor about the size of a stopwatch) is surgically implanted to deliver electrical stimulation that disrupts pain signals that travel from the spinal cord to the brain. This can be used to treat pain in many locations of the body.

•**Surgery.** This is an option if the cause of your pain is identified and can be surgically corrected.

Example: A herniated disk pressing on a nerve may be surgically removed. Of course, nonsurgical methods should be tried first. Surgeries can cause short-term pain and fail to provide the desired level of pain relief and function. Talk to your doctors so that you understand the risks of surgery and have realistic expectations for your outcome.

CHAPTER 14

Men's Health

4 Dangerous Myths About Testicular Cancer

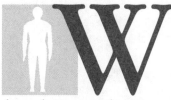

Women learn early about breast cancer. It's got ribbons and races. But men tend to know almost nothing about testicular cancer…and some of what they think they know is actually wrong—which could be putting their health and even their lives in danger. *Here's the truth regarding four common myths about this male cancer…*

MYTH #1: **Testicular cancer is mostly a problem for older men.**

Truth: Not even in the ballpark. Even though prostate cancer rates rise with age, especially after age 60, the majority of the approximately 8,850 cases of testicular cancer diagnosed each year in the US are found in men ages 15 to 40. It's the most common cancer to strike young men. It does occur in older men, though—about 7% of new cases are in men over age 55.

MYTH #2: **Testicular cancer is less "serious" than other types of cancers.**

Truth: Testicular cancer does have a relatively high cure rate—even if the cancer has spread. The five-year survival rate is 95%. When caught early and localized to the testicles, it's 99%. If it has spread to nearby tissue and/or lymph nodes, the survival rate is 96%. Even if the cancer has spread to other parts of the body, the five-year survival rate is 73%.

But these reassuring statistics mask the bigger truth that this is indeed a serious cancer. For starters, testicular cancer can't be easily diagnosed via a biopsy—the removal of a tiny piece of a potentially cancerous tissue for testing—because it could cause the cancer to spread.

Note: Biopsies do not cause most other types of cancer to spread.

So if symptoms (see next page) or a physical exam lead to a suspicion of testicular cancer,

Ajay Nangia, MD, professor of urology at University of Kansas Medical Center, with a practice at the University of Kansas Hospital, both in Kansas City. He is a leading male infertility specialist.

and serum tumor marker blood tests and testicular ultrasound also point to cancer, an accurate diagnosis often involves removing the entire affected testicle—a procedure called radical inguinal orchiectomy.

That's traumatic enough…leaving men self-conscious about their altered appearance. Then there's chemotherapy or radiation, and sometimes a second surgery to remove nearby lymph nodes.

What's more, both the cancer itself and treatment (especially chemotherapy) can lead to infertility—even in the 97% of cases in which only one testicle is removed. As a result, men who may wish to father children in the future are advised to bank sperm before treatment—or if they haven't, to wait for a year or two after chemo before attempting impregnation to reduce the likelihood of having DNA-damaged sperm.

Finally, sexual performance may be affected. Treatment often leads to low testosterone levels, which can increase the risk for high cholesterol and high blood pressure—and erectile dysfunction.

***MYTH #3:* Injuring your testicles ups your chances of getting testicular cancer.**

Truth: There's no evidence that a swift kick or some other assault you-know-where impacts your testicular cancer risk. Nor will certain sexual practices, having a vasectomy or infection with human papillomavirus (HPV) increase your risk.

What are the risk factors? There's a strong genetic link, so family history matters. Being born with an undescended testicle also is a risk factor. Sophisticated new genetic tests can help identify, for example, the risk that a man born with undescended testicles actually has of developing the cancer. Unfortunately, there are no preventive steps a man can take.

***MYTH #4:* Testicular self-exams are a waste of time and effort.**

Truth: This is where there's some disagreement. The US Preventive Services Task Force (USPSTF), an independent panel of national experts that makes recommendations about health-screening practices, has concluded from a review of studies that the benefit of self-exams

is small. But I, along with many other doctors in the field, disagree. The USPSTF's rationale is that there's no evidence that self-examination is effective at reducing mortality. Even without screening, if testicular cancer is discovered, "current treatment options provide very favorable health outcomes." But I see men who are dealing with the aftermath of testicular cancer, chemotherapy and/or surgery, and who are infertile and regret not having frozen their sperm. Plus, what harm is there in doing something that's free and can be handled, so to speak, in the shower?

HOW TO DO A TESTICULAR SELF-EXAM

Testicular self-exams are easy and painless. The hardest part is remembering to do it once a month. *Here are some guidelines from the Testicular Cancer Society…*

1. Do the exam during or right after a warm shower or bath, when the scrotum is most relaxed and easy to examine by hand.

2. Use both hands to examine each testicle. Place your index and middle fingers on the underside and your thumbs on top. Firmly yet gently roll the testicle between your thumbs and fingers to check for surface or texture irregularities (see below).

3. Find the epididymis, a rope-like structure on the back of the testicle. Become familiar with how it feels so you won't mistake it for a lump.

4. If you do the exam outside the shower, stand in front of a mirror and check for any visible swelling of the skin on your scrotum. It's not essential but provides an additional check.

5. If you notice irregularities or changes in your testicles, make an appointment to see your doctor as soon as possible.

TESTICULAR CANCER SYMPTOMS

Testicular cancer is often diagnosed when a man notices something unusual and goes to his doctor. *If you have any of these signs, it's best to get checked out…*

•**A painless lump or swelling,** usually hard, on the surface of either testicle.

•**A dull ache in the lower abdomen or in the groin—**especially if it lasts for more than an hour. It could be something else such as an infection or a physical twisting, but it's worth checking out, even going to the ER. Most guys wait too long—hours, days or even months!

•**A sudden buildup of fluid in the scrotum,** forming a soft or hard swelling.

•**Pain or discomfort in a testicle or in the scrotum.**

Dangerous Birthday

Sita Slavov, PhD, professor of public policy at George Mason University in Fairfax, Virginia.

If you're a retired male over 62, you've beaten the odds. In an analysis from Boston College's Center for Retirement Research, researchers discovered a 2% jump in male mortality at age 62. That early death risk was almost entirely concentrated in the 10% of men who quit working at age 62—early retirement. (Women are less likely to quit work at 62 and didn't face increased risk of dying at that age.)

Of course, one reason that some people stop working early is because they're in poor health, so their risk of dying young is higher. But other factors were at play, too. Leaving the workforce can be risky all by itself—men tend to drive more after retiring early, and there's a spike in fatal traffic accidents…some men become more sedentary…and smokers tend to smoke more, so deaths from lung cancer and COPD go up.

So is retirement unhealthy? Sita Slavov, PhD, professor of public policy at George Mason University in Fairfax, Virginia, has researched that topic.

Key finding: Ultimately, retirement increases both life satisfaction and health. Indeed, after retirement, people tend to get more physical activity, spend less time in sedentary pursuits—and finally get enough sleep. But not right away. Those healthy habits are actually stronger four years after retirement than in the first year.

What's tricky is the transition. Leaving the workforce—whether you're 62 or 72—is a time of enormous personal change, and many of us don't prepare for it enough.

Bottom line: The first year of retirement is a dicey time for your health and safety, so consciously use that year to take better care of yourself—so you can enjoy the fruits of your labor for many years to come.

It's Not Only the Most Powerful Men Who Commit Sexual Abuse of Power

Dacher Keltner, PhD, psychology professor at University of California-Berkeley and founding director of The Greater Good Science Center, a nonprofit organization that studies the psychology, sociology and neuroscience of well-being. He is author of *The Power Paradox: How We Gain and Lose Influence*. GGSC.Berkeley.edu

Public accusations of sexual harassment, lewd behavior and outright sexual assault by powerful men have now stretched from Hollywood to Washington, DC, to New York City and many points in between. They have shaken the worlds of entertainment, politics, media and others. What they all have in common is men wielding and abusing some form of great power. But if you are a man who doesn't have such great power—even a good man—don't assume that you are immune from abusing even the limited power you have. The fact is, research suggests that the abuse of power, including the sexual abuse of power, is not just the result of bad people rising to powerful positions. It also occurs because having power can alter the way the human brain works. And it's not just the very powerful who engage in sexual misconduct—even modest amounts of power can distort behavior, and we all wield at least modest amounts of power over others from time to time.

Of course, men who wield power don't necessarily abuse it.

We asked Dacher Keltner, PhD, professor of psychology at University of California-Berkeley and author of *The Power Paradox*, to help our readers understand why power so often leads to abuse of power, including inappropriate sexual behavior, and what we all can do to avoid letting this happen to us...

POWER CAN DISTORT THINKING

Some people behave as though they don't care about other people's feelings or opinions... or about the rules of polite society. But in many cases, it's not that they don't care—they don't even notice.

Brain scans of people in power reveal reduced activity in the orbitofrontal lobe, a region of the brain that helps us determine what other people are thinking and that reminds us of societal rules. In fact, the brain activity of powerful people is strikingly similar to the brain activity of people who have experienced brain damage to the orbitofrontal lobe, an injury that can cause rude and impulsive behavior.

And when a powerful person fails to sense what someone else is thinking or feeling, his brain often fills in this blank by projecting his own thoughts and feelings onto that person.

This can lead to boorish or pushy behavior, such as ignoring other people's opinions or cutting to the front of a line...and it also can lead to sexually inappropriate behavior. According to a 2010 study published in *Journal of Personality and Social Psychology*, in many cases when a powerful person feels sexually aroused, he may project that feeling onto the person who is the source of his desire—in other words, he concludes that this other person is sexually aroused as well. If that happens, this powerful person might truly—but wrongly—believe that his sexual advances are justified by the circumstances. That doesn't make the behavior any more appropriate, of course.

Meanwhile, the other people in these situations—those who are less powerful—often struggle to tell the high-power individuals what they really think in a straightforward way. Instead, they try to send subtle clues and hint at what they feel in hopes that this will get their message through without offending, angering or directly contradicting the powerful people. But while the attempted clues might seem clear to the person giving them, they might not get through to a powerful person who has reduced orbitofrontal lobe activity.

None of this excuses the abuse of power, but it does help explain why it happens so very often. And as discussed below, it should serve as a wake-up call to every one of us who has some power over another individual.

EVEN MODERATE POWER CAN BE ABUSED

People who have great power sometimes get away with blatant sexual misconduct (or other abuses of power) for years, as recent revelations amply show. These people have protectors and enablers to sweep their transgressions under the rug. Their victims often are afraid to come forward or are paid to remain silent. But if you think this problem involves only the very powerful, you're wrong. Whenever a person has the capacity to alter someone else's condition by providing or withholding resources, that person has power enough to exploit—and almost everyone has that amount of power at times.

Examples: A midlevel manager has power over entry-level employees...a member of a homeowner's association board has power over the home owners in the neighborhood...a popular member of any group has power over a less popular person who wants to join the group.

If you don't think this minor power affects behavior, consider that when researchers arbitrarily elevated one person in a group to a leadership role over his/her fellow participants in a study, this "leader" became more likely to flirt in overt ways...to make risky choices...and to make potentially inappropriate physical contact. And these people didn't even have any real-world power—they were just called powerful for the purposes of a psychology experiment.

HOW TO BREAK THE CYCLE—NO MATTER WHO YOU ARE

Whenever you are in a position of power—even if your power is modest—assume that you will be at a neurological disadvantage when it comes to figuring out what other people are thinking. To counteract this, make a conscious effort to speak less, listen intently and always respond politely. If you sense that someone over whom you have power is sexually attracted to you, consider that there's an excellent chance that this is just your mind playing tricks on you. Do not act on the sexual signals you think you are receiving unless they seem unequivocal—and even then, if you are interested, proceed only with great respect and caution.

Warning: Despite what you might have heard about power being an aphrodisiac to others, your power is not a turn-on for people who have less power than you—it's probably a turn-off. According to a 2006 study published in *Journal of Experimental Social Psychology*, when women (and men) sense that they have little power, their anxiety and self-consciousness increase and their pleasure—including sexual pleasure—declines sharply.

What about your behavior when you have power over someone and are not attracted to that person? Your best course is to avoid making any physical contact or comments that could possibly be construed as sexual. Such contact or words could cause discomfort and distress even if you have no sexual intent.

Example: John Lasseter, head of the Walt Disney Company's animation division, is taking a six-month leave of absence, reportedly because he gave coworkers unwanted hugs. It is possible that Lasseter truly did not realize that his hugs were unwanted—though, of course, he still was responsible for his actions.

If you have a say in who has control over a group, include women on the leadership team. Sexual misconduct seems to be most likely when men have virtually all the power—such as in Hollywood, where female producers and directors are rare. It's not that women do not abuse power (though they seem to be somewhat less likely to do so than men), but rather that a dramatic power imbalance between the sexes increases the odds that power will be abused in sexual ways.

If you are subjected to inappropriate sexual behavior from someone who has more power than you, immediately share what occurred with other people in the group or organization—in this current environment, there's an excellent chance that you will find allies, even fellow victims. You might feel relatively powerless, but there is power in numbers.

Be very specific when you describe what occurred. Victims of sexual abuse of power often speak in general terms if they speak up at all, in part because social norms frown on the public discussion of sexual topics. But the more vague your description of the misbehavior, the easier it will be for people to doubt that anything inappropriate occurred.

Example: Rather than say, "He made inappropriate contact," say, "He grabbed my butt." That leaves no room for doubt that a line was crossed.

Testosterone Warning

US Food and Drug Administration, Silver Spring, Maryland.

Abuse of testosterone can cause heart attacks, personality changes and infertility. Testosterone supplements are prescribed for men whose testosterone levels are low. But millions of others use testosterone and other anabolic steroids to try to boost physical health or libido. Athletes and body builders are especially likely to take these substances at high levels. This can hurt the heart, brain, liver and endocrine system and can have an impact on mental health as well. The FDA plans to revise labeling guidelines on all prescription testosterone products to make warnings of their dangers clearer.

TV Ads and Testosterone

J. Bradley Layton, PhD, research assistant professor, department of epidemiology, University of North Carolina, Chapel Hill.

Direct-to-consumer TV ads for testosterone therapy, used to treat hypogonadism (a condition marked by low libido, fatigue and depression in men), were linked to more testing…new use of the therapy…and use of the therapy without testing.

Why it matters: The study suggests that when ad-influenced men ask doctors for treatment, doctors comply…and sometimes without a clinical diagnosis.

If you see an ad for a treatment you'd like to try: Be sure to ask your doctor if you would truly benefit.

Men: Time to "Man Up!"

David Sherer, MD, a board-certified anesthesiologist who is president and CEO of Consolidated Medicine, a medical practice and consulting group in Chevy Chase, Maryland. He is coauthor of *Dr. David Sherer's Hospital Survival Guide: 100+ Ways to Make Your Hospital Stay Safe and Comfortable.* His blog on BottomLineInc.com is titled "What Your Doctor Isn't Telling You."

Here we are...it's almost 2020. Why is it that men are still so stubborn about taking care of themselves?

Recent articles put out by *The Huffington Post* and The American Heart Association have focused on the reasons why this is so. The former publication has pointed out that men die earlier than women and are more likely to die from the top 10 causes of death in the United States. (These are, according to the Center for Disease Control: heart disease, cancer, lung disease, accidents, stroke, Alzheimer's, diabetes, flu and pneumonia, kidney disease and suicide.) Part of this, they say, may be due to men taking more risks than women, as well as smoking and drinking to excess more than women. Men's relative social isolation and more dangerous jobs also put them at risk for earlier death. However, as foolish as some of these seem, *The Huffington Post*'s major reasons why men avoid the MD were...

- **"too busy to go."**
- **fear of finding out bad news.**
- **discomfort of examination (prostate, rectal, etc.)**
- **the doctor's "personal" questions**
- **getting weighed!**

Do visits to the doctor really save lives? You bet! Blood pressure screening, blood sugar tests and skin and testicular examinations are but a few of the easy interventions that can prevent or help treat diseases before they have gone too far. Lifestyle changes, medical and surgical therapies, as well as psychiatric counseling can literally save lives. But symptoms have to be heard and signs of disease have to be seen to be recognized and treated, and the only way that gets done is to visit the doctor. There is no substitute (short of telemedicine if that's the only option) for a face-to-face visit with the physician. So why is this still an issue?

Well, men appear to have no shortage of dumb reasons. "I don't want to ask for directions." "I don't want to show that I have no knowledge of a particular topic." These are typical foolish sentiments that Dr Glenn Good, an expert on masculinity and the psychology of men at The University of Florida, highlighted in a statement to *The Huffington Post.* The American Heart Association expanded on this issue, exploring other bird-brained but genuine excuses for not taking proper medical care of oneself. *These include...*

- **"I don't have a doctor."**
- **"I don't have insurance."**
- **"I don't have time."**
- **"I don't want to spend the money."**
- **"I'd rather 'tough it out'."**

So here we are, in 2018, and men are still playing the stoic Marlboro Man of decades ago. Along with this machismo BS, the lame justifications listed above may seem silly and trivial, but they stand up to scrutiny. Indeed, men will say and do just about anything to avoid the doctor's office. What is a spouse, girlfriend, friend or other loved one to do to combat this foolish and bone-headed behavior? *I have a few suggestions...*

- **Show him this blog post and read to him how lives have been saved** and countless suffering (physical, emotional AND financial) has been averted by a simple visit to the doctor.

- **Get on the web and research "Why Men Avoid the Doctor"** and show your XY chromosomal friend the potential disasters in not going.

- **Play on his conscience.** If he won't do it for himself, at least he can do it for his life-partner, his children, his friends, coworkers and community.

•**Read to him that hypertension, diabetes, prostate cancer, colon cancer and cardiovascular diseases** are relatively common in Western-society men and that these conditions can often be cured or effectively treated if recognized early.

•**"Scare him straight."** Tell him about someone you know who avoided the doctor only to learn that a condition has gone too far or, worse yet, caused an unexpected death to occur in a guy who appeared to be "healthy as a horse."

Most men, I believe, when pushed will listen to reason. But there will still be some guys out there that, despite your best efforts, will resist. At that point radical measures may be needed. You might have your doctor call him (if the doc is willing) to stress the importance of a physical. You might have a friend (preferably male), clergy member, trusted relative or grown child work him over as well. You can also play the "don't you want to dance at 'fill in the blank's' wedding?" (Insert child or grandchild's name there.)

It's going to take a cultural shift for men to "man-up" and take control of their health. I fear it is an uphill battle, but one well worth fighting. Men: It's time to drop the macho act and drop your pants for the doctor. It's the right thing to do!

MRIs Reduce Prostate Biopsies

Giving men suspected of having prostate cancer an MRI can reduce unnecessary biopsies by 27%. Compared with a surgical biopsy, which relies on random tissue samples, an MRI covers the entire gland, making it easier to spot a cancer, determine its size and density, and assess how aggressive the malignancy appears. If findings are suspicious, a surgical biopsy will then be needed.

Hashim Ahmed, PhD, professor and chair of urology, division of surgery, Imperial College, London.

The Best Prostate Cancer Treatment...for You

Ronald C. Chen, MD, MPH, associate professor of radiation oncology, University of North Carolina School of Medicine, Chapel Hill.

Since the latest treatment options for early-stage prostate cancer are thought to be similar in their effectiveness, choosing the best treatment can come down to side effects. A recent study sheds new light on those side effects.

Study details: Researchers looked at more than 1,100 early-stage prostate cancer patients whose treatment was either active surveillance (frequent monitoring to check for cancer growth but no immediate treatment)...complete removal of the prostate (radical prostatectomy)...external beam radiation...or brachytherapy (the implanting of radioactive seeds).

Finding: Prostatectomy was linked to a higher incidence of sexual dysfunction (characterized by difficulty achieving and maintaining erections and the ability to achieve orgasm) and urinary leakage than the other options. The two radiation treatments caused worse short-term urinary obstruction and irritation, with external beam radiotherapy causing worse bowel symptoms. But at the two-year mark, the differences in side effects were negligible between active surveillance, external beam radiation and brachytherapy—indicating that urinary obstruction, irritation and bowel symptoms associated with external beam radiation and brachytherapy improved over time. However, after two years, 57% of men undergoing radical prostatectomy who had normal sexual functioning prior to surgery reported poor sexual function after, as well as more urinary leakage than men who chose the other options.

This is the first comparison of quality-of-life outcomes since major advances have been made in both surgical and radiation therapies. Aware that the modern techniques are roughly equal in efficacy, researchers from the University of North Carolina's Lineberger Comprehensive Cancer Center wanted to study the side effects of the improved therapies so patients and doctors could select the most appropriate treatment. Patients were studied within five weeks of diagnosis and followed for two years, reporting on a quality-of-life index measuring sexual dysfunction, urinary obstruction and irritation, urinary incontinence and bowel problems. Results were published in *JAMA: Journal of the American Medical Association*.

Bottom Line: If you're diagnosed with prostate cancer, consider your options carefully and discuss both short-term and long-term side effects with your doctor so that you can choose the treatment that aligns best with your priorities.

Prostate Tumors Can Differ

Hannelore V. Heemers, PhD, is associate staff in the department of cancer biology at Lerner Research Institute, Cleveland Clinic. She is lead author of a study published in *European Urology*.

Prostate tumors can differ significantly even within the same patient. When a patient has multiple tumors and only the largest one is analyzed using genomic fingerprinting, a smaller but more aggressive tumor may go undetected. Your doctor should consider this when using genomic fingerprinting for prostate cancer treatment.

Mammograms for Men?

David R. Gruen, MD, codirector, Stamford Health Breast Center, and director, Women's Imaging, Stamford Health, Connecticut.

Since men can get breast cancer, should men get mammograms?

No. Routine mammograms are not recommended for men, since breast cancer in men is quite rare. Still, your husband should be aware of the risk factors, which are the same as for women. If he has a first-degree relative with

breast cancer…if he has inherited the BRCA gene mutation…or if he has a history of radiation to the chest, his chances of developing breast cancer are higher than average.

There are no definitive recommendations for men to do regular breast self-exams. If you (or the man in your life) notices a lump or has changes to breast tissue such as enlargement, swelling or pain, he should see his doctor. Most likely, a diagnosis will be made after a mammogram and/or an ultrasound or a needle biopsy. Treatments are similar to those used in women with breast cancer—surgery, radiation and/or chemotherapy.

New Treatment for Advanced Prostate Cancer

Nicholas D. James, MBBS, PhD, honorary professor of clinical oncology at Institute of Cancer and Genomic Sciences, University of Birmingham, UK.

Adding the medication *abiraterone acetate* (Zytiga) plus *prednisolone/prednisone* to standard treatment (androgen-deprivation therapy, ADT) lowers the risk for death by 37%. Abiraterone already is used to treat some men whose disease has spread, but the new findings mean that more men could benefit by using abiraterone with ADT as soon as they are diagnosed.

How a Quick Massage Can Help You Live Longer

Mark Tarnopolsky, MD, PhD, professor of pediatrics and medicine, director of Neuromuscular and Neurometabolic Clinic, McMaster University Medical Center, Ontario, Canada.

You might want to make massage, especially after a workout, a regular part of your life. Even a 10-minute massage leads

Prostate Cancer Treatment and Heart Disease

Prostate cancer treatment may increase risk for certain heart diseases. Androgen deprivation therapy (ADT) reduces male hormones to stop them from stimulating prostate cancer cells to grow.

Recent finding: Men on ADT with early, localized prostate cancer had an 81% higher risk for heart failure and a slightly increased risk for heart rhythm disorders, compared with those not on ADT. If you are on ADT, be monitored closely for heart disease.

Reina Haque, PhD, MPH, research scientist in the department of research and evaluation at Kaiser Permanente Southern California, Pasadena.

to physiological changes that may be protective, according to recent research. A mini-massage may even help reduce insulin resistance, a key driver of diabetes.

MASSAGING YOUR MUSCLES TO FIGHT DISEASE

Researchers were interested in studying massage immediately after exercise for two reasons. For one thing, practically speaking, that's a common time for people to get a massage, since many people say that massage helps reduce muscle soreness from exercise. Another reason is that, biologically, it's easier to measure differences in the effect of massage on cells after exercise because exercise puts the body into a state of temporary stress.

Volunteers in the study included 11 healthy, active men in their 20s who provided a bit of muscle tissue from one thigh for a baseline biopsy. Then researchers had the volunteers do 70 minutes of fast-paced cycling on a stationary bike. The volunteers rested for 10 minutes and then had a 10-minute massage on one thigh only. Immediately after the massage, researchers took second muscle biopsies, but this time from both thighs in order to compare massaged tissue versus nonmassaged tissue. Two and a half hours after the second biopsies, the volunteers underwent a third set of biopsies on both

thighs to capture any changes that might have occurred a bit later after their massages.

STOP THE DAMAGE!

Researchers found two very interesting differences in the muscles that had been massaged...

A gene pathway that causes muscle inflammation was "dialed down" in these muscles both immediately after the massage and 2.5 hours after the massage. (Specific genes can be present in our tissues but not always active.) This is helpful knowledge because muscle inflammation is a contributor to delayed-onset muscle soreness, so it confirms biologically what we've always believed through anecdotal observation—a post-exercise massage can help relieve muscle soreness. Inflammation also contributes to the development of diabetes.

Conversely, another sort of gene was "turned on" by the massage—this is a gene that increases the activity of mitochondria in muscle cells. You probably know that mitochondria are considered the "power packs" of our muscles for their role in creating usable energy. Better mitochondrial functioning has been shown by other studies to help decrease insulin resistance (a key risk factor for type 2 diabetes) and obesity and even to slow aging. And "mitochondrial dysfunction" is now being recognized as a potential contributor to diabetes.

Is it a stretch to link post-exercise massage to these benefits? They were not specifically studied, but since the question is posed, my reply is that it's not unreasonable—there is a potential connection, and future research will need to be done to confirm it. One thing is clear: Stress, especially the way our minds react to stress, is increasingly being recognized as a diabetes risk. Anything you can do to break the stress cycle is a healthy thing.

TREAT YOURSELF TO MASSAGE

The massage type that the researchers used was a standard combination of three techniques that are commonly used for post-exercise massage—effleurage (light stroking)...petrissage (firm compression and release)...and stripping (repeated longitudinal strokes). It's easy to find massage therapists in spas, salons, fitness centers and private practices who use these techniques.

Or you could ask your spouse or a friend to try some of these moves on you. Even if his/her technique isn't perfect, there's a chance that it could still provide the benefits.

Massage after exercise was studied, but it's possible that massaging any muscles at any time may have similar benefits—more research will need to be done to find out.

Remember, you don't have to break the bank on a prolonged 60-minute massage—a simple 10- or 20-minute rubdown (which usually costs $10 to $40) can do the trick.

CHAPTER 15

Natural Cures

The Healing Effects of Proper Breathing

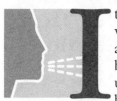

It's the first and last thing we do in this world—take a breath. But somewhere in between, far too many of us lose touch with how to breathe naturally, fully...and correctly. Though we inhale and exhale about 20,000 times each day, most of the time we take short, shallow breaths that I call "stress breaths."

Why does our innate sense of how to breathe properly slip away from us? Whether we're fighting traffic or multitasking, our fast-paced lives often throw us into a stress-driven spiral that interferes with our ability to optimally fuel our bodies with life-sustaining oxygen. People who are suppressing feelings such as anger or emotional pain tend to hold their breath. *Fortunately, a few simple strategies can help us reclaim our breathing skills...*

MORE THAN "BELLY BREATHING"

We have all heard the term "belly breathing," but the real key to proper breathing is not so much your belly but your diaphragm. Deeply breathing from this dome-shaped sheet of muscle at the bottom of the rib cage is vital for respiratory function.

True diaphragmatic breathing uses the entire respiratory system—starting with the belly, then moving on to the midsection and into the chest.

Try it: Inhale through your nose, directing your breath into your stomach. Allow your diaphragm to drop downward and the rib cage to expand, thus creating space for the lungs to inflate. Pause for a moment, then exhale through your mouth and feel the rib cage contract. The motion of breath should go in and out like a wave. To adopt this healthier way of breathing, practice for a minute or two several times a day until it feels natural.

Rebecca Dennis, a breath coach and founder of BreathingTree.co.uk, a website that's dedicated to health-promoting breathing strategies. Based in London, she is author of *And Breathe: The Complete Guide to Conscious Breathing for Health and Happiness.*

This form of breathing stimulates the parasympathetic nervous system (PNS), which slows your heart rate and breathing, lowers blood pressure and diverts blood toward the digestive system.

THE HEALING EFFECTS

Proper breathing offers a number of powerful health benefits, including…

•**Reduced anxiety and depression.** Deep breathing is believed to help elevate levels of serotonin and endorphins, naturally occurring "feel-good" chemicals. A study by Harvard Medical School psychiatrists showed that those who meditated daily for four years—a practice that relies heavily on conscious breathing—had longer telomeres, the protective "caps" on the ends of chromosomes that serve as biomarkers of longevity and slower aging.

•**Protection against viruses.** Our lymphatic system, which moves cleansing, vital fluids through our muscles and tissues, relies on breathing, movement and gravity to continue flowing. By promoting a healthy lymphatic system, deep breathing can play a crucial role in protecting the body from viruses, bacteria and other health threats.

•**Less constipation.** Deeper breathing (and the stress reduction that goes along with it) promotes intestinal action and stimulates overall digestion. This can improve conditions such as constipation and irritable bowel syndrome.

•**Improved sleep.** The relaxation that occurs with deep breathing is likely responsible for its positive effect on sleep quality.

BEST BREATHING FIXES

Targeted breathing exercises can help you deal more effectively with stress…and day-to-day health challenges such as indigestion, insomnia and fatigue. The best part is that you can do these exercises anywhere. Among my favorite quick breathing fixes—they can also help with respiratory conditions such as asthma and chronic obstructive pulmonary disease (COPD)…

•**Alternate nostril breathing.** This breathing exercise helps put you in a calm and centered state.

What to do: Breathe in deeply through your right nostril while pressing the left nostril closed with your right index finger…then exhale through the left nostril while pressing the right nostril closed with your right thumb. Next, inhale through the left nostril (right nostril still closed)…then close the left nostril and exhale through the right. The exhalations should take about twice as long as the inhalations. Repeat the cycle 10 times.

•**4-7-8 breathing.** If you are plagued by insomnia, this breathing exercise can put you to sleep within minutes.

What to do: Exhale completely through your mouth, making a "whoosh" sound. Close your mouth and inhale quietly through your nose to a count of four. Hold your breath for a count of seven. Exhale completely through your mouth, making a "whoosh" sound, to a count of eight. This is one breath.

Now inhale again and repeat the cycle three more times. Do this exercise when you need help going to sleep or if you awaken and want to get back to sleep.

Medicinal Mushrooms: They Fight Cancer, Heart Disease, Arthritis, More

Mark Stengler, ND, a naturopathic doctor in private practice at Stengler Center for Integrative Medicine in Encinitas, California. He is author of more than 30 books, including *The Health Benefits of Medicinal Mushrooms* and *The Natural Physician's Healing Therapies*. He is co-author of *Bottom Line's Prescription for Drug Alternatives*. He is host of the PBS program *Supercharge Your Immune System* and author of the daily e-newsletter *House Calls* and the monthly newsletter *Health Revelations*. Mark Stengler.com

Mushrooms may not seem like a big health deal—most people think of them simply as earthy additions to meals and salads.

What most people don't realize: Dozens of varieties of mushrooms are medicinal. Rich in unique carbohydrates (polysaccharides) called beta glucans, they can energize the body's disease-fighting immune cells.

Here's what you need to know about three effective medicinal mushrooms…

Note: Mushroom supplements generally are safe, but because they activate the immune system, they should not be taken by organ-transplant recipients on immunosuppressive drugs. Also, look for a hot-water (or hot-water/ethanol) extract. This may be stated on the supplement label—if not, check the company's website. I typically recommend that patients take one mushroom supplement at a time, rather than two or three.

MAITAKE

I consider the maitake mushroom (*Grifola frondosa*)—native to northern Japan and called the "King of Mushrooms" throughout Asia—to be one of the most powerful allies in the battle against cancer. It can be used for immune enhancement in addition to conventional cancer treatment.

Compelling research: Chinese doctors studied more than 300 people with bladder cancer after they had surgery for the disease, tracking the effectiveness of five standard and natural therapies, including supplements of a maitake mushroom extract. After an average of seven years, those taking maitake had the lowest rate of cancer recurrence (35%). And in a study of 36 cancer patients published in *Alternative Medicine Review*, maitake supplements improved symptoms and decreased the size of tumors in 69% of breast cancer patients, 63% of lung cancer patients and 58% of liver cancer patients. The supplements also boosted the cancer-killing power of chemotherapy by up to 40%—doses ranged between 50 milligrams (mg) to 150 mg daily (some patients received chemotherapy and some did not).

Decades of research from Japan show that one "fraction" or extract of maitake—the D-fraction—is most effective in boosting the immune system and fighting cancer. Specifically, D-fraction boosts the number and power of natural killer cells, immune cells that can "recognize" and kill cancer cells and viruses.

Best product and dose: For my patients with cancer, I often prescribe the over-the-counter product MaitakeGold 404, used in many studies on cancer. I prescribe a daily dose of 0.5 mg to 1 mg per kilogram (2.2 pounds) of body weight. For everyday immune-strengthening, I often recommend 5 mg to 15 mg daily taken 20 minutes before meals or on an empty stomach.

You can find maitake mushrooms in your supermarket, farmers' market or gourmet market—and add them to your diet to help prevent cancer. The mature mushroom—also called "Hen of the Woods"—has large, fleshy grayish-brown caps. Cut off the tough white base, then slice and sauté the caps for 10 to 15 minutes with salt, pepper and garlic. They're great in pasta, risotto, eggs and other dishes. I recommend two to three servings of maitake mushrooms weekly.

TURKEY TAIL

The turkey tail mushroom (*Trametes versicolor*) grows around the world and has a fan-shaped, brown-and-tan cap that resembles turkey feathers. Used for centuries in folk and traditional medicines in China and Japan, this mushroom can treat lung infections, hepatitis (liver infection) and cancer. Modern medicine has focused on cancer.

Compelling research: More than 400 studies show that turkey tail can fight cancer. Nearly all the studies on people have been with PSK (krestin), a proprietary extract that has been used as a supportive therapy by thousands of cancer patients in Japan. In one study published in *Anticancer Research*, Stage 1 and 2 lung cancer patients taking the extract had a five-year survival rate of 39%, compared with 16% for patients taking a placebo. Other studies show higher survival rates in people taking PSK for colorectal, esophageal and stomach cancers.

Best product and dose: For those with cancer, I often recommend 1,000 mg to 1,500 mg, twice daily, taken in the morning and evening on an empty stomach. Look for a product that has 20% beta glucans. As for your diet—turkey tail is not an appetizing mushroom.

REISHI

Reishi (*Ganoderma lucidum*)—a shiny fan-shaped mushroom with colors ranging from reddish brown to black—has been used for thousands of years by traditional healers in Japan and China. (Chinese healers call this the "Mushroom of Immortality.") Among mushrooms, it's your best choice for an everyday tonic to boost the strength of your immune system. And it also strengthens the rest of the body. *Proven benefits include...*

•**Reversing fatty liver disease.** Fatty liver afflicts an estimated 25% of Americans and can lead to liver disease and liver cancer. In a new study published in *Pharmaceutical Biology,* the livers of people with fatty liver completely normalized after they took reishi for six months. And their levels of cell-damaging oxidants fell by 42%. The participants made no other changes in diet, exercise or anything else.

•**Improvement in fibromyalgia.** In a recent study by Spanish researchers published in *Nutrición Hospitalaria*, people with the pain, stiffness and poor fitness typical of fibromyalgia saw improvements in flexibility, strength and endurance after taking reishi for six weeks.

•**Eliminating oral HPV virus.** Oral infection with some strains of human papillomavirus (HPV) can cause throat cancer. In a study of 61 people with cancer-causing oral HPV, published in *International Journal of Medicinal Mushrooms*, 88% of people who took reishi for two months had complete clearance of the virus.

•**Easing rheumatoid arthritis pain.** In a study of people with rheumatoid arthritis published in *Arthritis & Rheumatism*, people who took reishi had less inflammation and pain compared with those taking a placebo.

•**Raising HDL "good" cholesterol in people with diabetes.** In a study published in *British Journal of Nutrition*, people with diabetes who took reishi had an increase in "good" HDL cholesterol.

•**Preventing altitude sickness.** Reishi is a favorite natural remedy of travelers and trekkers to prevent altitude sickness. Start taking the supplement 10 to 14 days before you travel to a higher altitude.

Best product and dose: Look for an extract product containing a minimum of 10% polysaccharides (beta glucans) and 4% triterpene (another active ingredient). Take 800 mg two to three times daily.

Reishi is bitter and woody-tasting and not ideal for culinary use.

6 Natural Fixes for Neuropathy

Janice F. Wiesman, MD, FAAN, associate clinical professor of neurology at New York University School of Medicine in New York City and adjunct assistant professor of neurology at Boston University School of Medicine. She is author of *Peripheral Neuropathy: What It Is and What You Can Do to Feel Better.*

Nerve damage can be both mysterious and maddening. It's mysterious because about one-third of those with neuropathy never discover what's causing the pain, tingling and numbness. It's maddening because damaged nerves recover slowly—if they recover at all. Even when an underlying cause of neuropathy is identified (diabetes, for example, is a big one) and corrected, the symptoms may persist for months, years or a lifetime.

MORE THAN PAIN

About one in every 15 American adults has experienced some form of neuropathy, also known as peripheral neuropathy. The symptoms vary widely—from sharp, shooting pains that feel like jolts of electricity...to burning sensations, tingling...numbness...muscle fatigue...and/or a lack of muscle strength in the feet. Symptoms typically start first in both feet, then slowly move up the legs and to the hands. Nerves that control functions such as sweat, blood pressure, digestion and bladder control can be affected as well.

There are hundreds of different causes of neuropathy. Diabetes, mentioned above, accounts for about one-third of all cases. Elevated blood sugar damages nerve cells and blood vessels and can cause numbness and other symptoms.

Other common causes of neuropathy: Heavy alcohol use, rheumatoid arthritis, vitamin deficiencies (including vitamin B-12) and certain medications, especially some chemotherapy drugs.

Important finding: One-third to one-half of patients with neuropathies of unknown origin have inherited neuropathies—that is, they're genetically susceptible to nerve damage, even in the absence of a specific disease/injury, according to research conducted at Mayo Clinic.

A few medications are FDA-approved for neuropathy, but the side effects may be more uncomfortable than the condition itself. Fortunately, there are some surprisingly effective nondrug therapies.

NATURAL TREATMENTS

It can be a challenge for doctors (usually neurologists) to identify what is responsible for neuropathies. But it's worth making the effort because treating the cause early can stop ongoing damage and potentially allow injured nerves to regenerate. When nerves repair there may be some increased sensitivity, but this is usually temporary.

When the cause of neuropathy can't be identified, the symptoms can still be treated. If your symptoms make you very uncomfortable, there are medications that can help. The drugs that have been FDA-approved for neuropathic pain include *pregabalin* (Lyrica), also often used for seizures…and *duloxetine* (Cymbalta), also used for depression. Lyrica can cause drowsiness and weight gain…and Cymbalta can cause drowsiness as well as sweating in a small number of people. *Gabapentin* (Neurontin) and tricyclic antidepressants, such as *amitriptyline* and *nortriptyline* (Pamelor), are used off-label for neuropathy. Neurontin is similar to Lyrica with the same side effects…and the antidepressants can cause sedation, dry mouth and, in high doses, arrhythmias.

My advice: If you'd describe your symptoms as uncomfortable and annoying—but not debilitating—you might want to start with nondrug treatments. They probably won't eliminate the discomfort altogether, but they can make it easier to tolerate. Plus, if you do decide to use medication, these treatments may enable you to take it for a shorter time and/or at a lower dose. *Try one or more of the following at a time…*

•**Natural fix #1: Vibrating footbath.** Most patients will first notice tingling, numbness or other symptoms in the feet. Soaking your feet in a warm-water vibrating footbath (available in department stores, pharmacies and online) for 15 to 20 minutes dilates blood vessels and increases circulation in the affected area. More important, the vibrations are detected and transmitted by large-diameter sensory nerve fibers. Because of their large size, these fibers transmit signals very quickly. The sensations of vibration reach the spinal cord before the pain signals from damaged nerves, which blunts the discomfort.

The pain relief is temporary but reliable. You can soak your feet as often as you wish throughout the day.

Helpful: Soak your feet just before bed—the pain relief you get will help you fall asleep more easily.

For discomfort in other parts of the body, you can get similar relief from a whirlpool bath or a pulsating showerhead.

Important: Some people with neuropathy are unable to sense temperatures and can burn their feet in too-hot water. Test the temperature with your hand first (or have someone else test it).

•**Natural fix #2: Menthol cream.** The smooth muscles in arterial walls are lined with receptors that react to menthol. When you rub an affected area with menthol cream (such as Bengay), the blood vessels dilate, create warmth and reduce discomfort. Creams labeled "menthol" or "methyl salicylate" have the same effects. These creams can be used long-term as needed.

•**Natural fix #3: Transcutaneous electrical nerve stimulation (TENS).** This therapy delivers low levels of electric current to the surface of the skin. It's thought that the current stimulates nerves and sends signals to the brain that block the discomfort from damaged nerves.

How well do the devices work? The research is mixed. In 2010, a meta-analysis of TENS in patients with diabetic neuropathies found that the treatment led to a decrease in pain scores. Other studies, however, have shown little or no benefit.

Battery-powered TENS units cost about $30 for low-end models. The treatment is largely without side effects, and some people have good results. Treatments are typically done for 30 minutes at a time and can be repeated as needed throughout the day. Treatments should not be done on skin that is irritated.

My advice: If you want to try TENS at home, start using it under the direction of a physical therapist so that he/she can suggest the appropriate settings and amount of time for treatment.

•**Natural fix #4: Percutaneous electrical nerve stimulation (PENS).** Percutaneous means that the electric current is delivered under the skin, using short needles. Studies have shown that the treatments, done in rehabilitation/physical therapy offices, decrease pain, improve sleep and may allow patients to use smaller doses of painkilling medication. After each treatment, the pain relief can potentially last for weeks or longer.

The treatments take about 30 minutes per session and are generally repeated three times a week, until the patient achieves the desired amount and duration of pain relief. The risks are minimal, although you might have mild bruising or a little bleeding. Infection is possible but unlikely. Most patients have little or no pain during the treatments. PENS is not advised for those with pacemakers and should not be done on areas of irritated skin. The treatments might or might not be covered by insurance—be sure to ask.

•**Natural fix #5: Self-massage.** Firmly rubbing and/or kneading the uncomfortable area is another way to block pain signals. You don't need to learn sophisticated massage techniques—but you (or a loved one) must use enough pressure to stimulate the big nerves that carry the pressure sensations. A too-light touch won't be helpful.

Caution: If you have a history of deep vein thrombosis, ask your doctor before massaging your legs.

•**Natural fix #6: Relaxation techniques.** Stress and anxiety do not cause neuropathy, but patients who are tense may feel pain more intensely. A multiyear study found that patients with chronic pain who completed a mindfulness/stress-reduction program reported significantly less pain—and the improvement lasted for up to three years.

Helpful: Meditation, yoga and other relaxation techniques. Most large medical centers offer programs in anxiety/stress management. Excellent guided meditations are also available on YouTube.

Hypnosis Works! How to Make It Work for You

Roberta Temes, PhD, a psychotherapist, hypnotist, former faculty member, SUNY Downstate Medical Center, Brooklyn, and member of the Society for Clinical and Experimental Hypnosis. Dr. Temes has a private practice in Scotch Plains, New Jersey, and has been practicing hypnosis, treating thousands of clients, for more than 35 years. She is author of *The Complete Idiot's Guide to Hypnosis*. DrRoberta.com

---

Hypnosis is powerfully effective mind-body medicine. But it's underutilized—partly because of confusion about what hypnosis can and can't do…and because it's too often misused and abused.

Hundreds of scientific studies show that hypnosis can help with a wide range of physical and emotional issues, including pain, depression, phobias, unwanted habits, performance enhancement and much more. But not everything called "hypnosis" is helpful.

A hypnotic trance is nothing extraordinary. In fact, when you've been so intensely focused—maybe in a book, a TV program or a craft project—that you're unaware of your surroundings, you've been in a hypnotic trance. If someone asked you for a dollar bill, you would probably hand it over—because the power of suggestion is uniquely effective during a hypnotic trance.

However, since anyone can call himself/herself a hypnotist, you need to know what to look for and what to avoid. Pitfalls to watch for…

•**The "hypnotist" is unqualified.** There are no state or national certifications nor any formal licensing required to call yourself a hypnotist. "Training" can be a YouTube video or a three-hour course. Instead, look for training from the American Society of Clinical Hypnotists or the Society for Clinical and Experimental Hypnosis. Both offer programs and workshops that are open only to health professionals.

Better: In my opinion, word-of-mouth is the only way to find a competent hypnotist. If a friend has used hypnosis and it worked, ask if he would recommend his hypnotist. A good endorsement might be, "I was afraid of flying, and now I can get on a plane with no problem" or "I smoked two packs of cigarettes every day, and now I cannot stand the thought of cigarettes." If none of your friends have tried hypnosis (or would recommend theirs), ask your doctor or dentist for a recommendation.

•**Hypnosis masks an underlying health problem that requires medical care.** Many people (and unqualified "hypnotists") believe hypnosis can fix any problem, but it's important to know when hypnosis should not be the first thing you try.

Example: I can easily hypnotize someone with a headache to relieve the pain. But if the cause of the headache is an undiagnosed brain tumor, what the person needs most is a neurologist.

Better: A doctor visit—not hypnosis—should be the first response to a new symptom. Make sure that any underlying medical condition is appropriately addressed first.

•**The hypnotic suggestions are inappropriate.** Many years ago, asthmatic patients in a hospital in North Wales in the UK were hypnotized to not panic, remain calm and slowly and carefully seek help when having asthma attacks. These turned out to be terrible suggestions. Some of the asthmatics were so calm and deliberate when they had a life-threatening asthma attack that they almost died!

Better: Both hypnotist and client should evaluate the safety of the suggestions that are going to be used and write them down so that there is no ambiguity—before the client is brought to a hypnotic state.

•**The hypnotist recommends long-term treatment.** Some psychotherapists offer "hypnotherapy" as an adjunct to standard treatment—sometimes for a year or longer—usually as a way to uncover "repressed" material to help achieve psychological health. I don't endorse this approach.

I believe hypnosis works rapidly and should be used for changing habits and attitudes, not for delving into the unconscious. For instance, a patient undergoing psychotherapy might benefit from one session of hypnosis to deal with a particular issue—such as unhealthy eating habits, fear of public speaking or reluctance to meet a certain person—that is preventing him from moving forward with therapy.

Better: A good hypnotist should need to see you only one or two times.

Helpful: Hypnotic suggestions can "wear off." Ask if you can record the session on your phone to replay later if you need it. Some of my clients play their recording once a week…others never, but like to keep it as a "security blanket."

•**The hypnotist helps you to "recover" a repressed memory.** A memory "recovered" during hypnosis, especially a new memory about a past supposedly traumatic event, is almost always a false memory. In fact, there's a name for this common phenomenon—false memory syndrome.

Problem: Such memories are usually "recovered" by a therapist with an agenda, such as proving that you're a victim of childhood sexual abuse, something that's too easy for a hypnotist to create and reinforce.

Better: If you don't remember an event when you're not in a hypnotic trance, it probably didn't happen.

•**You're hypnotized on stage—and feel anxious afterward.** I love stage hypnosis! But I never volunteer to be hypnotized, and I don't think you should either. A stage hypnotist rapidly induces a hypnotic state and rapidly ends it. If your mental state is at all fragile—if you're stressed or didn't sleep well the night before—such rapid transition into and out of a hypnotic state could create a few days of mental imbalance and anxiety.

Better: Enjoy the show, but don't participate!

HOW I DO HYPNOSIS WITH MY CLIENTS…

I start a session by informally chatting with a client to establish a comfortable rapport.

We then decide together on verbal suggestions—the words I will say, slowly and deliberately, while he/she is in a hypnotic state.

Example: For a claustrophobic client scheduled for an MRI, we agreed that I would suggest that the cramped quarters of the MRI machine were a protective womb…and that the loud noise was a lullaby that would put her to sleep.

Finally, I help the client enter a hypnotic state. A typical session takes about one hour, although the actual hypnosis portion is usually about 20 minutes. I suggest that my clients record their sessions, but some of my clients prefer instead to return to my office for another session when or if they feel they need reinforcement.

This "Weed" Is a Healthy Healer

Jamison Starbuck, ND, is a naturopathic physician in family practice and writer and producer of *Dr. Starbuck's Health Tips for Kids*, a weekly program on Montana Public Radio, MTPR.org, both in Missoula. DrJamisonStarbuck.com.

Stinging nettle, with its odd-sounding name, grows throughout the US and is thought by some to be nothing more than a weed. This deep green, leafy plant can indeed grow to six feet tall or more. And if you're hiking in a damp forest or taking a stroll past a weed-filled, untended lot, you'll likely happen upon nettle. But don't be deceived—stinging nettle is a nutritious spring food and is widely considered to be one of the most useful of botanical medicines. As a food, stinging nettle is often eaten like spinach. It contains calcium, potassium, iron and plant protein. The irritating needles are destroyed by steaming. Some people harvest stinging nettle on their own or buy it at a local farmer's market.

As a medicine, I frequently recommend stinging nettle to treat…

•**Seasonal allergies.** When allergy season begins (or up to a month before, if possible), patients who suffer from annoying seasonal allergy symptoms can start using nettle in tea or tincture form. The typical dose is 16 ounces daily of nettle tea or one-quarter teaspoon of tincture in two ounces of water, twice a day— taken at least 15 minutes before or after eating. The herb helps strengthen the body's immune system to reduce common allergy symptoms such as runny nose, watery eyes, sneezing and fatigue.

For prompt allergy relief: Freeze-dried nettle in capsule form is an effective and convenient way to help fight symptoms. A typical dose is two capsules three or four times a day when you have allergy symptoms. Many of my patients find that they need more nettle at the beginning of allergy season and that they are able to reduce the dose after a few weeks. Once allergy season is over, you can stop taking this herbal medicine.

•**Cough.** Nettle also acts as an expectorant, a medicine that helps push mucus out of your throat and lungs. For patients who have a simple cough or cough due to bronchitis, for example, I often recommend nettle tea or tincture. A typical dose is four ounces of tea, four times a day…or one-quarter teaspoon of tincture in two ounces of water, four times a day.

•**Enlarged prostate.** Men with enlarged prostate experience urinary frequency—especially at night—and difficulty initiating and/or maintaining urination. Nettle root is frequently found in men's prostate formulas, which contain other herbs such as saw palmetto and pygeum africanum.

Scientists aren't entirely sure how stinging nettle works, but because it has multiple medicinal uses, it continues to be studied in North America and Europe. Because the plant is considered generally safe to use as medicine, you can purchase it over-the-counter and follow the manufacturer's instructions. But if you want to try nettle, it's wise to visit a health-care practitioner who is knowledgeable about botanical medicines. This includes naturopathic physicians. To find one near you, consult The American Association of Naturopathic Physicians, Naturopathic.org.

Caution: If you are allergic to any type of weed, don't use stinging nettle. If you have diabetes, high blood pressure, kidney disease or take a blood thinner, lithium or a sedative, talk to your doctor before taking nettle. This herb can interact with certain medications—especially those listed here and used for the conditions above. Pregnant women should not use nettle.

7 Days to Switch Your Brain to Calm

Andrew B. Newberg, MD, director of research at the Marcus Institute of Integrative Health of Thomas Jefferson University in Philadelphia and the lead author of a study titled, "Effect of a 1-week Spiritual Retreat on Dopamine and Serotonin Transporter Binding: A Preliminary Study," published in *Religion, Brain and Behavior*.

Remember your last vacation? Maybe you burned out trying to see every attraction in the guidebook or you landed in a noisy hotel room by the elevators. Next time, a meditative spiritual retreat could be a soothing alternative that goes beyond merely taking time to chill. A new study shows that a weeklong spiritual retreat can reroute brain chemicals to bolster feelings of calm and well-being that can be lost in the everyday hustle and bustle.

Background: Yoga and spiritual retreats have become popular escapes from work and life's day-to-day routine. People who've attended extended retreats often come back feeling relaxed and content—and some say that they've been through a life-altering experience. But is that just talk from proponents of these retreats, or is there a biological reason for feeling better?

Study: In 14 men and women ranging in age from 24 to 76, researchers compared brain scan results before and after they attended the same seven-day spiritual retreat. The retreat took place on the serene grounds of a Pennsylvania Jesuit center. After attending morning mass, the participants spent the rest of the day in prayer and reflective silence. They ate meals in a common dining area. Before the scans, participants were injected with a specific tracer that follows the movements in the brain of two neurotransmitters (chemical messengers)—dopamine and serotonin. Dopamine is involved in reward pathways by inducing positive, feel-good emotions. Serotonin affects how we regulate emotions and mood.

Results: After the retreat, the scans revealed significant decreases in a process that essentially absorbs dopamine and serotonin in certain regions of the brain. With less of that absorption, greater levels of dopamine and serotonin should be available to circulate throughout the brain. Higher levels of the circulating neurotransmitters are associated with positive emotions, such as those reported by the people who attended the retreat.

Bottom line: Those feel-good responses to extended meditative practice are rooted in biological changes in your brain. How long will they last? This study didn't follow the retreat participants over the next few weeks or months, so it can't answer that question. Because there was no comparison group, it also can't tell us whether similar changes might occur after, say, a seven-day African safari—or a beach vacation. But it does reinforce the benefits of a sustained "digital detox" and the brain-changing benefits of meditation. Intrigued? Find out how to plan your own spiritual retreat. Pressed for time? Check out this 12-minute meditation.

Surprising Benefits of Acupuncture: It Works for Asthma, Stroke, More

Stephen Chee, MD, MPH, MA, MTOM, LAc. He is dual-trained and dual-licensed as a medical doctor and acupuncturist. He is quadruple-board-certified in family medicine, integrative medicine, medical acupuncture and acupuncture, and Traditional Chinese medicine. Dr. Chee has a private practice in Beverly Hills, California. DrSteveChee.com

A recent *Vanity Fair* cover story about actress Angelina Jolie revealed that she had suffered from Bell's palsy (temporary weakness or paralysis and drooping of one side of the face). But Jolie said she no longer had the disorder—and credited acupuncture for her full recovery.

It took acupuncture a very long time to move from its roots as an ancient Chinese therapy to being accepted as "real medicine" in the West—and even today, most people, including most doctors, think of acupuncture mainly as a treatment for pain such as low-back pain, headaches and pain from arthritis. And acupuncture does treat pain effectively, probably because its placement of very fine needles into the skin in particular spots blocks the transmission of pain signals to the brain and also releases the body's natural endorphins.

What most people don't know: Acupuncture also is an excellent treatment for a wide variety of other illnesses and conditions.

Research shows that acupuncture reduces inflammation…improves circulation…regulates the autonomic nervous system (which controls heart rate, breathing, digestion and other body functions)…and balances the production of neurotransmitters, brain chemicals that control mood—all therapeutic keys to treating many health problems.

Here are surprising conditions that acupuncture can treat…

OVERACTIVE BLADDER SYNDROME (OAB)

This problem afflicts one in six Americans and becomes more common with age. You feel a sudden, uncontrollable urge to urinate (which can lead to incontinence), and you may have to urinate many times a day and even several times overnight.

How acupuncture helps: When medications can't control the problem, electroacupuncture—in which the needles conduct a very mild, nonpainful electric current—often can. The proven approach is using electroacupuncture to stimulate a point in the ankle along what Traditional Chinese medicine practitioners call the "kidney meridian." This also happens to be the location of the posterior tibial nerve, which controls the bladder.

Recent finding: A team of researchers from several major institutions—including Johns Hopkins School of Medicine, Columbia University Medical Center and Brown University—reviewed studies on nondrug treatments for OAB, publishing the results in *American Journal of Obstetrics Gynecology.* The researchers found that electroacupuncture was effective for the problem and improved quality of life.

What works best: Weekly electroacupuncture for 12 weeks. Discontinue the treatment if it isn't improving the condition after four or five weeks. Patients who respond to the treatment may require additional therapy at individually defined treatment intervals (for example, every three weeks) for sustained relief of symptoms.

Acupuncture may help for incontinence as well: Stress urinary incontinence—passing urine inadvertently when you cough, sneeze, laugh, exercise or lift a heavy object—afflicts an estimated 35% of women, most of them older. A recent study of about 500 women with this condition, published in *JAMA*, showed that electroacupuncture decreased urine leakage after six weeks. (Using electroacupuncture to treat stress urinary incontinence is still being researched.)

DIABETIC PERIPHERAL NEUROPATHY

An estimated 50% of older people with diabetes develop this nerve disorder, which can cause numbness, burning, tingling and pain in the feet, legs, hands and/or arms—and also increases the risk for infected diabetic foot ulcers and the need for amputation.

Recent finding: A study published in *Journal of Acupuncture and Meridian Studies* showed that 10 weekly sessions of acupuncture improved the symptoms of diabetic peripheral neuropathy in three out of four patients.

Another recent finding: Acupuncture also may help control high blood sugar itself. In a study published in *Nutrition & Diabetes*, treatment with a diabetes medication (metformin) and acupuncture controlled high blood sugar more effectively than the medication alone.

What works best: Electroacupuncture and scalp acupuncture weekly for 10 weeks. (Scalp acupuncture utilizes advanced acupuncture needling techniques and points on the scalp that have been identified not by Traditional Chinese medicine but by neuroanatomy. In my clinical experience, it often is the most effective type of acupuncture for treating neurological problems such as neuropathy, stroke and mental decline and usually requires additional training by the acupuncturist.)

ASTHMA

I have used acupuncture to treat a number of patients with asthma, helping them decrease the frequency and severity of asthma attacks—and reduce the dosage of their asthma medication. (As with all the medical problems discussed here, I almost always use acupuncture in combination with other medical and nondrug treatments—in the case of asthma, those nondrug treatments include certain supplements, conscious breathing, meditation and eliminating environmental and potential food triggers.)

Recent finding: In a study published in *The Journal of Alternative and Complementary Medicine*, German and Swiss researchers added acupuncture (15 sessions over three months) to standard asthma treatment in 184 patients, comparing them with people who had asthma but did not receive acupuncture. Compared with those not getting acupuncture, those receiving it had a 70% greater improvement in asthma symptoms and in limits to their daily activity. They also had two to four times greater improvement in perceived physical and mental health.

What works best: Any style of acupuncture can be effective for asthma, with treatments once a week for 10 to 15 weeks. Patients who respond to the treatment may require additional therapy at regular intervals (for example, every three to four weeks) for sustained relief of symptoms.

POST-STROKE REHABILITATION

Research shows that acupuncture can treat a variety of post-stroke symptoms including pain, depression and insomnia—and can help restore the basic nerve and muscle function that strokes rob from patients.

Recent finding: Researchers from Australia and China analyzed the results from 22 studies on 1,425 stroke patients, publishing their results in *Archives of Physical Medicine and Rehabilitation*. They found that electroacupuncture reduced spasticity (in which muscles involuntarily shorten or flex, causing stiffness and tightness) by more than 40% and improved everyday functioning.

What works best: Scalp acupuncture combined with either electroacupuncture or standard acupuncture.

FINDING AN ACUPUNCTURIST

Word-of-mouth is the most effective way to find a competent acupuncturist. Ask your doctors, family members and friends for recommendations. You also can use the "Find a Practitioner" feature at the website of the Na-

tional Certification Commission for Acupuncture and Oriental Medicine (NCCAOM.org).

Talk to the acupuncturist before your treatment to see whether you feel comfortable with him/her, which, I think, is a key element of healing. (Avoid treatment from any acupuncturist who is not willing to talk to you or answer your questions before charging you or starting treatment.)

Some Like It Hot: Saunas Cook Up Sizzling Health Benefits

Jari A. Laukkanen, MD, PhD, cardiologist and professor in the School of Medicine at the University of Eastern Finland's Institute of Public Health and Clinical Nutrition, Kuopio. He has published numerous articles about the long-term health effects of sauna use.

E very now and then something that feels great turns out to be great for your health. This time, it's the modern sauna—a room that radiates dry heat.

Saunas have had a healthy reputation for a long time, to be sure, but scientific evidence has been scant—mostly small, short-term studies. Now there's compelling new research that has tracked the long-term health of thousands of sauna-taking men and women over a period of more than 20 years—and it found wide-ranging benefits for the heart, the respiratory system and the brain.

Not surprisingly, the new studies are coming from Finland, where the sauna has been a part of home life for millennia. But even in the US, there's a sauna at many gyms, and new kinds of home saunas are increasingly affordable and popular—imagine taking a relaxing dry sauna any time you want! *Here's a look at the proven benefits of dry sauna—and how to get them for yourself…*

FOUR WAYS SAUNAS MAKE YOU HEALTHIER

Saunas are such a part of Finland's culture that nearly everyone uses one. So rather than comparing people who use them frequently with those who never use them, researchers compared frequent users with infrequent ones.

They then took steps to control statistically for the fact that people who use saunas often might live healthier lives in other ways as well, such as exercising more or smoking less. *Among the health benefits of taking saunas regularly…*

•**Healthier heart.** A 20-year study published in *JAMA Internal Medicine* found that people who took saunas four to seven times a week were 50% less likely to develop cardiovascular disease than those who took saunas only once a week or less. Regular sauna use increases blood flow and heart rate in much the way that cardiovascular exercise does—and improves the function of the inside layer of blood vessels in ways that are beneficial for blood pressure.

•**Protection from dementia.** Research published in *Age and Ageing* found that middle-aged men who took 15-minute saunas four to seven times per week were 66% less likely to develop dementia than men who took one sauna per week or less. One reason may be the cardiovascular benefits that improve blood flow to the brain.

•**Less respiratory disease.** A study published in *European Journal of Epidemiology* found that middle-aged men who took at least four saunas per week were 41% less likely to develop certain serious respiratory conditions over time including chronic obstructive pulmonary disease (COPD), asthma and pneumonia.

•**Longer life.** A healthier heart, brain and lungs may add up to preventing premature death. The study published in *JAMA Internal Medicine* also found that middle-aged men who took saunas four to seven times each week were 40% less likely to die from any cause during the 20-plus-year study than were men who used the sauna only once a week or less.

YOUR SAUNA STRATEGY

Taking the occasional sauna when you visit a hotel or spa is not enough to derive significant health benefits. The secret to saunas is to use them often—ideally every day or every other day.

How long you spend in the sauna and how hot the sauna is matter as well.

Example: Studies show that sauna use is associated with a lower overall risk for sudden cardiac death—and that risk was 52% lower for men who habitually spent more than 19 minutes in the sauna than for those who spent 11 minutes. Various studies confirm that the best sauna temperature for health is about 175°F at head level.

Spending that much time in a hot sauna is likely to make your heart rate accelerate, and it might no longer feel completely comfortable—but maybe that's the point. With cardiovascular exercise, our bodies derive the greatest benefits when we push ourselves beyond the point where the exercise is easy. That's true with saunas, too.

Warning: People who have high or low blood pressure or other cardiovascular problems should speak with their doctors before taking saunas—and in fact, that's a good idea for everyone just to make sure that the heat won't be risky for you.

So far, almost all of the research on health benefits has been done on the traditional "dry" sauna—often called a "Finnish" sauna in the US. This type of sauna features very little steam and humidity levels of just 10% to 20%. Popular "infrared" saunas, which also are dry but work on a different principle to heat the body, have been shown to reduce blood pressure and have other short-term health benefits, but there is no long-term data. Nor do we know much about the health effects of steam rooms, although they, too, create a passive cardiovascular workout.

SAUNA BEST PRACTICES

For safe, effective use of a sauna…

The best temperature is around 175°F, although you'll get benefits over 160°F. Avoid going as high as 195°F—that's unsafe for everyone.

Twenty to 30 minutes is ideal.

After a sauna, let yourself cool down for a few minutes by sitting in a normal-temperature room—and drink two to four eight-ounce glasses of water.

Saunas are places where people sit or stand and perspire—so they should be cleaned regularly.

Don't drink alcohol an hour or two before a sauna—or during. The combination of heat and alcohol can make blood pressure drop too low.

Doctors Said There Was No Cure, but These People Didn't Give Up

Susannah Meadows, author of *The Other Side of Impossible: Ordinary People Who Faced Daunting Medical Challenges and Refused to Give Up*. The book is based on her family's quest to find a way to help her son's arthritis when they were told he was unlikely to recover. She is a former senior writer for *Newsweek*. SusannahMeadows.com

A professor of medicine in Iowa was told that her multiple sclerosis (MS) would confine her to a wheelchair for the rest of her life. A girl in Washington State endured seizures for years—doctors could not pinpoint a cause, much less propose a solution. A boy in New York was diagnosed with a rare form of debilitating arthritis and given little hope of recovery.

But despite these seemingly hopeless prognoses, these people were able to improve their health and their lives. How did they do it?

When people are told that medical science has no solution for their health problems, some give up and accept their fates. Others, in their desperation, fall victim to quacks and con artists peddling ineffective and potentially dangerous fake cures. But a few manage to find treatments outside traditional medicine that seem to work. Some of these approaches may not have gone through rigorous clinical trials, so they have not earned the approval of mainstream medicine, but they are rooted in science.

There are no guarantees, of course. In fact, unproven medical treatments often turn out to be ineffective. But despite the unfavorable odds, unproven treatments still might be worth trying when doctors have no solution to a health problem…and the unproven treatment itself poses no health risks.

Journalist Susannah Meadows recently wrote *The Other Side of Impossible*, a book about people who overcame daunting diagnoses after trying unproven treatments and other strategies. She also is the mother of the boy from New York who, at the age of four, overcame polyarticular juvenile idiopathic arthritis.

We asked Meadows what we can learn from these stories about how to search for solutions when doctors offer no hope. Because she is a journalist, not a doctor, she is not offering medical advice. Instead she is sharing her observations and some of the steps she took that could be helpful to others…

•**The people I wrote about in my book sought unproven solutions that have attracted the attention of researchers.** People facing difficult illnesses often hear about unproven medical treatments, perhaps in illness support groups or on websites—and a smart response is to then investigate whether the treatments have received any interest from the scientific community.

It can take many years for the medical community to test and accept a new treatment. The people whose stories I tell in my book felt that they didn't have time to wait. When my son was lying sick on the couch after taking his medication, which wasn't helping his arthritis much, I couldn't accept that this was our only choice. People in this position sometimes look into joining a trial to get access to cutting-edge therapies.

The Internet has made a lot of this work possible. You can look for websites, articles or press releases citing the newest research. For example, at PubMed, the National Institutes of Health's free online medical research database, you can see whether anything favorable has been published about a possible treatment in a medical journal (NCBI.nlm.nih.gov/pubmed). Websites of nonprofits associated with various diseases also are good resources. They often will issue press releases regarding studies that they are currently funding to explore an intervention's effectiveness.

Example: The Iowa professor I write about in my book recovered from MS after she changed her diet. It may sound unlikely that such an intervention could have such a powerful effect, but the National Multiple Sclerosis Society (NMSS) recently committed more than $1 million to studying her protocol—and someone searching online could learn this by visiting the NMSS website (search for "Dietary Approach").

Search tip: When looking for trials of treatments relating to a given condition, search the names of the scientists who you see have produced recent research on the topic—because individual medical researchers often pursue the same topic of research in multiple studies.

•**We talked over everything with our doctor to make sure that we were safe.** Doctors are unlikely to advocate any solution that has not yet been put through clinical trials and been accepted by the medical community—but it still is important to keep your doctors in the loop if you want to try an unproven treatment. Doctors can't offer much guidance about whether an unproven treatment will help you, but they can weigh in about risks.

Example: When I learned of another child whose juvenile arthritis appeared to have improved dramatically after gluten and dairy were removed from his diet—and fish oil, probiotics and Chinese herbs were added to it—I asked my son's doctor whether these herbs and dietary changes were risky. We tried them only after we were assured that they were not. Our doctor's main concern was that we keep our son on medication, which we did. (I already was aware of the risk that Chinese herbs can contain toxic heavy metals, so we found a source of herbs that were subjected to third-party testing. All supplements come with some risk because they are not regulated in this country—manufacturers don't have to prove that the supplements work or even that they won't hurt you.)

Some doctors are more accepting of these complementary treatments than other doctors. If my family faced a difficult illness again and found that our doctor was not open-minded, I probably would seek another opinion. One thing I've learned is that good doctors know that they don't know everything.

•**It's right to be especially wary of cures that are being pushed by those who stand to make a profit.** I always think like a journalist when approaching medical issues. A good source is not someone with a conflict of interest—in medicine as well as in reporting. In the alternative medicine world, there are plenty of scammers because there are a lot of people who are desperate for treatment that works.

•**Diet-related solutions are promising.** The microbiome, the population of bacteria that lives in and on our bodies, is among the hottest fields of medical research these days.

These microbes are fed by the food we eat. If we don't treat our population well—if we take unnecessary antibiotics and we don't eat a variety of fiber, which our bacteria thrive on—we can end up with a compromised population. And an unhealthy microbiome is linked to all kinds of diseases.

Researchers also are investigating the potential connection between having a hyper-permeable gut lining, also called a leaky gut, and autoimmune disease. Eating gluten, for example, can cause the lining of the gut to become more permeable, which could allow proteins from food to escape into our bloodstreams, triggering immune-system–related health problems.

If the gut and its bacteria are indeed involved in a wide range of poorly understood health problems, changing one's diet could potentially solve or reduce some of those problems. But because research into these issues is in its early stages—and because few physicians have much training in nutrition—there's a good chance that your doctor will have little or no knowledge of possible dietary solutions.

Example: As noted earlier, our son's arthritis treatment included removing gluten and dairy from his diet. Another child I wrote about saw a dramatic improvement in his ADHD symptoms after he changed his diet—under his doctor's supervision, he tried an elimination diet, taking out eight foods and adding them back in one at a time to see which ones gave him a problem. A little girl's autistic traits were less pronounced after she removed grains, starches, milk and any added sugar.

•**The search itself may be good for your health.** Trying unproven treatments could improve your health even if the treatments you try are found not to hold water. The placebo effect is well-established—when people believe that they are receiving medical treatment, their health often improves and/or their pain lessens. In one study, 62% of irritable bowel syndrome patients reported that their symptoms improved when they received a sham treatment from a doctor who projected compassion and confidence.

Also, the longer you keep up the search for a solution, the greater the odds that you will stumble upon one—and it even could be something completely backed by science. The mother of the girl in Washington who suffered seizures tried treatment after treatment, both mainstream and outside the box, without success. Eventually, in desperation, she took her daughter to a third pediatric neurologist. He suggested an MRI. The imagery showed a benign brain tumor—the likely cause of the seizures. In almost 10 years, no other doctor had suggested doing an MRI. The tumor was removed in the spring of 2016, and the girl hasn't had a seizure since. If she is cured, it wasn't just that neurologist who saved her—it was her mother's determination to keep searching for a solution.

4 Natural Therapies for Adult ADHD

James M. Greenblatt, MD, psychiatrist and chief medical officer and vice president of medical services at Walden Behavioral Care in Waltham, Massachusetts. He is author of *Finally Focused*, which covers the integrative treatment of ADHD.

If you hear about someone suffering from attention deficit hyperactivity disorder (ADHD), you'll probably assume that it's a child or adolescent. That's understandable—more than six million youngsters have been diagnosed with the disorder. But that's only part of the ADHD story.

Surprising statistic: More than 10 million adults may have ADHD, according to research published in *The American Journal of Psychiatry*.

What's more, research shows that less than 10% of adults with ADHD have ever received a diagnosis to explain their symptoms—problems such as an inability to focus and/or impulsivity…traits that may have led to marriage troubles, a stalled career or depression. The majority of adults with ADHD have struggled since childhood.

Even worse, many adults who suspect they have ADHD may forgo diagnosis and treatment because the go-to therapies include stimulant prescription drugs, such as *methylphenidate* (Ritalin) or *dextroamphetamine* and *amphetamine* (Adderall), with many possible side effects such as irritability, agitation, anxiety, insomnia and facial tics.

A better approach: Science-based natural therapies that restore biochemical balance to the brain. Over the past three decades, I have treated thousands of adults and children with these therapies—and found them highly effective.

Important: If you think you have ADHD, seek out a professional (such as a psychologist, psychiatrist or social worker) who has experience treating people with the problem. If you are diagnosed with the condition, talk to your doctor about using one or more of these natural treatments before taking a prescription drug. If you and your doctor determine that you do require a prescription medication, these nondrug therapies may help such drugs work more effectively.

Among the best natural therapies, based on research and my clinical experience, for adults with ADHD…*

OPCS

Nutritional supplements known as oligomeric proanthocyanidins, or OPCs for short, are usually made from grape seeds, pine bark and/or green tea.

What OPCs do: These plant extracts appear to regulate brain waves, as I've observed using an electroencephalograph (EEG), a device that records electrical activity of the brain. My patients using OPCs become more focused in conversation, and I've even seen illegible handwriting become readable.

Good advice: The best supplements combine several OPCs. One such product is CurcumaSorb Mind, made by Pure Encapsulations. It contains pine bark extract, green tea extract, blueberry extract and grape extract. Another good product is OPC-3 from Isotonix.

MAGNESIUM

At least half the people in the US don't get enough of this nutrient, which is involved in more than 300 biochemical reactions in the body.

What magnesium does: Low magnesium can undercut the functioning of glutamate re-

---

*These therapies are generally safe and best tried in the order they appear here, but check with your doctor first, especially if you take medication or have a chronic medical condition.

ceptors, areas in brain cells that assist the movement of neurotransmitters. The possible results include poor concentration and irritability, anxiety, depression, mood swings, fatigue and sleeping problems.

Good advice: Ask your doctor whether you should be taking a magnesium supplement.

Also: Add magnesium-rich foods to your diet, including nuts, seeds, dark chocolate, leafy greens, such as spinach, and avocado.

OMEGA-3 FATTY ACIDS

Sixty percent of your brain is fat, which means that this vital organ depends on a steady supply of essential fatty acids, the building blocks of fat, for its health and function.

What omega-3s do: Just about every aspect of neurotransmission—the movement of information from brain cell to brain cell that supports every thought, emotion and action—is affected by omega-3s. Fatty fish and fish oil supply two of the most important omega-3 fatty acids—EPA (eicosapentaenoic acid) and DHA (docosahexaenoic acid).

Good advice: Eat at least two weekly servings of omega-3-rich fish and take a high-quality (molecularly distilled and tested for environmental contaminants such as heavy metals and PCBs) fish oil or krill oil supplement (1 g to 2 g daily).

LOW-DOSE LITHIUM

If your symptoms of ADHD include irritability, anger and impulsivity, low-dose lithium may help.

What low-dose lithium does: High doses of this mineral are prescribed for bipolar disorder. But very low doses of lithium can be a safe and effective nutritional treatment for ADHD when taken to calm the turbulent emotions that may agitate people with the disorder.

Good advice: Ask your doctor whether it makes sense for you to take 5 mg of lithium orotate, available over the counter, each day.

Also helpful: A diet that limits refined sugar and carbohydrates and emphasizes protein, which promotes the production of dopamine—

one of the neurotransmitters that aids focus and attention.

DO YOU HAVE ADHD?

Adults who have attention deficit hyperactivity disorder (ADHD) often experience difficulty paying attention, feelings of restlessness and impulsive behavior. These symptoms can result in dangerous driving, poor financial decisions, missed deadlines and substance abuse, among other issues. If you have one or more of the following symptoms that is ongoing and severe enough to negatively impact your life, talk to your doctor…

Impulsiveness…lack of focus…mood swings…easily frustrated…inability to cope with stress…problems planning, prioritizing, multitasking or completing tasks…restlessness…quick temper…disorganization.

Avoid Jet Lag—3 Natural Remedies That Work!

Michael J. Breus, PhD, clinical psychologist based in Manhattan Beach, California, diplomate of the American Board of Sleep Medicine and fellow of the American Academy of Sleep Medicine.

Wendy Bazilian, DrPH, RD, founder of Bazilian's Health Clinic in San Diego, where she has been helping clients with their health, nutrition and fitness goals for more than a decade. She is author of *Eat Clean, Stay Lean* and *The SuperFoods Rx Diet.*

Robin DiPasquale, ND, RH (AHG), doctor of naturopathic medicine and registered herbalist (American Herbalist Guild), in private practice at Red Lotus Healing Arts, Fort Collins, Colorado. Dr. DiPasquale has been practicing the healing arts for more than 30 years.

It's fun to see distant, exotic places, but if you're zoned out from jet lag, it's not nearly as much fun as it could be. Yes, eventually you adjust. But why lose precious vacation days (or productive workdays)? You don't have to.

Here are three top experts' favorite techniques to quickly sync your body clock to a new local time.

Bonus: You can use these strategies again when you get back home…

TRY MELATONIN—THE RIGHT WAY

On average, our bodies tend to naturally adjust to time zones at a rate of one or two per day—so recovering from flying from Miami to Paris, six time zones away, can take up to five days. To shorten the recovery time, sleep specialist Michael J. Breus, PhD, recommends melatonin…taken in the right dose.

How it works: Melatonin is a sleep-enhancing hormone produced in the brain in step with Earth's 24-hour cycle of daylight and darkness. Levels are naturally highest at night (even if your body doesn't think it's night) and lowest upon exposure to sunlight in the morning (ditto). When you travel long distances, your body's rhythm gets confused by the external light and dark signals of your new location. The effect is especially pronounced when you travel more than three time zones eastward.

Try this: Melatonin is widely available as an over-the-counter supplement. To reduce jet lag, take 0.5 mg on the plane 90 minutes before bedtime in the place you're traveling to. A similar protocol was found to be remarkably effective in reducing jet lag for airline passengers, airline staff and military personnel who crossed five or more time zones in a UK study that compared oral melatonin with a placebo or medication.

Important: Although melatonin is sold in much higher doses than the 0.5 mg mentioned here, the smaller amount is just as effective—and less likely to cause side effects such as headache, dizziness or stomach irritation. (You might have to buy a 1-mg form and split it in half, which is fine.) Because melatonin can have side effects, such as those described above, and can interact with other medications, such as antidepressants and blood pressure drugs, check with your health-care provider before taking melatonin.

CHERRY REMEDY

Would you rather eat a natural source of melatonin to reset your body clock? If so, tart cherries are one of the few foods known to contain the hormone and can be an effective remedy that is also tasty (albeit tart). Juice made from tart cherries also works. A study reported in *Journal of Nutrition, Health & Aging* found that, compared with a placebo drink, drinking tart cherry juice was better at increasing total nighttime sleep and reducing the number of awakenings.

Superfoods expert Wendy Bazilian, DrPH, RD, has found that staying hydrated, avoiding alcohol right before and during travel and getting regular daily exercise during your trip combined with the following protocol works against jet lag…

•**During the two days prior to departure,** drink six ounces of 100% tart cherry juice three times a day during each day. It doesn't matter whether you drink the juice straight or add it to another drink such as a smoothie, green tea, chamomile tea or sparkling water (all good combinations).

Another option: Instead of drinking cherry juice on these two days, eat three-quarters cup of dried tart cherries over the course of the day. These can be added to salad, cereal, trail mix, yogurt—or just eaten on their own. Fruit-juice-sweetened dried cherries are best, but whether sweetened with fruit juice or sugar, dried tart cherries have a total amount of sugar that's comparable to most dried fruits, such as raisins.

•**On the day of travel,** if your flight leaves at 2 pm or later, drink six ounces of juice or eat one-quarter cup of dried tart cherries three times during the day, spaced out until your flight. For a flight earlier than 2 pm, drink six ounces of juice or eat one-quarter cup of tart cherries in the morning before leaving for the airport.

•**Once on board the plane,** eat one-quarter cup of dried tart cherries with at least eight ounces of plain or sparkling water.

Continue snacking on one-half to three-quarters cup of dried cherries each day in the days after landing. Also remember to stay well hydrated—which you can do not only by drinking water but also by eating water-rich foods such as soups and salads.

HELP FROM HOMEOPATHY

Homeopathy uses tiny, diluted doses of substances that in larger amounts typically cause particular symptoms but in tiny amounts provoke a healing response to those same symptoms. There is not enough scientific evidence to say with certainty that homeopathy is an effective treatment for jet lag, yet many users say it has worked for them.

For jet lag, naturopathic doctor Robin Di-Pasquale, ND, RH (AHG), typically prescribes for her patients Blatta orientalis, also known as Indian Cockroach. Homeopathic practitioners use the remedy prepared from this nocturnal insect to help diminish the effects of jet lag. Although homeopathic remedies are sold at many health-food stores, natural-food markets and drugstores, they are best prescribed by knowledgeable practitioners.

What to do: Regardless of what time of day or night it is when you land at your destination, take five pellets of 30c-potency homeopathic Blatta orientalis, placed under your tongue. Don't chew the pellets. Let them dissolve, and don't eat or drink anything for 10 minutes before and after. Repeat twice a day for two to three days.

Note: While homeopathic Blatta orientalis is indeed derived from insects, the pellets themselves are tiny, white, sugary-tasting pills. There are no legs or antennae anywhere!

If you travel long distances frequently, the homeopathic remedy Cocculus indicus, made from the root of a climbing plant called Indian Cockle, may be more appropriate to address the extreme fatigue and exhaustion from continuous jet lag. Follow the same protocol as above.

Can't Sleep? Try Tai Chi

Michael Irwin, MD, professor of psychiatry, University of California, Los Angeles.

Practicing the slow-moving Asian martial art on a weekly basis for three months was just as effective at improving sleep quality and total sleep time as cognitive behavioral therapy (a form of talk therapy), the treatment of choice, a new study of 90 breast cancer survivors with insomnia has found. Other research has shown that cognitive behavioral therapy is as effective in the long term as medication.

Theory: Tai chi relaxes the body, slows breathing and reduces inflammation. It's also a form of meditation, so it eases anxiety. Practicing tai chi can help anyone with trouble sleeping, not just cancer survivors.

CHAPTER 16

Optimum Aging

The End of "Old Age"—Change Your View to Live Longer

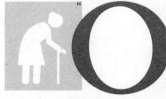

"**O**ld age" has long gotten a bad rap. The conventional thinking has been that it's a time for rocking chairs, fading memory, illness and decrepitude.

Now: As an increasing number of Americans are living—and thriving—into their 80s and beyond, it's more important than ever to cast aside those outdated and harmful attitudes.

What the new thinking can mean for you: Older adults who see aging as a positive stage of life have fewer cardiovascular problems and actually outlive those with gloomier self-perceptions by more than seven years, according to landmark research conducted at Yale University.

So what are you waiting for? There are simple steps you can take to make sure that you aren't missing out on the richness of aging—and this uniquely positive life stage.

THE GIFTS OF AGE

As a geriatric psychiatrist, I have worked with hundreds of older adults who have developed life skills and perspectives that, in many ways, enable them to live more successfully than younger adults.

Of course, we can't kid ourselves. Old age does bring some challenges. We become more susceptible to disease. Our brains and bodies slow down. Daily life gets harder in many ways. The flip side is that some of the traits that come with age make us more adept at dealing with adversity and finding purpose in our lives.

Don't believe the myth that older adults get stuck in the past and can't handle new challenges. For example, research has shown that

Marc E. Agronin, MD, vice president, behavioral health and clinical research, Miami Jewish Health Systems, and an adult and geriatric psychiatrist and affiliate associate professor of psychiatry and neurology at University of Miami Miller School of Medicine. He writes about senior health for *The Wall Street Journal* and is author of *The End of Old Age.* MarcAgronin.com many older adults excel at divergent thinking, the ability to generate different solutions to particular problems. A lifetime of experiences helps them sort through complexities and explore novel ideas.

Other significant benefits that come with growing older—and what you can do to cultivate them in your own life…

•**A reserve of wisdom.** You can be smart and capable at any age, but wisdom is something different. It's an amalgam of all the knowledge, skill and attitudes that you've gained over time.

Wisdom is a trait that we often attribute to the world's great thinkers, but it also has a smaller, day-to-day scope.

Example: Mary, a woman in her 90s, had no earth-shattering life experiences. She wasn't known by anyone outside her small circle of family and friends. But within that circle, she had tremendous influence.

She had two Sunday rituals that gave her a sense of purpose—Catholic Mass in the morning and a family dinner in the afternoon. Her son-in-law would take her to church. After that, she would spend hours with her daughter and other family members preparing a multicourse Italian meal. She was the glue that held the family together—the one who shared recipes…passed along family stories…and overflowed with love. These are powerful forms of wisdom.

My advice: People sometimes ask, "How do I achieve wisdom?" The answer: You already have it. Think of wisdom as your life's résumé. It might consist of knowledge from previous careers…military experience…being a good listener…a tolerance for different ideas, etc.

•**Resilience.** Hurricane Katrina, which devastated the Gulf Coast, was one of the deadliest hurricanes in history. Older adults were among the most vulnerable and suffered disproportionately. Thousands lost their homes, support networks and even their lives.

Yet subsequent research found that many of them coped just as well with the chaos as younger adults—and, in many cases, even better. Decades of experience increased their stores of resilience, the ability to manage life's obstacles without feeling helpless.

Examples: They didn't sweat the storm-related loss of cell-phone service or the Internet because they tended to view these things as luxuries, not necessities. Shortages of food and water? People who have lived through tough times know how to be resourceful when things are scarce. They could see beyond the chaos and find glimmers of acceptance and hope.

Resilience has physical benefits, as well. Not getting overwrought about difficulties allows the body to quickly recover from stress-related changes—muscle tension, increased heart rate, elevated stress hormones, etc.

Remarkable finding: A study of hundreds of older victims after the storm found that they often had the emotional and psychological strength to deal with the widespread loss of electricity and other basic services. In a way, it's not surprising—these were the same people who went through the Great Depression and World War II. Unlike younger victims, they already knew how to be resourceful in these types of situations.

My advice: Even resilient adults will eventually hit what I call an "age point," in which their resources and coping skills are temporarily overwhelmed. It's important to get help—from a therapist and/or friends and family members—when you suffer such a potentially serious setback. The ultimate resolution can bring growth and greater resilience.

For example, one of my elderly patients had a blood test that indicated abnormal liver enzymes. She was convinced that she had a terminal disease and would be unable to care for her husband who had Alzheimer's disease. Her emotional state started to rapidly deteriorate.

Along with therapy, I treated her with a short-acting tranquilizer, which allowed her to get out of bed, leave the house and function more normally overall. She eventually recovered and was able to go off the medication—and, in some ways, grew stronger.

After further tests showed that she was fine, she recognized that she'd had a turning point that clarified what she wanted from life. She felt that she had been given a second chance to do what really mattered—to care for her husband, be a guide for her son, be active in the community and form a close network of friends.

•**Reinvention.** Older adults can do some of their best work late in life. After a serious illness, the French painter Henri Matisse turned his attention, in his 70s and 80s, to the paper cutouts that appeared in the influential book *Jazz* and eventually revolutionized the world of art. He brought a lifetime of experience to the new medium, along with a sense of freedom that's often missing in the young.

Gene Cohen, MD, a well-known psychiatrist, describes an encore phase that starts in the late 70s and continues until the end of life. People often take up new activities during this phase. It can be artistic endeavors…more reading…landscape design…or even real estate investing!

Important: You can reinvent yourself even if you're dealing with physical/cognitive issues. In fact, these issues mean that you should reinvent. You can shape your interests to circumvent otherwise detrimental changes.

My advice: Start small. Manage your expectations to match your current reality.

For example, one of my clients, a retired professor, suffered from memory loss that made it difficult to keep up with the high-powered, distinguished people she had always spent a lot of time with. She was deeply depressed.

We decided that she should find new intellectual opportunities that didn't require her to be on stage or to "compete." She started taking art and adult-education classes. Family members helped her get used to a computer and an iPad. She was able to pursue her intellectual interests in new (and more comfortable) ways. The opportunities are endless!

These Habits Make You Look Older

In a study of more than 11,500 adults living in Copenhagen, smoking and/or heavy drinking were strongly linked to four visible signs of aging, including earlobe creases, eye discoloration, yellow eyelid plaques and hair loss.

Journal of Epidemiology & Community Health.

The Older You Are, the Happier You Can Be

David Mischoulon, MD, PhD, a psychiatrist and director of the Depression Clinical and Research Program at Massachusetts General Hospital and an associate professor of psychiatry at Harvard Medical School, both in Boston.

The image of a "grumpy old man" (or "grumpy old woman") is pervasive in movies, TV shows and other media. Perhaps it's because we assume that as we grow older, our lives will be filled with aches and pains, sickness and depression. But it turns out that this age-old stereotype isn't usually true.

Game-changing finding: In a 2016 study published in *Journal of Clinical Psychiatry*, researchers found that happiness increases with age. While those in their 50s, 60s and beyond reported more cognitive impairment and physical ailments, they were happier, more satisfied, less depressed and anxious and experienced lower levels of perceived stress than younger adults.

How could this be? While the study did not determine exactly why older people tend to be happier, greater experience and wisdom most likely contribute to one's superior mental health in later life. Plus, as we transition from building careers and raising families to having more personal time, we're under less daily pressure and have more time to engage in meaningful activities that make us happy.

Our brains help out as well. The amygdala, an almond-shaped section of the brain that controls our emotional responses to stress, has been shown in brain scans to be less active in older people than in younger individuals when both are presented with upsetting images. This could be another reason why seniors deal with negative events more calmly and positively.

COULD YOU BE HAPPIER?

It's worth noting that some people who have experienced tragedy and misfortunes may have less capacity for happiness than others. But for almost everyone, there are ways to improve the way you feel about yourself and your life—no matter what your age or circumstances.

Strategies to boost your mood, happiness and satisfaction with life…

Happiness booster #1: Foster the right kind of connections. More than fame, career success, money, IQ or genes, close connections are what promote happiness throughout life, according to a 75-year study from Harvard. In fact, study participants with the most satisfying relationships at age 50 were found to be the healthiest at age 80.

What to do: Make it a priority to spend time with friends, family and colleagues whose company you enjoy. And don't assume that just because you're married and/or have children you're automatically covered when it comes to close connections. You need to regularly assess whether your relationships are having a positive impact on your psychological well-being. If not, do something about it.

Also: If you are married or in some other type of romantic relationship, you need to make time for each other to fan the flames of love. Travel, have sex and/or take up a new hobby together. Remember birthdays and anniversaries. Don't take each other for granted!

Happiness booster #2: Fake it 'til you make it. Whether you feel like it or not, putting on a happy face can actually lift your spirits.

Evidence: In a 2012 study, researchers at University of Kansas found that those who smiled while performing stressful tasks had lower heart rates and self-reported lower stress levels afterward.

What to do: When you are in social situations, practice smiling…even when you don't feel like it. Flexing the facial muscles that form a smile tells the brain you are happy. And conveying a positive demeanor attracts others to you, which boosts your mood.

Happiness booster #3: Show up on a regular basis. This could be at your job…or if you are retired, some other activity or hobby that you enjoy and do regularly. The sense of accomplishment from a job well done improves mood and life satisfaction.

What to do: If you have a fulfilling job, activity or hobby, stick with it. If you are in a job that causes you anxiety—or creates a toxic environment—it may be too difficult to derive pleasure from it no matter how positive you try to be. If so, request a transfer to a different department, look for a new job or change your expectations so that you are less affected by the negativity.

If you are retired, cultivate an existing interest by joining a club or starting a hobby. For example, if you enjoy bird-watching, join a bird-watching group that meets regularly for outings.

Happiness booster #4: Be grateful. It may sound trite, but it's true—people who are grateful for what they have lead healthier and more contented lives.

What to do: Even if this strikes you as a little hokey, make a list of what you are grateful for. Doing this makes you appreciate what you have, instead of worrying about what you don't have. Then take a few minutes each day to review/update the list at the same time every day. Do it first thing in the morning…on your commute to work…while brushing your teeth…or before you turn out your light at night. After a few weeks, ask yourself if you're feeling any happier. Chances are, the answer will be yes!

HOW HAPPY ARE YOU?

No measures of happiness apply to everyone, but some basic questions can give you an idea. Using the 1-to-7 rating scale that follows, indicate how much you agree with each of the five statements below. Total the numbers for your results.

1. In most ways, my life is close to my ideal ____
2. The conditions of my life are excellent ____
3. I am satisfied with my life ____
4. So far, I have gotten the important things I want in life ____
5. If I could live my life over, I would change almost nothing ____

Rating scale:
7: Strongly agree
6: Agree
5: Slightly agree
4: Neither agree nor disagree
3: Slightly disagree
2: Disagree
1: Strongly disagree

The higher your score, the greater your life satisfaction...

31-35	=	Extremely satisfied
26-30	=	Satisfied
21-25	=	Slightly satisfied
20	=	Neutral
15-19	=	Slightly dissatisfied
10-14	=	Dissatisfied
5-9	=	Extremely dissatisfied

Credit: The Satisfaction with Life Scale was created by Ed Diener, Robert A. Emmons, Randy J. Larsen and Sharon Griffin.

Muscle Weakness Is Not Inevitable: How to Fight Sarcopenia

John E. Morley, MD, director of the division of geriatric medicine and the Dammert Professor of Gerontology at Saint Louis University School of Medicine. He is coeditor of the textbook *Sarcopenia* and editor of the professional publication *Journal of the American Medical Directors Association.*

If you're age 50 or older, you've probably noticed that your suitcases and grocery bags have gotten mysteriously heavier. It's hard to admit it, but your muscle power is not what it used to be.

Unfortunately, far too many people assume that this age-related condition known as sarcopenia, which literally means "loss of muscle or flesh," is an inevitable part of aging. But that's simply not true. New and better ways to prevent and diagnose this condition now are available—and there's more reason than ever to not ignore it.

The dangers of sarcopenia are more serious than experts once thought—and may involve other crucial elements of your health such as your risk for diabetes, dementia and other chronic conditions.

MORE THAN MUSCLE LOSS

With advancing age, our muscles shrink because the body loses some of its ability to convert protein into muscle tissue. By age 50, the average adult loses about 1% to 2% of muscle mass every year.

That's bad enough, but the real problem is what results from this muscle loss. Over time, it becomes more difficult to stand up from a chair...climb a flight of stairs...or even open a jar. People with sarcopenia are far more likely than stronger adults to suffer falls and/or bone fractures. They're also more likely to be hospitalized or admitted to a nursing home—and even die during a given period of time.

An increasing body of evidence shows that people with weak muscle strength have a higher risk of developing type 2 diabetes—a disease that can also double your risk for heart attack and stroke.

Recently discovered danger: People with sarcopenia are at increased risk for cognitive decline, including brain atrophy and dementia, according to research published in *Clinical Interventions in Aging*. In this study, people with sarcopenia were six times more likely to suffer from physical/cognitive impairments than those without this condition.

What this means to you: Collectively, the risks associated with sarcopenia are so great that clinicians from a variety of disciplines assess signs such as weight loss (from shrinking muscles)...fatigue...and a loss of strength to determine which patients are at highest risk for frailty and to work toward intervention.

THE 4-STEP PLAN

As scientists learn more about sarcopenia, the better your odds are of fighting it—if you take the appropriate steps. *What works best if you have sarcopenia...*

STEP 1: Load up on protein. Everyone needs protein to increase muscle size/strength. People with sarcopenia need a lot of protein. The recommended daily allowance (RDA) for protein is 0.8 g per kilogram of body weight. (That's about 54 g for a 150-pound woman.) If you've been diagnosed with sarcopenia, you need much more (about 1.2 g per kilogram of body weight).

My advice: Whenever possible, get most or all of your protein from natural foods rather than from protein-fortified foods—the nutrients in natural foods work synergistically to provide greater benefits than supplements. (For example, a small, 3.5-ounce serving of lean pork has about 26 g of protein…one-half cup of pinto beans, 7 g…and a large egg, about 6 g.)

Note: If you have kidney disease, you may have been told to limit your protein intake. Ask your nephrologist for advice on optimal protein levels for you.

Helpful: If you find it difficult to get enough protein from food alone, try whey protein supplements. You can buy these milk-based supplements in powder and liquid forms. Products such as Ensure typically provide 12 g to 20 g of protein per serving, while some protein powders deliver up to 60 g in two scoops mixed in a smoothie, for example. An advantage of whey protein supplements is that they contain leucine, an amino acid involved in muscle synthesis. If you can't have dairy, ask your doctor about taking an essential amino acid supplement enriched with leucine.

STEP 2: Get enough vitamin D. You need vitamin D for both muscle and bone strength. Depending upon the time of year and where you live, you can get all you need from 10 or so minutes of daily unprotected sun exposure. But many older adults don't spend that much time in the sun…and those who do are probably covering up or using sunscreen to protect against skin cancer.

My advice: Consume at least 1,000 international units (IU) of vitamin D daily. You can get some of this from D-fortified cereal, milk or juice. If you don't eat a lot of these foods, you may find it easier to take a 1,000-IU vitamin D supplement.

STEP 3: Eat fish. There's good evidence that two-to-four weekly meals of fatty fish (such as salmon, mackerel or sardines) will improve blood flow to all of the body's muscles, including the heart. In theory, this should help people with sarcopenia maintain or gain muscle mass, but the evidence that it helps isn't conclusive. Even so, I still recommend fish because it's a good protein source and has many other health benefits.

STEP 4: Exercise the right way. Exercise is the only way to build muscle, even if you consume plenty of protein. Aerobic exercise (such as brisk walking) is good—everyone should get some because it improves both muscle and cardiovascular health. But strength training is the real ticket for building muscle. As an added bonus, it also appears to promote brain health.

Important recent finding: When Australian researchers had 100 people age 55 or older with mild cognitive impairment (a condition that often precedes Alzheimer's) do weight-lifting exercises twice a week for six months, the stronger the study participants' muscles got, the greater their cognitive improvement, according to a study published in 2016 in *Journal of the American Geriatrics Society*.

Even if you are not able to use weight-lifting machines at a gym, there are plenty of ways to do strength training. The American College of Sports Medicine recommends lifting weights (hand weights are fine) or using elastic resistance bands two to three days a week. Unfortunately, that's too ambitious for many people.

My advice: Just do some exercise, whether it's 10 minutes every day or an hour once a week. If you feel too weak to start with "real" exercise, you can keep things simple. Example: A chair-stand exercise, in which you sit in an armless chair…extend your arms in front of you…slowly stand up…then slowly lower yourself back down. Do this five to 10 times, twice daily.

For arm strength: Hold the ends of a large elastic resistance band in each hand, and stand with both feet on the middle of the band. Keeping your body straight and your elbows by your side, slowly curl your hands up toward your shoulders. You can raise both hands together or one at a time. Try to repeat the movement eight to 12 times, twice daily.

For leg strength: Sit on a chair. Keeping your back straight, slowly extend your right leg straight out in front of you and hold for several seconds before lowering it slowly back down. Repeat with the left leg. Do 10 repetitions on each leg. When this becomes easy, strap on an ankle weight that's heavy enough so that you cannot do more than 15 repetitions per leg.

If you tend to get bored with exercise…

Research shows that people who work with an exercise coach or personal trainer—at home or at a health club—are more likely to stick with regular exercise. In a program that my colleagues and I supervise, patients with sarcopenia first attend physical therapy to help restore flexibility, balance and endurance, then attend weekly sessions led by exercise coaches who are enthusiastic and keep people motivated.

My advice: Consider using an exercise coach. It may be one of the best things you do for your overall health! To find an exercise coach near you, consult the American Council on Exercise, ACEfitness.org.

Your Bones Are in Danger

Neil Binkley, MD, professor in the divisions of geriatrics and endocrinology at University of Wisconsin (UW) School of Medicine and Public Health, Madison. He is director of the UW Osteoporosis Clinical Research Program and associate director of the UW Institute on Aging. Aging.wisc.edu

---

We've been told that the best way to prevent fractures is to prevent or treat osteoporosis—diet, exercise and, if needed, medications. But that approach has not been successful.

For people with osteoporosis, medications do prevent many spinal fractures—but fewer than half of hip and other fractures, according to a major study published in *The New England Journal of Medicine.* And many people who fall and break bones don't even have osteoporosis.

Example: An overweight or obese person may have good bone density (from carrying that extra weight) but still get fractures. Unless he/she has the muscle strength to carry that extra weight, mobility issues—such as difficulty getting up off the toilet or climbing stairs—can lead to falls that cause fractures. Rather than hip fractures due to weakened bones, they tend to get ankle or lower-leg fractures.

In the end, it's preventing fractures—from any cause—that really matters. Many of us think that if we break a bone, our friendly orthopedic surgeon will put it back together and life will go on as usual. But after age 50—and especially after age 65—a fractured bone can threaten independence and quality of life. And that's what we fear most about aging—losing independence…not being able to drive…and winding up in a nursing home. The classic example is a hip fracture, which often sends people to nursing homes and is linked to a shorter life span. But breaking an ankle, an arm or even a wrist can make daily life harder at home…and make it tougher to be mobile.

To find out what is really needed to prevent fractures, we spoke with geriatrician and endocrinologist Neil Binkley, MD. He started with a simple question—"What causes most fractures in older people?"

The answer: Falling.

Here's how to prevent falls—and the fractures that could end your independence…

•**Eat for muscle strength, not just bones.** Getting enough calcium and vitamin D—standard elements of osteoporosis prevention—still is important. But pay close attention to calories and protein, too. These are essential to maintaining muscle strength—and that's as important as strong bones in preventing fractures. After all, when our muscle strength declines, we fall. And when we fall on weak bones, guess what? They break.

Protein needs are based on your body weight. To calculate your individual needs, multiply your body weight by 0.45. For a 150-pound woman, that's 67 grams a day…for a 185-pound man, 83 grams. To get a sense of what that looks like, a three-ounce serving of tuna or salmon contains about 22 grams of protein and an egg contains six grams, on average. Aim to include good sources of protein—seafood, lean meat, poultry, eggs, nuts, seeds, soy and legumes such as beans and peas—at every meal.

For some older people, a waning appetite also can mean that they just don't eat enough calories. If you're not eating enough, a registered dietitian can help find practical ways to help you get enough protein and calories each day.

•**Get strong—and balanced.** Now that you're nourishing muscles, make them work. Exercise helps keep your bones and muscles strong, so it's vital for lowering your fracture risk. The best exercise is the one that you'll actually do, whether it's walking, biking, swimming or team sports. Beyond general fitness, exercises that improve core strength and balance are key to fall prevention. Suggestions…

•**Join a tai chi class.** This ancient Chinese set of gentle, slow-moving exercises strengthens lower limbs and improves balance. Several studies have found that practicing tai chi regularly significantly reduces fall risk in older adults.

Yoga may help, too. It can strengthen bones, and while it is less well-studied for fall prevention, it has been shown to improve balance and mobility in older people.

•**Take fall-prevention classes.** One popular, evidence-based program is Stepping On, a seven-week, two-hours-per-week workshop, first developed in Australia, that now is offered in 20 US states. It is geared to healthy adults over age 65. One study, published in *Journal of the American Geriatrics Society*, reported that people who participated in Stepping On had 31% fewer falls over the next 14 months, compared with a similar group of people who didn't go through the program. To find programs like this in your area, check with the National Council on Aging's Fall Prevention website (NCOA. org/healthy-aging/falls-prevention).

•**Consider physical therapy.** If you've fallen and have been injured—even if you didn't break a bone—you're waving a red flag that a fracture could be in your future. A physical therapist can do a formal strength-and-balance assessment…show you exercises to strengthen muscles, bones, walking posture and balance… and help you find classes in your community.

•**Make your home safer.** *A key part of fall prevention is taking a look at what you can do to make it less likely that you'll trip and fall…*

•Do you have night-lights in your home? Consider putting a night-light in your bathroom for those middle-of-the-night trips.

•Are there throw rugs that you might slip on? Get rid of them!

•Is there clutter on the floor or stairs that you could stumble on? Declutter!

•Do you need to get on a chair or step stool to reach things on high shelves? Put everyday items on lower shelves that are easy to reach.

•Is it hard to get in and out of your bathtub without slipping? Consider installing grab bars or replacing your tub with a walk-in shower.

Some of your safety changes may need to be in your own behavior—such as drinking less alcohol. That's a fall risk that many older people don't consider.

And don't forget to get your vision checked regularly. If you can't see it, you can trip on it.

•**Review your medications.** Some medications (prescription or over-the-counter) or medication interactions can cause dizziness, light-headedness or low blood pressure, which can increase the risk of falling. Key medications to be aware of include antihistamines, sleep aids, pain pills, antidepressants and antianxiety medications. In addition, some medications, such as glucocorticoids (steroids taken for inflammatory and autoimmune conditions) contribute to bone loss. If you are taking medications that increase your fall risk, talk to your doctor to see if you can reduce the dose, find an alternative—or modify how you take it, such as only at bedtime.

It's not that strong bones aren't important —they're a key part of a fracture-prevention plan…but only one part. If your doctor has prescribed a diet, exercise program or medication for you to prevent or treat osteoporosis, continue following those instructions. Osteoporosis medications often are prescribed based on an individual's estimated risk for fracture. For individuals at high fracture risk, the benefits of reducing that risk far outweigh the risk of side effects. But just taking medications is not enough.

Now you know what else you need to do to protect yourself.

THIS EXERCISE PREVENTS FALLS

One of the simplest and most effective exercises—and one that you can do almost anywhere—is the Chair Rise. *Do this daily to strengthen the muscles in your thighs and buttocks, which can help keep you steady on your feet and prevent falls…*

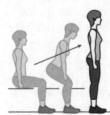

•**Sit toward the front of a sturdy chair,** with your knees bent and feet flat on the floor, shoulder-width apart.

•**Rest your hands lightly on the seat on either**

side of you, keeping your back and neck straight and chest slightly forward.

•**Breathe in slowly.** Lean forward and exhale as you stand up—feel your weight on the front of your feet.

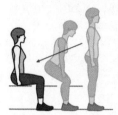

•**Pause for a full breath in and out.**

•**Breathe in as you slowly sit down.** Try not to collapse down into the chair. Rather, control your lowering as much as possible.

•**Breathe out.**

Repeat for a total of 10 to 15 stand/sits. Rest and breathe for a minute, then do another set of 10 to 15. You may need to work up to this level over several days or a few weeks. The goal is to get to the point where you can complete two sets without using your hands at all.

You Could Have a Spinal Fracture and Not Know It

Vinil Shah, MD, assistant professor of clinical radiology and associate program director of the neuroradiology fellowship program at University of California, San Francisco. Dr. Shah's areas of academic interest include assessing clinical outcomes of spine intervention.

Did you know that you can get a spinal fracture from simply stepping off a curb, sneezing, lifting a small pet or even just getting out of bed?

Fractures due to osteoporosis are much more common than many people realize. In fact, after age 50, one in two women and one in five men will have an osteoporosis-related fracture in their lifetimes.

The most common type of fracture linked to osteoporosis is a vertebral compression fracture (VCF)—a break in a vertebra of the spine. VCFs are more common than hip or wrist fractures… often are painful…and can lead to loss of height and a stooped back. So why do a shocking two-thirds of VCFs go undiagnosed and untreated?

Osteoporosis can weaken the bones so much that even routine activities or seemingly innocuous movements can cause a spinal fracture.

Sudden, nonradiating pain ranging from mild to severe is typically the first sign. But the pain is often mistaken for arthritis or a pinched nerve. And because many people with osteoporosis don't even know they have it, VCFs simply aren't on their radar.

QUICK ACTION IS VITAL

An undiagnosed VCF will often heal on its own, with the pain diminishing in six to eight weeks. But you don't want this fracture to go undiagnosed! One VCF increases the risk for a subsequent VCF fivefold. And multiple fractures result in a loss of height and stooped posture. With each additional untreated VCF, the spine can get a few millimeters shorter. If the vertebrae in the upper back fracture and become wedge-shaped, the spine curves abnormally causing kyphosis, a rounding of the back better known as a dowager's hump.

If you're a woman or man over age 50 or a postmenopausal woman under age 50 who is experiencing new, unexplained mild-to-severe midline back pain that doesn't go away in a day or two, you need to see a doctor. Your primary care physician will perform a physical exam to check for back tenderness and will likely order an X-ray to confirm the diagnosis, following up with a CT scan or MRI to evaluate the problem further. Your doctor will then advise you on the best treatment for your specific situation.

TREATING THE FRACTURE

If the pain and loss of function from a VCF are mild, conservative treatments are usually recommended…

•**A few days of bed rest.** VCF pain tends to worsen when sitting or standing and improves when lying down.

•**Pain relievers.** Over-the-counter pain relievers, such as *ibuprofen* (Advil) or *acetaminophen* (Tylenol), help reduce mild pain.

•**A hyperextension back brace.** Wearing a rigid hyperextension back brace for a few weeks can help relieve pain and improve function in some patients. Ask your doctor for guidance.

•**Physical therapy (PT).** PT helps strengthen back muscles and can improve posture and prevent the development of chronic pain. It also has a beneficial effect on bone mineral density in osteoporosis patients and may prevent future fractures. Note: PT can be started once the patient's pain is under control.

Conservative treatment of a VCF is not recommended for more than a few weeks or for those with more severe pain or limited function. Prolonged bed rest may lead to loss of bone mass (up to 1% loss each week) and muscle strength (10% to 15% loss each week). Bed rest can also increase risk for blood clots and bed sores, and painkillers should only be used short term.

OTHER TREATMENTS

Patients whose pain doesn't resolve in two to three weeks with the treatments above may be candidates for a minimally invasive procedure called vertebroplasty. Guided by computed tomography and/or fluoroscopy (a continuous X-ray "movie"), the doctor injects bone cement into the fracture. The outpatient procedure takes about 45 minutes while the patient is typically conscious but sedated. The cement not only stabilizes the fractured vertebra, it also prevents nearby nerve endings from causing pain.

Studies show that 75% to 100% of patients enjoy good-to-moderate pain relief and increased mobility quickly after vertebroplasty, often the next day. The procedure usually doesn't restore much height loss, but it can prevent further height loss and additional fractures.

With kyphoplasty, a modification of vertebroplasty, a balloon is inflated in the fractured vertebra to create a cavity that is then filled with cement. This procedure may offer a better chance of restoring height loss. However, kyphoplasty is more expensive than vertebroplasty, and there is mixed data on its benefit over vertebroplasty.

In general, vertebroplasty and kyphoplasty are safe when done by an experienced doctor. Interventional radiologists and neuroradiologists often do these procedures. Look for a doctor who has experience in using image guidance for spine procedures. Like all invasive medical procedures, these treatments do have risks—such as infection or bleeding. And in rare cases, the cement can leak into the spinal canal, causing nerve compression, or travel into adjacent veins, which can lead to blood clots in the lungs or heart.

The best candidates for these procedures are patients who have pain of at least moderate intensity (rated a five or greater out of 10) that impacts their mobility and daily quality of life. Additionally, those who have fractures that have occurred recently (within a few months prior to the procedure) tend to have more success with vertebroplasty and kyphoplasty than those who have older fractures. The age of a fracture can be determined by an MRI.

PREVENTING FUTURE FRACTURES

Treating the underlying osteoporosis to help prevent future fractures is crucial. Ask your doctor for a bone mineral density test called a DXA (or DEXA)—this low-dose X-ray measures bone density in the hip and spine and can guide your physician in choosing the best course of action for your case. Options include prescription medications such as bisphosphonates (patients should weigh the risks versus benefits of these drugs with their doctors)...calcium and vitamin D supplementation...and weight-bearing exercise to improve bone strength and other exercises to build core strength. Multiple clinical trials have shown that early treatment of osteoporosis can increase bone mineral density by 5% to 15%, reducing vertebral fracture rates by 40% to 70%.

The Cataract Fix: What Are You Waiting For?

David F. Chang, MD, clinical professor of ophthalmology at University of California, San Francisco, and past president of the American Society of Cataract and Refractive Surgery. He is an international authority on cataract surgery who frequently lectures surgeons about advanced cataract techniques and the newest lens implants. He is coauthor of Cataracts: A Patient's Guide to Treatment.

No one wants to have surgery—any surgery. But once you have had cataract surgery, you'll probably wonder why you waited so long.

Recent developments: Cataract surgery now takes about 20 minutes for most people. You'll go home soon after the procedure...serious, vision-threatening complications, such as infection, are extremely rare…and it's successful in about 99% of cases, making it one of the most effective of all surgeries.

The benefits are undeniable. Within days, you'll see better—with sharper vision, better nighttime eyesight and fewer bright-light "halos." But that's not all.

The procedure, which usually is done on one eye at a time, is performed while you're awake and while your eye is numbed with eye-drop anesthesia, so it's not even painful. Most health insurance plans pick up the tab.

To learn more about the latest advances in cataract surgery, we spoke with David F. Chang, MD, a noted authority on cataract techniques.

IS IT YOUR TIME?

Most people are familiar with the telltale signs of cataracts—the normally clear lens within your eye becomes cloudy and/or discolored. Because the lens focuses incoming visual images and transmits them to the retina, these changes, though generally gradual (occurring over a period of years), can cause significant vision loss if untreated.

Important: The lens sits behind the iris and pupil, so you can't self-diagnose cataracts by looking in a mirror. Only an eye doctor using a special microscope can actually see cataracts.

That's why it's important to see an eye doctor (in addition to having routine eye exams) if you're experiencing vision problems, including blurred vision, difficulty seeing details (such as small print or road signs) and glare or poor night-driving vision.

Age is the main risk factor for cataracts. When you're young, the proteins that form the lenses of your eyes are arranged in a way that makes the structures crystal-clear. Over time, these proteins eventually start to clump together and reduce the amount of light that passes through.

By your 60s and 70s, these changes will have gradually begun to occur. Most people, if they live long enough, will develop cataracts that are advanced enough for them to consider surgery.

Earlier-onset of cataracts has been associated with such risk factors as smoking, diabetes, prior retinal surgery, severe nearsightedness, excessive sun exposure and prolonged use of certain medications such as steroids.

WHAT ARE YOU WAITING FOR?

Cataracts can affect one or both eyes, either simultaneously or at different times. In the past, doctors advised patients to delay surgery until a cataract was "ripe"—meaning that it was so advanced that the benefits justified the lengthy recovery and the potential for complications due to the large incision that was used at that time. Unfortunately, many people are still operating under this misconception.

Newer thinking: You don't need to wait so long. If the cataract is impairing your daily activities, such as reading and/or driving, it makes sense to have cataract surgery sooner rather than later because of the procedure's exceptionally high success rate.

Now the lens is broken up into many small pieces using ultrasonic vibrations within the eye, then suctioned out. The incisions are so small that stitches aren't required—and cataracts can be safely removed at an earlier stage. The replacement artificial lens lasts a lifetime and is folded so that it can pass through the tiny (about one-eighth inch) incision.

The timing is important because cataracts can get so bad that they increase a person's risk for falls and auto/pedestrian accidents, as well as contribute to depression.

These factors may have something to do with the recent research regarding cataract surgery that was published online in the journal *JAMA Ophthalmology*.

Key findings: This study of more than 74,000 women ages 65 and older found that those who had undergone cataract surgery had a 60% lower risk of dying over the 20-year study period than those who did not get treated.

BETTER VISION WITHOUT GLASSES

You'll obviously see better once a cataract is removed. What some people don't realize is that they might see better than they ever did.

The surgeon will remove the cloudy lens and replace it with a clear, artificial lens that comes in more than 50 different powers.

Suppose that you have always worn glasses to see well in the distance. When you have cataract surgery, a replacement lens can be chosen to correct your particular type/degree of optical error. For example, some lenses correct for astigmatism (blurred vision that is caused by incorrect corneal curvature). Certain artificial lenses function like bifocals and reduce how frequently people must rely on reading glasses.

In most cases, cataract surgery won't completely eliminate the need for glasses. Most people will have excellent distance vision without glasses following cataract surgery. However, most will need reading glasses—but can perhaps use them less often and/or get by with a lower-power prescription.

WHAT ELSE CAN YOU DO?

Surgery is the only treatment for cataracts, and it is a permanent solution—the new lens will remain transparent forever. Unfortunately, there is no medication that can halt or reverse cataract formation. What can one do to prevent cataracts?

•**Wear sunglasses outdoors.** The UV radiation in sunlight damages eye proteins and can lead to cloudiness. A large study that reviewed data from more than a half million people found a strong association between cataracts and skin cancer—more evidence that UV exposure is a major risk factor.

What to do: Wear sunglasses with UV protection whenever you plan to spend prolonged periods of time outdoors. Virtually all sunglasses today are UV-protected.

•**Wear a broad-brimmed hat to block UV radiation.** It will reduce your risk for eyelid skin cancer as well as cataracts.

•**Eat a nutritious diet.** Many studies have found an association between a healthy diet and fewer cataracts—but that's not the same as proof.

For example, several studies have suggested that particular nutrients—alone or in combination—can help prevent cataracts. The large Age-Related Eye Disease Study (AREDS) reported that people with cataracts who got the most lutein and zeaxanthin (antioxidants that are found in leafy greens and other fruits/vegetables) were 32% less likely to need cataract surgery.

Other research has looked at the effects of fish oil supplements (or regular meals including fatty fish)…vitamin C…vitamin E…and other nutrients.

It's common sense to eat a nutritious diet. If you want to take one of the AREDS formulations, check with your doctor first if you are a current or former smoker. Certain versions of these supplements (with lutein and zeaxanthin) also contain beta-carotene, which has been linked to increased risk for lung cancer in current and former smokers.

Stop Neglecting Your Eyesight: 4 Eye-Health Secrets Can Save Your Vision

Jeffrey D. Henderer, MD, professor of ophthalmology and the Dr. Edward Hagop Bedrossian Chair of Ophthalmology at the Lewis Katz School of Medicine at Temple University in Philadelphia. Dr. Henderer is the Secretary for Knowledge Base Development for the American Academy of Ophthalmology and has authored numerous articles and textbook chapters on glaucoma and growth.

When it comes to staying on top of our health, far too many people take their eyesight for granted. It's obvious that we should get regular eye exams (see next page), but there are other steps that often slip under the radar. *Here are the strategies that ensure you're doing all you can to protect your vision…*

Eye-health secret #1: **Use the right eyedrops.** Older adults and those of any age who are heavy users of computers and/or electronics know that they're more likely to suffer from dry eye. Lubricating drops, sometimes called artificial tears, are effective for this condition. But when you're in the store, it's easy to mistakenly pick up redness-reducing eyedrops, which temporarily constrict the blood vessels. These drops do not help with dry eye.

In fact, daily use of redness-reducing drops can cause rebound redness and set off an unhealthy cycle of using more eyedrops. For this reason, redness-reducing drops should be used only occasionally—and if the redness persists, see your eye doctor to find out why.

Best for dry eye are lubricating drops such as Refresh, Systane, GenTeal, Bion Tears and even pharmacy brands.

Caution: If the preservatives they contain irritate your eyes, look for preservative-free brands.

Lubricating drops come in three viscosities— liquid, thicker gel-like formulas and ointments. The thicker drops and ointments last longer but can temporarily blur vision.

Eye-health secret #2: **Watch your medication.** Steroids—taken orally, inhaled or in eye-drop form—can cause cataracts and glaucoma. Cataracts can start to develop within months of regular steroid use, while glaucoma is slower and subtler. If you must take a steroid, ask your doctor for the lowest dose possible, schedule an eye exam one to two months after starting any form of the drug, then return every six to 12 months for monitoring. *Other drugs that can affect the eyes…*

•***Tamoxifen,*** used to treat and prevent recurrences of breast cancer, can cause eye irritation and dryness…lead to cataracts (usually after five years of use)…and accumulate in the retina, weakening color vision and central vision. Fortunately, as oncologists have started prescribing lower doses of tamoxifen, these side effects happen less often. Self-defense: Have an annual dilated eye exam with a retina specialist while you are taking tamoxifen and have him/ her examine your retinas to be sure there is no accumulation in the retina.

•***Tamsulosin*** (Flomax), used to treat an enlarged prostate, can make the iris, which is normally fairly rigid, turn floppy. Ordinarily, this shouldn't lead to vision complications, but if the patient undergoes cataract surgery, it can cause a condition called intraoperative floppy iris syndrome (IFIS), possibly complicating the procedure by preventing the pupil from dilating well and causing the iris to herniate out of the incision. Self-defense: If you plan to undergo cataract surgery, let your eye surgeon know if you are taking tamsulosin or have in the past.

•**Erectile dysfunction drugs** such as *sildenafil* (Viagra) and *tadalafil* (Cialis) can, in rare instances, cause irreversible damage called nonarteritic anterior ischemic optic neuropathy (NAION), which is like a stroke of the optic nerve. Incidences are not dose-related and can happen after a single use of the drug. Self-defense: Avoid erectile dysfunction medications if you have hypertension or diabetes (which put you at greater risk for NAION), and/or if you take nitrates to lower blood pressure—erectile dysfunction drugs can lower blood pressure even more.

Eye-health secret #3: **Keep diabetes well-controlled.** People with diabetes tend to develop cataracts at an earlier age than people without diabetes. They also have an elevated risk for visual impairment and blindness due to diabetic retinopathy, when high blood sugar levels damage blood vessels in the retina.

What to do: Get a dilated eye exam annually or more often if recommended by your doctor, particularly if you struggle to keep your sugar under control. Early treatment can prevent an astonishing 95% of diabetes-related vision loss!

Also important: The better you are able to control your blood sugar with diet, lifestyle changes and medication, the better your chances of delaying the onset of cataracts and diabetic retinopathy.

Eye-health secret #4: **Take this eye supplement.** If you're at high risk for advanced age-related macular degeneration (AMD)—that is, you have intermediate AMD or advanced AMD in one eye only—taking high levels of certain antioxidants plus zinc can reduce the risk of developing an advanced form of AMD by about 25%, according to a major National Eye Institute clinical trial called the Age-Related Eye Disease Study (AREDS). A leading cause of blindness among Americans age 50 and older, AMD causes damage to the retina that may lead to central vision loss.

What to do: Look for a supplement labeled "AREDS formula" (such as Bausch & Lomb PreserVision AREDS 2 Formula). It's not an AMD cure, but it may help preserve vision in susceptible individuals. Ask your ophthalmologist if it's right for you.

WHEN WAS YOUR LAST EYE EXAM?

Adults between the ages of 55 and 64 who are risk-free and have no eye symptoms should have eye exams every one to three years, but nearly half of those recently surveyed have not.

People who are over age 65 or of any age with a risk factor, such as high blood pressure, diabetes or a family history of eye disease, should have an eye exam at least every one or two years, according to the American Academy of Ophthalmology.

Because your eyes offer an unobstructed view of your blood vessels, nerves and connecting tissue, any abnormalities that show up in an eye exam may indicate similar changes elsewhere in the body. This means your optometrist or ophthalmologist can give you crucial information about your risk for serious conditions such as stroke, high blood pressure, diabetes and autoimmune disease, such as Graves' disease, a thyroid disorder. Insurance should cover these exams.

How to Protect Your Eyesight

Mrinali Patel Gupta, MD, a retina specialist and assistant professor of ophthalmology at Welll Cornell Medicine in New York City. Her research has been published in many professional journals, and she was a recipient of the Howard Hughes Medical Institute-National Institutes of Health Research Fellowship for her work on AMD at the National Eye Institute.

How would you feel if you lost your eyesight? When asked this question, nearly half of Americans recently surveyed by researchers at Johns Hopkins University said that it would be the worst possible thing that could happen to their health. Ironically, half of the respondents in the same survey were completely unaware of age-related macular degeneration (AMD), a leading cause of blindness in the US.

THE BASICS OF AMD

The word "age" in AMD doesn't mean that the condition affects only the elderly. Rather, it means that the incidence of AMD rises with age. The exact causes of AMD are unknown, but some risk factors are well established—such as age, gender (women get it more often than

Teatime for Eye Health

In a survey of 1,678 people, those who drank hot tea at least once daily were 74% less likely to develop glaucoma—a potentially blinding condition due to a buildup of pressure in the eyeball—than those who drank no hot tea.

Theory: Black and green teas contain polyphenols, antioxidants with anti-inflammatory properties that help fight glaucoma.

Anne L. Coleman, MD, PhD, professor of ophthalmology, David Geffen School of Medicine, UCLA, California.

men) and race (whites face a higher risk than other races). Other risk factors: Having blue eyes...obesity...and high blood pressure. A healthy lifestyle that includes not smoking and a nutritious diet are the best ways to help reduce the risk for AMD.

DRY AND WET AMD

AMD affects and damages the macula of the retina—the region of the retina responsible for central vision (seeing what's right in front of us) and fine acuity vision (seeing fine details).

There are two forms of AMD—dry and wet. The dry form accounts for 90% of people with AMD. In the early stages, dry AMD may cause no visual symptoms, which is why routine eye exams are important for diagnosis. As dry AMD progresses, patients may start to notice subtle changes or distortions in central vision such as straight lines that appear wavy or written words that seem to be missing letters. In the late stages of dry AMD, patients may have severe vision loss. In general, however, the progression of dry AMD is slow and occurs over many years, and some patients may never have vision loss.

Wet AMD is characterized by abnormal blood vessels that grow under and into the retina. The blood vessels can leak blood and fluid that reduce vision and damage the retina. Wet AMD causes the majority of cases of AMD-related blindness and can progress rapidly.

The dry form of AMD can progress to the wet form—risk of conversion from dry to wet AMD is approximately 14% to 20% over five years. There may be no symptoms early in the conversion of dry to wet AMD. Subsequently, patients may notice subtle vision changes such as those described above. Severe vision loss, such as dramatic reduction in overall vision or a large dark area in central vision, can develop, especially if wet AMD goes untreated.

DIAGNOSIS OF AMD

Because most people with dry AMD may have no symptoms, regular eye exams are important to identify the early signs of the disease. AMD can be diagnosed during a routine dilated eye exam done by an ophthalmologist or optometrist. The American Academy of Ophthalmology advises a baseline eye exam at age 40 (earlier if you have eye disease or are at risk for developing eye disease) and an exam every year or two at age 65 and older. However, your doctor may advise more frequent exams based on your specific situation.

If you experience any slowly progressive (over weeks or months) vision changes, get promptly evaluated by an ophthalmologist. And if you have severe and sudden vision loss, see an eye doctor immediately, preferably on the same day, for an evaluation to determine if you need emergency treatment.

TREATMENT FOR DRY AMD

If you have dry AMD, there are currently no medical treatments, but it can be effectively managed to prevent progression. *What to do…*

•**Maintain a healthy lifestyle**—don't smoke and eat a nutritious diet.

•**Get an eye exam once or twice yearly,** including an optical coherence tomography scan to check for progression from dry to wet AMD. This noninvasive imaging test allows doctors to examine the retina to detect the abnormal blood vessels of wet AMD at very early stages. Your doctor may repeat the test at every visit. The test is also used to monitor wet AMD.

•**Self-monitor.** Use the Amsler grid—with horizontal and vertical lines—at least a few times a week to check for subtle vision changes in each eye. If there's any change in the grid when looking at it, such as straight lines that appear crooked/wavy or parts of the grid are missing, you should contact your eye doctor. A downloadable Amsler grid is available at Amsler Grid.org, and grids are also available as a smartphone app.

Also: For some patients, getting the right nutrients may prevent dry AMD from worsening. An eye doctor can tell you if your situation warrants vitamins for your eyes.

What the research shows: A large clinical trial led by the National Institutes of Health found that patients with intermediate or advanced AMD in only one eye who took an antioxidant mix—500 mg of vitamin C…400 international units (IU) of vitamin E…15 mg of beta-carotene…80 mg of zinc…and 2 mg of copper (known as the AREDS formula)—were less likely to have progression of AMD.

Note: Current or former smokers should use the newer AREDS2 formula, which has lutein and zeaxanthin instead of beta-carotene—beta-carotene is associated with increased risk for lung cancer in smokers.

These mixes are available over-the-counter in pharmacies.

BREAKTHROUGH INJECTIONS

Previously, the average patient with wet AMD quickly lost significant vision (two to three lines on the vision chart in the first two years alone). But with the advent of anti-vascular endothelial growth factor (VEGF) therapy, vision can be stabilized or improved in roughly half of patients.

Multiple large clinical trials have demonstrated that intravitreal injection (into the eye) of medications that block VEGF, such as *bevacizumab* (Avastin) and *aflibercept* (Eylea), dramatically reduce vision loss in wet AMD.

The procedure is done with local anesthesia in the ophthalmologist's office. It's quick and usually painless. The injections are often given monthly…or on a less frequent basis, depending on how the patient is doing. Some people need long-term therapy, while others can over time reduce or discontinue it but are monitored closely as many patients subsequently need additional treatments (when the wet AMD becomes active again). The treatment controls wet AMD but is not a cure. The risk associated with injections is very low but includes cataracts, retinal detachment, bleeding or infection/inflammation in the eye.

Hearing Aids Help More Than Hearing

Larry Humes, PhD, distinguished professor in the department of speech and hearing sciences at Indiana University, Bloomington. Dr. Humes served on the editorial board for several audiology journals, and his research has been published in more than 200 scholarly publications.

Hearing aids are smaller, sleeker and cheaper (see below) than ever before, yet about 80% of people with hearing problems don't get them—and all too often because of vanity.

Allowing hearing loss to go untreated is a mistake. The parts of the brain associated with hearing need stimulation to stay active. People who wait too long before getting a hearing device can permanently lose some of their capacity to hear.

And there's more than your hearing that's at risk. The ears are involved in balance, so people who don't hear well are more likely to fall. Hearing loss also has been linked to depression and social isolation. One study found that moderate hearing loss can triple the risk for dementia.

Of course, vanity isn't the only barrier. A pair of hearing aids costs, on average, more than $4,000. Insurance usually doesn't cover the cost, but it's worth checking.

Good news: Congress recently approved a bill that would allow hearing aids to be sold over the counter, which will increase competition and reduce costs. Another option: Personal sound- amplifying products, sold online and in retail stores. They're not "official" hearing aids, but they are far less expensive—and, for some people, just as effective.

Life is better when you can hear!

A New Twist on Hearing Aids

Larry Humes, PhD, a leading expert on speech and hearing.

Imagine if getting a hearing aid were as simple as picking out a pair of reading glasses at the drugstore. Sounds like music to your ears, right? This scenario may not be such a pipe dream.

Latest development: The FDA is being urged to create a new category of "over-the-counter (OTC) hearing devices" for adults with mild-to-moderate hearing loss. This recommendation comes from a recent report released by a committee convened by the National Academies of Sciences, Engineering, and Medicine, an independent, nonpartisan body of experts who advise the federal government on matters related to science, technology and health policy.

THE APPEAL OF OTC

Statistics show that 86% of people who would benefit from hearing aids do not get them. The main deterrent is cost. Since the average retail price for a pair of hearing aids is almost $5,000, hearing aids are a big purchase for most people—especially since they are not covered by Medicare or most private insurers. (Hearing aids may be eligible for reimbursement from health savings accounts or flexible spending accounts.)

OTC hearing devices, on the other hand, are expected to be much more affordable than traditional hearing aids. They will likely come in a range of prices but will probably be closer to several hundred dollars per pair...not several thousand. There will also be easier access to the OTC devices (in drugstores and online, for example).

And OTC hearing devices are likely to be just as unobtrusive as the latest high-end traditional devices.

An important distinction: OTC hearing devices are not to be confused with personal sound amplification products (PSAPs), also OTC products, which are approved by the FDA for people with normal hearing who may need sound amplification in certain situations. PSAPs are commonly used, for example, by birdwatchers and hunters to hear animal calls. The FDA prohibits these devices from claiming to actually improve hearing.

ARE THEY EQUAL?

Hearing aids are not just expensive. They also require going to an audiologist or a hearing aid dispenser to get advice on the right model for you, fittings and instructions on their use. It typically takes one to two visits until a new hearing aid user is tested, fitted and fully set to go.

Because OTC devices are expected to be easier to access, those with hearing loss will likely treat their problem much sooner. Hastening this process could reap real health benefits, since research shows that untreated hearing loss—even if mild—is socially isolating and is linked to increased risk for serious conditions such as depression and dementia.

OTC hearing devices remove barriers—without sacrificing hearing improvement. In a double-blind, placebo-controlled, randomized clinical trial published in the *American Journal of Audiology*, researchers analyzed data from 154 adults ages 55 to 79 with mild-to-moderate hearing loss. One group received preprogrammed hearing aids with the help of an audiologist, while the other group followed an OTC-style process by choosing a similar high-end set without a professional fitting and instructions.

Both groups reported that the devices had similar levels of effectiveness, as measured by self-report surveys of hearing aid benefits. Those in the OTC group, however, were somewhat less likely to say that they would purchase the devices—perhaps because they lacked confidence in their own choices compared with those whose hearing aids were chosen for them by professionals.

THE PROS AND CONS

It's important to note that no standard definition or design has yet been established when it comes to OTC hearing devices. So you should be clear-eyed when it comes to expectations.

Among the most significant pros and cons…

Pro: Easily accessible. In a best-case scenario, you will try on a few versions of OTC hearing devices at your local drugstore and go home with your choice the same day. For some people, these devices may be an entry-level product—and a way to bridge the gap before having a professional fitting for traditional hearing aids later.

Con: That choice might be trickier than you think. Choosing OTC hearing aids essentially requires a self-diagnosis of your hearing ability, which could be more complicated than it seems. It's possible that a consumer would be able to see an audiologist and take his/her test results to a retailer to then purchase OTC hearing devices. There are also online hearing tests now available, including the FDA-cleared at-home hearing test iHEAR, available for $69 at iHearMedical.com.

Also: Varying levels of hearing loss may affect each ear, confounding the process. However, many OTC models will likely have a volume control (manual or automatic) that will enable different volumes for each ear.

Important: Medical clearance is not required or recommended for OTC hearing devices. In fact, the FDA recently removed this requirement for adults with mild-to-moderate hearing loss who are purchasing hearing aids because the evidence does not support a need to consult a doctor first.

Good news: Congress recently approved a bill that would allow hearing aids to be sold over the counter, which will increase competition and reduce costs.

When All Else Fails for Overactive Bladder, Botox—or a "Pacemaker"

Cheryl Iglesia, MD, director, section of female pelvic medicine and reconstructive surgery (FPMRS), MedStar Washington Hospital Center, Washington, DC.

If you suffer from an overactive bladder (OAB), you're no stranger to those alarming gotta-go-now moments that can strike day or night.

Lifestyle approaches are often effective and should always be your first line of defense. If these fail, there are medications—but they have lots of drawbacks, including dry mouth, constipation and dizziness. So what if lifestyle approaches don't work for you and medications either don't provide relief or you can't stand the side effects?

Then it's time for what doctors call "third-line" treatments. One is Botox, which was approved for this condition in 2013. Another is a kind of bladder "pacemaker" called sacral neuromodulation (SNM). It has been available since the 1990s, but the technology has improved and it's gaining adherents among patients and doctors.

Is either approach right for you? And if so, which one? The good news for women struggling with this serious problem is that there is now a head-to-head clinical comparison of Botox and SNM. To learn more, we spoke with Cheryl Iglesia, MD, director of the female pelvic medicine and reconstructive surgery division at MedStar Washington Hospital Center in Washington, DC.

OAB—WHEN YOUR BLADDER SENDS THE WRONG SIGNALS

Before looking at the pros and cons of SNM and Botox, it's important to understand OAB. Bladders are considered overactive when the muscles contract to squeeze out pee when you're trying to hold it in. Sometimes nerves mix up the signals the bladder sends to the brain, so your bladder contracts when it should be relaxed and filling up with urine.

For people with OAB—slightly more women than men are affected—social gatherings, traveling and sitting through a meeting or movie can become an ordeal even when you know where to find the nearest bathroom. OAB goes hand-in-hand with incontinence—involuntary leakage—which just compounds the embarrassment. For women, menopause makes both conditions more likely.

THIRD-LINE TREATMENTS: WHEN ALL ELSE FAILS

The best first approach is to try lifestyle changes, including Kegel exercises to strengthen the pelvic floor and help stop leaks. Diet changes (such as cutting out caffeine) and mind-body approaches such as visualization may also help. While lifestyle changes work for many patients, those who can't find relief from their symptoms with medication—or who can't tolerate the side effects—have two other options, both of which are covered by insurance…

•**Botulinum toxin (often sold under the brand name Botox).** Given as a series of injections directly to the bladder, Botox tem-

porarily paralyzes your muscles so that they no longer contract involuntarily. For many patients, Botox works at reducing OAB symptoms. But success comes at a price. There's an increased risk for urinary infections. And for about one in six patients the bladder becomes so relaxed that they have problems emptying it completely. They require catheters to drain their urine—at least for a few weeks. You'll also need to get another shot every six to nine months, on average.

•**Sacral neuromodulation (SNM) works like a bladder pacemaker.** Doctors implant a device at the base of your spine that sends a mild electric current to nerves that control the bladder. The current restores the normal signals between the brain and the bladder so you'll only feel the need to go to the bathroom when your bladder is actually full. While SNM has been around for 20 years, the two-step treatment has become easier and less invasive than it used to be.

The first step is a "testing phase." During an outpatient procedure, a temporary electrode is placed under the skin near the tailbone. The electrode is attached to a wire that leaves the body through the skin over your tailbone and hooks up to a stimulator the size of a battery pack that you carry around. During this two-week phase, you'll be asked to keep a diary describing how often and how urgently you have to urinate. You'll also have to stay hooked up most of the time, except for when you bathe.

If the trial is a success—you're making much fewer runs to the bathroom—a surgeon will replace the temporary electrode and stimulator and implant permanent ones. This part of the process takes less than one hour and is generally performed under local anesthesia with sedation. Once the surgery is over, you or your doctor can adjust the device with a hand-held controller to maximize its effectiveness and comfort level. Then you'll need to check in with your doctor every six to 12 months to make sure that the device is working well. Depending on the settings, the device will need to be replaced about every five years.

For many women and men, SNM can be a game-changer. One long-term study found that significant improvement in OAB symptoms

Time to Take Up Drawing?

Art can help your brain become more resilient. Recent retirees who made time to paint or draw once a week for 10 weeks were better able to handle the pressures of everyday life than people who did not take the time to create art.

Possible reason: Creating visual art may improve the connections among brain regions associated with resilience.

Study of retired adults by researchers at University Hospital Erlangen-Nuremberg, Germany, published in *PLOS ONE*.

was sustained over two-and-a-half years—of the 96 women followed, 85 chose to keep the devices implanted. The results are comparable to medications but without the side effects of the drugs.

HOW SNM STACKS UP TO BOTOX

When researchers compared the two treatments in a recent clinical trial, they found that both worked equally well in reducing symptoms and the Botox injections were slightly better at reducing daily leaking. But unlike Botox, if SNM isn't treating your OAB, you can simply have the device removed without any lingering side effects.

That doesn't mean SNM is risk-free. Medtronic, maker of the InterStim System used for SNM, did its own clinical study. Results: Out of the 219 men and women in the study, 52% experienced adverse effects ranging from temporary pain at the site of implantation (the most common) to occasional electric shocks (reprogramming the device usually fixes this problem).

What's best for you? The choice is yours, of course, but it's worth noting that in one study of 272 patients using SNM for one year, only seven chose to have the devices removed. If your battle with OAB has made you desperate and nothing else seems to help, SNM may be a way to get your life back.

Medication Fights Dangerous UTIs

Brad Spellberg, MD, is professor of clinical medicine at the Keck School of Medicine, University of Southern California, Los Angeles, and author of *Rising Plague*.

Vabomere combines two existing products—the antibiotic *meropenem* and *vaborbactam*, which inhibits certain mechanisms that bacteria use to resist antibiotics. The elderly, those who are immunocompromised and patients with cancer or other serious conditions are especially at risk for an antibiotic-resistant urinary tract infection (UTI) caused by a strain of bacteria known as carbapenem-resistant enterobacteriaceae (CRE). Vabomere is given intravenously.

This Alzheimer's Imposter Is Treatable

Michael A. Williams, MD, director of adult and transitional hydrocephalus and CSF disorders at University of Washington Medical Center and professor of neurology and neurological surgery at University of Washington School of Medicine, both in Seattle.

If you're over age 65, it's common to feel that you're slowing down a bit. Simply walking to your mailbox could take longer than it used to, and you may have even started shuffling as you walk. Getting out of a chair could be getting harder, too.

On top of that, your bladder might not be cooperating, so you have started to wear pads for incontinence. Your thinking isn't quite as clear as it used to be, and you are now having trouble keeping your checkbook.

Don't make this mistake: While these changes all may seem to point to the fact that you're simply growing older, having all three of these symptoms could actually be a red flag for a treatable brain disorder.

As many as 700,000 people in the US are believed to have idiopathic (with no known cause) normal pressure hydrocephalus (iNPH), an often-misdiagnosed brain condition. Of the 5.2 million individuals diagnosed with dementia, estimates show that 10% to 15% actually have this treatable condition.

WHEN IT'S NOT NORMAL AGING

A shuffling gait, incontinence and memory problems may prompt a person to see his/her doctor, but these symptoms are also among the most common in older adults. For that reason, your doctor may chalk up these problems to "normal aging"—when, in fact, they are not normal.

If the patient is savvy and doesn't accept that answer, he/she will find another doctor and get a more extensive workup.

The turning point comes when the doctor orders a CT scan or an MRI—a test usually included in a dementia evaluation. If the imaging test shows that the brain's ventricles—normal cavities within the brain that contain cerebrospinal fluid (CSF)—are enlarged, that should trigger consideration of iNPH.

What's gone wrong: Hydrocephalus results from a defect in circulation of the CSF, which surrounds and cushions the brain. Normally, the choroid plexus (vascular tissue in the ventricles) produces up to 2.5 cups of CSF daily, which bathes the brain and is absorbed back into circulation, maintaining a constant volume of fluid inside the skull. If absorption slows down, then CSF accumulates, the ventricles enlarge and eventually symptoms (such as those described earlier) may appear.

GETTING DIAGNOSED

If the brain scan shows enlarged ventricles, indicating possible iNPH, the next step is to see a neurologist for a clinical exam. The first symptom a neurologist will probably look for is a gait disturbance, including difficulty getting in or out of a seat, trouble initiating gait, shuffling gait and instability on turns. The presence of a shuffling gait along with cognitive slowing and memory impairment and/or urinary incontinence raises the diagnosis to "probable iNPH."

Important: Because cognitive defects caused by iNPH are frequently mistaken for Alzheimer's disease, a neurologist is best qualified to distinguish between the two types of memory loss.

Unlike Alzheimer's, iNPH usually does not reach the stage where the individual fails to recognize family or close friends. In addition, those with early Alzheimer's rarely display the distinctive gait impairment characteristic of iNPH, such as difficulty standing or turning, as mentioned above.

Unlike arthritis, the gait disturbance caused by iNPH is due to a neurologic impairment rather than pain or stiffness. Normal walking should be effortless, but individuals with iNPH must concentrate to walk and often complain that their feet won't do what they want them to do.

The slowness and shuffling of iNPH may cause it to be mistaken for Parkinson's disease, but the tremor that is typical of Parkinson's is not a key feature of iNPH. Patients with iNPH may even be prescribed medications for Alzheimer's, Parkinson's or incontinence, but these rarely help.

Another disorder that iNPH may resemble is vascular dementia, which is caused by the cumulative effects of various risk factors, such as high blood pressure, a history of small strokes, elevated cholesterol and diabetes. Because vascular dementia and iNPH often affect the same areas of the brain, the conditions can produce similar symptoms and sometimes even occur at the same time.

GETTING THE RIGHT TREATMENT

It's important for iNPH to be treated. While there are no drugs for iNPH, the good news is that most cases can be treated by surgically implanting a shunt. The shunt consists of three components—a narrow tube that is placed in the ventricles…a valve mechanism to control the flow, which is usually placed beneath the scalp…and a narrow tube that transports excess CSF somewhere else in the body, usually to the abdominal cavity, where it's easily absorbed into the bloodstream.

To determine whether shunt surgery will help, tests of the patient's response to CSF removal are recommended. A spinal tap (also known as lumbar puncture) may be performed on an outpatient basis. With this procedure, approximately 30 milliliters (ml) to 40 ml, or nearly 1.5 ounces, will be removed. The patient's gait should be evaluated before the lumbar puncture and several hours afterward. If the gait improves significantly, then a shunt is very likely to help the patient.

If there's no improvement after the spinal tap, a more extensive test called external lumbar drainage (ELD) may be performed in the hospital. In this case, the doctor will insert a temporary tube into the spinal fluid to drain it for about four days, for an approximate total of 400 ml to 600 ml, or 13.5 ounces to 20 ounces, of CSF.

ELD is like a test-drive of shunt-like conditions for the brain, without actually having the shunt operation. If the patient shows improvement following prolonged drainage, he will then be referred for shunt surgery. If the patient does not respond to prolonged drainage, then the odds of a shunt helping are small—below 5%.

iNPH CARE LASTS A LIFETIME

Following shunt surgery, recovery rates for iNPH patients range from 60% to 90%, according to the medical literature. All symptoms can improve, but the extent of improvement may be limited if patients have other disorders that contribute to their symptoms.

It's important for people with shunts to visit the neurologist or neurosurgeon regularly following shunt surgery, initially to find the optimal setting for the shunt valve that controls drainage and on an ongoing basis to ensure that it's still operating correctly.

Too much drainage can increase the risk of bleeding within the skull, known as a subdural hematoma, and can cause symptoms such as headaches and nausea. Sometimes, therapy is useful to help patients regain balance and cognitive function.

FINDING THE BEST DOCTOR

To find a neurologist or neurosurgeon who has experience diagnosing and treating iNPH, consult the website of the Hydrocephalus Association, which provides a directory of neurologists and neurosurgeons throughout the US, HydroAssoc.org/physician-directory.

Drinking Coffee May Increase Life Expectancy

Drinking coffee may increase life expectancy. Researchers found that people who drank two to three cups of coffee a day were as much as 18% less likely to die over an average of 16 years than nondrinkers. Other studies already have associated coffee drinking with lower risks for diseases including heart disease, type 2 diabetes, liver cancer, Parkinson's and multiple sclerosis.

Study of nearly 186,000 Americans, ages 45 to 75, by researchers at University of Southern California's Keck School of Medicine, Los Angeles, published in *Annals of Internal Medicine*.

When You're Older, How Much Alcohol Is Too Much?

George Koob, PhD, director, National Institute on Alcohol Abuse and Alcoholism, Bethesda, Maryland.

How alcohol affects you does change greatly as you age. There are several reasons. First, you metabolize alcohol more slowly in your 50s, 60s and up than when you were younger. The result is that alcohol stays in your blood longer, increasing its sedating effect. And this effect can be obvious even with light drinking. When you're in your 30s or 40s, a glass of wine or beer at a party might relax you and help you feel more sociable. Once you hit your 50s, though, that same alcoholic drink is more likely to make you yearn for a nap!

Alcohol also affects balance and coordination more as you age, increasing your likelihood of falling and injuring yourself. And alcohol impairs attention and reaction time more with age—raising your risk of causing a car crash.

And it is not just drinking on its own that's a concern. If you're a senior, chances are that you're taking at least one medication, either prescription or over-the-counter (OTC). Many drugs, both prescription and OTC, should not be combined with alcohol. Drugs to watch out for include pain medications, sleeping pills, antidepressants and even such seemingly benign OTC drugs as aspirin, acetaminophen and allergy medicines. When combined with alcohol, these can cause side effects such as confusion, nausea or gastrointestinal bleeding, depending on the drug.

For women younger than 65, the National Institute on Alcohol Abuse and Alcoholism (NIAAA) considers moderate drinking, providing that you're healthy and do not take medications, to be no more than three drinks in a single day and no more than seven in a week. For men of that age, it's no more than four drinks in a single day and no more than 14 in a week. But once you reach age 65, the NIAAA's moderate drinking limit for both women and men is no more than three drinks in a single day or seven drinks in a week.

The Dietary Guidelines for Americans 2015-2020, issued by the US Department of Health and Human Services and the US Department of Agriculture, recommends no more than one daily alcoholic drink for women and no more than two for men. For reference, NIAAA identifies a drink as 12 ounces of regular beer (5% alcohol)…eight-to-nine ounces of malt liquor (7% alcohol)…five ounces of wine (12% alcohol)…or 1.5 ounces of gin, rum, tequila, etc. (80 proof, which is 40% alcohol). If the spirits you choose have higher alcohol content than that, then it takes less to count as "one drink."

But these guidelines are only averages, and for individuals, the safe amount of alcohol can be much less. Whatever amount of alcohol you're currently drinking, if it's affecting you to the point of causing problems, it's best to cut back.

Good idea: Include a discussion of your alcohol consumption during a regular doctor visit. Be sure to review any medications you may be taking—including OTC drugs and/or supplements—for potential interactions with alcohol. Your doctor may be able to prescribe an alternative medication if necessary.

Got Age Spots?

Valori Treloar, MD, CNS, a board-certified dermatologist in private practice at Integrative Dermatology in Newton, Massachusetts. A fellow of the American Academy of Dermatology, she is coauthor of *The Clear Skin Diet*. Dr. Treloar is also a Certified Nutrition Specialist, a credential awarded by the American College of Nutrition.

Soaking in the sun can leave you with more than just wrinkles. Age spots—those flat, roundish marks that appear on sun-exposed areas such as the face, chest and backs of hands—also result from exposure to ultraviolet (UV) light, which stimulates the production of pigment known as melanin. Sometimes called liver spots, these brown, tan or black marks actually have nothing to do with the liver…or with age, for that matter. Age spots are more common among fair-skinned and light-haired individuals, and they affect men and women about equally.

HARMLESS OR NOT?

True age spots, also called solar lentigines, are harmless. If you find them unsightly, you can significantly lighten them or, in some cases, render them almost invisible with the therapies described below.

Important: Some skin cancers can masquerade as age spots. That's why it's crucial that you show any new or changing growths or spots to a dermatologist. Be aware of the ABCDE signs of skin cancer—Asymmetry, Border irregularity, Color that is not uniform, Diameter greater than 6 mm (size of a pencil eraser) and Evolving size, shape or color.

A NATURAL APPROACH

Over-the-counter (OTC) topical products cost significantly less than prescription treatments…but they don't work quite as well. Even with consistent use and rigorous sun protection, it can take a month or so to see some improvement. *For an OTC product, consider one that contains one of these ingredients…* *

•**Niacinamide (vitamin B-3).** Topical niacinamide lightens age spots without irritation. Hundreds of skin creams contain this ingredient. Look for one with a 2% to 5% concentration for best results. This cream can be used on your face, chest, arms, hands, etc.

•**Glycolic acid.** Originally sourced from sugarcane, glycolic acid is used in varying concentrations in facial peels, cleansers, moisturizers and serums. Also called a fruit peel, it exfoliates the outer layer of dead skin cells. When purchasing a product, make sure glycolic acid is listed as an active ingredient…or look for a product with 5% to 10% glycolic acid. It can be used all over the body if it's tolerated—glycolic acid can be irritating for some people.

Niacinamide works better for some, but for others glycolic acid is more effective.

EAT TO BEAT AGE SPOTS

A plant-based diet, filled with antioxidant-rich produce, may help combat sun-induced skin damage by fighting harmful free radicals. Eat plenty of berries, dark leafy greens and tomatoes. Foods rich in beta-carotene may be particularly helpful—the carotenoids that give sweet potatoes and other orange produce their color get converted to vitamin A in the body, speeding cell turnover and perhaps helping the top layer of skin to shed more quickly.

These foods alone won't prevent age spots, but they may slow their growth and help prevent new spots from forming. My advice: Eat nine fist-size servings of vegetables that have a variety of colors each day.

PRESCRIPTION CREAMS

The following products, which can be prescribed by your doctor, are considered the most effective topical treatments for age spots. Note: Insurance companies generally will not cover age spot treatments as they are considered cosmetic.

•**Hydroquinone.** This bleaching cream interrupts pigment production. With a prescription-strength cream containing 3% or 4% hydroquinone, you may notice lightening within a few weeks…maximum effect occurs after a few months. Apply it twice daily to the spots only, not the surrounding skin. This cream can be used all over the body if it's tolerated.

*Caution: Products made outside the US may contain mercury. Use caution if buying online.

Note: Do not use if you are pregnant or breastfeeding or are using peroxide products.

•**Tretinoin.** This vitamin A–based product slows melanin production and increases skin cell turnover. Sunlight causes tretinoin to break down, so you should apply it only at night. I recommend applying it to your face or other affected area one to two times a week to begin. Then when any redness or irritation has subsided, use it nightly. For initial treatment of the face, dilute the tretinoin with a mild face cream. Tretinoin can take up to 40 weeks for noticeable results.

I like a combination hydroquinone/tretinoin product that includes a topical steroid, which helps calm possible irritation.

Topical treatments cost an average of $50 to $200 per tube. A course of treatment may require one or more tubes.

How Can I Make My Butt Look Younger?

Jill Miller, fitness therapy expert, cofounder of Tune Up Fitness Worldwide, creator of Yoga Tune Up and author of *The Roll Model.* She teaches at fitness and yoga conferences worldwide. Learn more at TuneUpFitness.com.

It can be discouraging when you're keeping yourself fit but your bum still looks like it suffered a landslide.

But here's good news for you: There are certain exercises that can not only strengthen your hip bones and spine, reducing your risk for falls and fractures—but also give you a better-looking derrière.

One reason buttocks flatten is from spending too much time sitting. Long periods of sitting cause butt muscles (specifically, one muscle called the gluteus medius) to weaken and sag—what physical therapy experts call "gluteal amnesia." An easy way to help counteract this butt slump is to just get up and walk around for a few minutes every hour.

Another effective way to strengthen and firm buttocks muscles is with yoga. The following three poses are especially good for butt firming. Do them daily for the most benefit—but even doing them a few times a week will help. (Check with your doctor before trying these if you have osteoporosis or are being treated for a medical condition.)

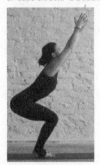

Chair pose (builds strength and endurance in glutes). Stand with your feet hip-width apart, and tighten your butt and abdominal muscles. Raise your arms up above your head, elbows straight, while you bend your knees and slowly lower your butt back—as if you were lowering yourself into an imaginary chair. Hold the "sitting" position while you take eight breaths. Then slowly lower your arms and straighten your legs back to standing position.

Locust pose (strengthens your lower back and tightens butt). Lie facedown with your arms stretched out in front of you, palms facing each other. (This is a variation of the traditional Locust pose, where your arms are at your sides.) Tighten your abdominal and butt muscles as you raise

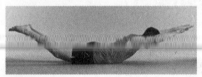

your legs, upper body and arms a few inches off the floor. Hold the position for six to eight breaths. Then lower your upper body, arms and legs to starting position. Rest for one or two breaths, and repeat the move three more times. *Note:* If you feel pinching or pain in your lower back while doing this move, lower your legs.

Bridge pose (helps counteract "gluteal amnesia"). Lie on your back, knees bent, feet flat on the floor with heels several inches from your butt. Tighten your abdominal and butt muscles, and raise your hips off the floor until your body

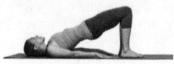

forms a straight line from your shoulders to your knees. Hold the position for four to eight breaths—don't let your hips sink!—then slowly lower your hips back to starting position. Rest for a few breaths, then repeat three times.

Note: If you feel any pain in your lower back while doing this move, lower your hips slightly.

Feet Getting Bigger???

Neil A. Campbell, DPM, FACFAS, DABFAS, staff podiatrist, Cuero Regional Hospital, Texas.

You may have had a recent panic when shopping for shoes. It might seem as if suddenly your usual shoe size is too small.

Here's the good news: Your feet are not growing.

Now the bad: As we age, we lose some of the elasticity in the ligaments and connective tissues in our bodies. This is the reason why various body parts start to "sag." In the foot, that means the supporting tendons and ligaments become lax and can't hold the bones and joints in the same position as when we were younger, causing the arch to flatten and the feet to expand. Pregnancy and weight gain also can cause your feet to spread, due both to hormones and the added pressure on the feet, and this change is generally permanent. An injury to the bones or tendons that causes a rupture or dislocation is another reason feet can change shape.

For all these reasons, it's normal for feet to become longer and wider, perhaps gaining a half size or more every decade or so. However, if change in size is also accompanied by pain, see a podiatrist to rule out a more serious foot problem such as arthritis, tendon dysfunction or nerve damage. And always try on shoes before purchasing them—you may also find you need a wider size.

CHAPTER 17

Pain Relief

Is Your Medication Causing You Pain?

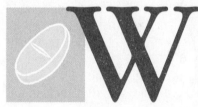**W**hen your foot goes numb after a few hours of couch time or you wake up at night with a tingling (or even painful) arm crooked beneath your head, you're experiencing what people with neuropathy live with…every day.

Peripheral neuropathy is a mysterious condition. Many patients never discover what is causing their nerve-related numbness, pain, tingling or other sensations.

Often-overlooked culprit: The medicine cabinet. After diabetes, medication is one of the most common causes of neuropathy. Dozens of medications—even those that you would think are totally safe—can cause nerve damage that's often slow to appear and equally slow to heal… if it ever does. What you need to know…

THE LEADING CULPRITS

Nerve-related side effects, known as drug-induced neuropathies, are tricky to identify because they often appear months or even years after starting a medication—although there are exceptions.

Example: Some of the drugs used in chemotherapy are notorious for causing neuropathy. These cases are easy to identify because the symptoms show up quickly—typically within a week or a few months of starting the chemotherapy. Up to 75% of cancer patients given the chemotherapy drug *vincristine* will experience neuropathy. Paclitaxel (Taxol), discussed later, is another common offender.

In general, about one-third of patients who have drug-induced neuropathy will completely recover when they stop—or at least lower the dose of—an offending drug. One-third will stay

Janice F. Wiesman, MD, FAAN, clinical associate professor of neurology at New York University School of Medicine in New York City and adjunct assistant professor of neurology at Boston University School of Medicine. She is author of *Peripheral Neuropathy: What It Is and What You Can Do to Feel Better.*

the same, and another third might get worse. *Drugs to suspect...*

•**Statins.** Cholesterol-lowering statins—including *atorvastatin* (Lipitor), *rosuvastatin* (Crestor) and *simvastatin* (Zocor)—are among the most commonly prescribed medications in the US. According to research published in *Neurology*, statin users were four times more likely to develop neuropathy than people not taking statins.

Experts aren't sure why statins often cause neuropathy. The good news, however, is that most people with statin-related nerve symptoms will recover when they stop taking the drug, though it may take months in some cases. But how do they manage their cholesterol without the medication?

My advice: Switching to a different statin might be the solution—but it's impossible to predict if (or when) a new drug will cause similar problems. To help control your cholesterol levels, your doctor should advise you to exercise more and eat a lower-meat (or even vegetarian) diet.

Even if you can't completely control cholesterol with lifestyle changes, diet and exercise can lower it enough that you might be able to take a lower statin dose—important because the higher the statin dose, the greater the risk for neuropathy.

Note: Case reports have shown that people taking supplements containing red yeast rice, a naturally occurring statin, have also developed neuropathy.

•**Antibiotics.** A number of antibiotics can lead to *neuropathy. Ciprofloxacin* (Cipro) is a widely used broad-spectrum antibiotic. Along with other drugs in this class, known as *fluoroquinolones*—such as *levofloxacin* and *moxifloxacin* (Avelox)—it's a common cause of nerve symptoms.

Important: If you notice neuropathy symptoms while taking one of these drugs, don't ignore them. The discomfort usually involves tingling and/or numbness that starts in the feet, moves up to the knees and then starts to affect the hands and fingers.

My advice: If you experience such symptoms, promptly contact your doctor. Ask him/

her whether you can switch to a safer antibiotic, such as penicillin, tetracycline or doxycycline. Neuropathy symptoms usually subside when a person goes off a fluoroquinolone but, in rare cases, may not.

In my opinion, Cipro or another fluoroquinolone antibiotic should be used only when you have an infection that won't respond to one of the safer antibiotics mentioned above.

Nitrofurantoin (Macrobid) is an antibiotic that's used both to treat urinary tract infections (UTIs) and to help prevent recurrent UTIs in patients who are particularly susceptible, such as nursing home patients and those with spinal cord injuries using urinary catheters.

Unlike most other drug-induced neuropathies, the ones caused by Macrobid usually occur quickly—within a week, in some cases. The discomfort usually begins in the feet and legs and moves upward (as described earlier) and can be irreversible if the drug isn't stopped quickly enough.

Most UTIs can be treated with newer, safer drugs or drug combinations, such as *trimethoprim* and *sulfamethoxazole* (Bactrim or Septra). Patients should tell their doctors immediately if they notice neuropathy symptoms, such as numbness, tingling, etc., to determine whether they can be switched to a different antibiotic.

•**Taxol.** About 30% to 40% of cancer patients who are treated with chemotherapy will develop neuropathy. Taxol, commonly used for breast cancer, is a common offender because many women take it for years after their initial diagnosis and treatments.

Important finding: More than 40% of women taking Taxol or similar drugs continued to experience numbness and/or tingling in their hands or feet two years after starting treatment...and 10% rated the discomfort as severe, according to a report in *Journal of the National Cancer Institute*. Neuropathy symptoms should subside when Taxol is changed or stopped, but this might take months or years.

You're more likely to get foot tingling/numbness (the so-called "Taxol toes") or other symptoms, such as sensations of burning in a hand or loss of touch sensation, if you're also obese... have a preexisting history of neuropathy...have had a mastectomy…or if a large number of your lymph nodes harbored cancer cells.

My advice: Be sure to tell your oncologist (if he doesn't ask) if you've had neuropathy in the past. You might be advised to undergo treatments that have about the same survival benefit but are less likely to have this side effect.

•**Amiodarone.** This drug is one of the most frequently prescribed for heart-rhythm abnormalities (arrhythmias).

Up to 10% of patients who take amiodarone over a period of years will develop neuropathy…and some will develop optic neuropathy, which can cause blurred vision, abnormalities in the visual field (such as "halo vision") or even progressive (and painless) vision loss.

Note: Certain other drugs, including Cipro, the cancer medication *tamoxifen* and the erectile dysfunction drug *sildenafil* (Viagra), also can cause optic neuropathy.

My advice: Tell your doctor right away if you notice visual symptoms after starting any of these medications. "Ocular toxicity" usually begins within one year, with vision changes occurring in as little as six months. The vision changes usually will clear up once you stop the drug and switch to a different one, but in rare cases they may not.

•**Phenytoin (Dilantin).** This antiepilepsy drug is sometimes used, paradoxically, to treat neuropathic pain. Up to half of patients who take Dilantin for 15 years will develop neuropathy. Many patients experience neuropathy sooner.

Neuropathies caused by the drug tend to be minor. These might include diminished (or absent) tendon reflexes in the legs that are barely noticeable, although some may observe that they're a bit unsteady when they walk.

My advice: Be sure to tell your doctor about your neuropathy symptoms. If they are mild, he may feel that the benefits of the drug outweigh the risks. More likely, your doctor will advise switching to one of the newer (but more expensive) antiepilepsy drugs, such as *lamotrigine* (Lamictal) or *topiramate* (Topamax), which do not cause neuropathy. If the medication is changed, neuropathy symptoms may or may not subside.

Better Than Opioids

Topical treatments for chronic pain can be as effective as opioids and prescription nonsteroidal anti-inflammatory drugs (NSAIDs) for some patients. Prescription topical treatments, such as diclofenac and ketoprofen, may work for the pain of moderately severe arthritis, neuropathic conditions and musculoskeletal disorders. Treated patients for whom the topical approach worked said that they favored topical treatments for their convenience.

Jeffrey Gudin, MD, director of pain management and palliative care, Englewood Hospital and Medical Center, New Jersey, and leader of a study published in Journal of Pain Research.

Pain Relief Without the Pitfalls

David Sherer, MD, a board-certified anesthesiologist who is president and CEO of Consolidated Medicine, a medical practice and consulting group in Chevy Chase, Maryland. He is coauthor of *Dr. David Sherer's Hospital Survival Guide: 100+ Ways to Make Your Hospital Stay Safe and Comfortable.* His blog on BottomLineInc.com is titled "What Your Doctor Isn't Telling You."

P ain…physical pain. We've all had it. None of us (except those who are masochists) like it or want it. From the mildest headache to the most excruciating kidney stone, pain comes in many forms and severity. It is estimated that 100 million Americans suffer some form of chronic pain, and when you add to this the number of us who suffer from acute pain (injuries, postsurgical pain, the common headache or toothache, etc.), it is easy to appreciate the magnitude of this problem.

Whenever possible, we all want and expect relief from pain, but few of us appreciate the potential dangers inherent in the way moderate-to-severe pain has been handled by the medical community in the last few decades. For pain that is moderate to severe—from whatever cause—there had been a prevailing view that brief, controlled use of narcotic medications such as Percocet (*oxycodone*) or *hydrocodone* was acceptable and appropriate. However, in light of recent studies and literature to the contrary, we now know that these medications and those similar to them have a far wider potential for abuse, danger and overdose than originally thought.

First, a little background. The human body contains untold receptors in the central and peripheral nervous system that react to a class of naturally occurring and synthetic drugs used to relieve pain. These opiates and opioid-type medicines, as opposed to the commonly known anti-inflammatory pain medicines (aspirin, ibuprofen, naproxen, etc.), interact with these receptors to cause a decrease in pain perception and an overall feeling of well-being. However, these medications not only cause side effects, including itching, constipation, slowed breathing and difficulty urinating to name a few, but they have the potential for addiction and tolerance (increasing doses are needed to achieve the desired pain-relieving effect). As a result, it is estimated by the National Institutes of Health that more than two million people in our country have become addicted to this class of medication after receiving prescriptions written to relieve pain. Alarmingly high rates of near-overdoses and overdose-related deaths are reaching the hundreds of thousands each year. The government is trying to tackle the problem of addiction in new and novel ways, but the end is nowhere in sight.

What can you, the average patient who wants relief from moderate-to-severe pain, do to get the pain in check without the inherent dangers of opioid therapy? I have a few suggestions…

• **When it comes to postsurgical pain,** consider skipping this class of medicine altogether. Now, this won't always be possible because of the severity of some types of pain. It is up to you to decide your own tolerance for pain and how to deal with it. Consider asking your doctor for the newer injectable forms of the standard anti-inflammatory painkillers. Ibuprofen and naproxen now are available in injectable forms (another med in this class, injectable ketorolac, has been around for decades). These medicines may be appropriate in some cases to give you the pain relief you need.

• **Consider the newer form of injectable acetaminophen,** better known as Tylenol in pill form. Ofirmev is the brand name of this newer agent and it has shown promise for post-surgical pain relief. Realize, though, that this drug will not have the anti-inflammatory properties of the others mentioned above.

• **A groundbreaking time-released form of the local anesthetic Exparel has emerged as a novel way to treat surgical pain.** This medication, injected by the surgeon or anesthesia provider, can result in longer-lasting pain relief with much fewer side effects as compared to the nonsteroidal anti-inflammatories or narcotic medicines.

• **Alternative pain relief can be achieved with the use of specific nerve blocks.** Ask the anesthesia provider if this is possible. Local anesthetics can be released over time in epidurals and other nerve blocks (for the arm, hand, leg or foot, etc.) with the use of infusion pumps and other devices.

• **Guided imagery and other modalities** (neuro-feedback, using brain imaging technology) are showing some promise.

• **The use of medical marijuana** is also gaining some traction for pain relief in some areas of the country.

Because of the addiction and abuse problem of narcotic pain medicines, the pendulum is starting to swing away from their automatic use and toward a more cautious approach. The root causes of the epidemic have been identified—cavalier prescribing, social acceptance and drug-company marketing efforts let the opiate genie out of the bottle decades ago. Getting the genie back in the bottle is going to be a struggle. Along with the alternative therapies I have mentioned, drugmakers are now looking at painkilling medicines that have less potential for addiction and tolerance. Also, drugs like Lyrica and Neurontin have emerged as useful players in relieving some forms of chronic pain. In 2018, the world of pain relief has never seen such concentrated research and innovation.

You need to communicate with your doctor to avoid the pitfalls of potential addiction and abuse. Ask your doctor about the alternatives available to handle your pain. Your body will thank you for the effort.

Acupuncture: The Go-To Pain-Fighter

Roger Batchelor, DAOM, LAc, doctor of acupuncture and Oriental medicine and associate professor of acupuncture at the National University of Natural Medicine in Portland, Oregon. He was the primary acupuncturist at the Hooper Detoxification Stabilization Center, a 54-bed public-health facility and regional detox center, also in Portland.

Got a backache? If you're like most people, you probably reach for a bottle of *ibuprofen* (Motrin). If the pain is more severe—say, a broken bone or a piercing ache after surgery—you, like millions of Americans, may be prescribed a highly addictive opioid, such as *oxycodone* (OxyContin) or *hydrocodone*.

Now: Acupuncture, an ancient form of healing that has been practiced and refined for centuries, is increasingly being used in the US as the go-to treatment for pain relief. About three million American adults receive acupuncture each year, with chronic pain being the number-one reason—whether it's back, neck or shoulder pain, chronic headache or osteoarthritis.

HOW ACUPUNCTURE EASES PAIN

If the thought of being stuck with needles sounds more pain-inducing than pain-relieving, there are a few details you need to know. It's true that acupuncture involves "needling"—or the insertion of needles through your skin. But it's worth noting that the typical acupuncture needle is sterile and no wider than a strand of hair.

When these needles are inserted by a skilled acupuncturist, it doesn't hurt. The most that some people feel is a mild tingling or pin-prick sensation at the outset. During a typical session for a pain-related condition, the acupuncturist might use 10 to 20 needles, often placed in such areas as the limbs, back and scalp.

The needles are inserted into specific "acupoints" throughout the body, based on the ancient Chinese philosophy that our health is governed by the uninterrupted flow of qi (pronounced "chee"), or bioenergy, through the body. According to the principles of traditional Chinese medicine, when one's bioenergy becomes blocked, it builds up like water behind a dam, leading to pain and/or dysfunction. Needling a combination of acupoints—there are thousands of them—can relieve qi blockages and elicit the body's natural healing response.

Needling also signals the brain and spinal cord to produce chemicals and hormones, such as endorphins, that function as the body's own pain relievers, as well as natural anti-inflammatory compounds.

The result: Less need for pain medication. Many patients also feel less stress and sleep better following acupuncture—benefits that also help them cope with pain.

So what happens when you go for acupuncture? You'll be asked to lie on an exam table for the treatment. You can usually remain clothed, though you may need to remove a shirt or your socks, for example, if they are covering an area that will be needled. In some cases, you may prefer to change into a gown provided by the practitioner. You can expect to see your acupuncturist once or twice weekly for five to 10 sessions that last about one hour each. Not all insurance (including Medicare) covers acupuncture. Check with your insurer.

What About Acupressure

For certain conditions, acupressure—applying pressure or massaging acupoints—can be as effective as acupuncture.

How it works: Massaging one point on the body can relieve symptoms in other parts of the body via pathways called meridians.

You can try acupressure for 30 to 60 seconds once or more daily on yourself or another person for...

Frontal headache: Massage the fleshy spot between the thumb and pointer finger with firm pressure. This point is known as Large Intestine 4.

Nausea: Massage the spot on the palm side of the forearm, three finger widths from the base of the palm, between the two tendons in the middle of the forearm. This point is known as Pericardium 6.

Note: During opioid withdrawal or after surgery, traditional acupuncture is more appropriate than acupressure.

ACUPUNCTURE FOR OPIOID WITHDRAWAL

On the heels of a shocking report that more than 64,000 Americans died from drug overdoses in 2016, the US Department of Health Human Services recently declared the abuse of pain-relieving opioids a public health emergency.

Not only does acupuncture lessen the need for opioids, it can help opioid-addicted individuals through the painful withdrawal process. When a person addicted to opioids first quits, he/she will experience unpleasant withdrawal symptoms, including insomnia, pain, leg cramps, irritability, nausea and constipation.

Medications such as *methadone* (Dolophine or Methadose) and *buprenorphine* are prescribed to ease withdrawal but tend to backfire. Methadone must be taken daily, with each dose providing pain relief for about four to eight hours. However, methadone is highly addictive, and misuse of this drug can be fatal. Buprenorphine can cause side effects such as muscle aches, nausea, constipation, sleep problems, irritability and more.

Acupuncture, on the other hand, has no side effects...may help prevent relapse...quells cravings...and does not require the patient to take yet another drug.

It's all about the ears: When treating people addicted to opioids, many acupuncturists follow an auricular, or ear-focused, acupuncture protocol endorsed by the US National Acupuncture Detoxification Association (NADA). Auricular acupuncture is based on the belief that points on the ears correspond to different areas of the brain and body. The NADA-approved protocol, also called acudetox or 5-Needle or 5NP ear acupuncture protocol, involves inserting three to five needles into each ear at specific points.

For opioids such as OxyContin, one to three months of daily acupuncture are needed to get through the worst of the detox process.

To get more information on the NADA-approved protocol, visit Acudetox.com. For general pain relief, you can find an acupuncturist with multiple years of training and certification at NCCAOM.org.

A NEWER APPROACH

With electroacupuncture (EA), a newer form of acupuncture that was developed in the 1950s, the needles may be connected to a small unit that provides painless mild electrical stimulation. The electricity mimics the act of a practitioner physically maneuvering the needle, sending a stronger signal to the body. Even though you may feel a mild electric tingle with electroacupuncture, it is not uncomfortable and should feel relaxing.

Numerous studies show that different types of naturally occurring pain-relieving hormones are released at different EA frequencies. Needles are typically left in for 20 to 40 minutes.

Important finding: In a study in the journal *Pain*, women who received EA prior to abdominal surgery needed 60% less morphine in the 24 hours following the operation. Besides reducing the need for addictive pain medications, acupuncture also counters the most common side effects of opioids—including nausea, dizziness, urinary retention, constipation and lethargy.

Note: People with pacemakers should avoid EA to prevent unnecessary interference with the device.

Dr. Levin's Anti-Migraine Plan

Morris Levin, MD, chief of the Division of Headache Medicine and director of the Headache Center at UCSF Medical Center in San Francisco. He is coauthor of *Understanding Your Migraines: A Guide for Patients and Families*. Dr. Levin is board-certified in neurology, pain medicine and headache medicine.

Medications can help prevent and treat migraine, but fortunately there are many lifestyle and other treatment options that can help dramatically—without drugs.

THE ADVICE I GIVE THE MIGRAINEURS I TREAT...KNOW YOUR TRIGGERS

Identifying your migraine triggers and avoiding them is key to preventing an attack. Triggers are highly individual, including particular smells, sounds, lighting, 3-D movies—even weather changes. *Common food triggers include...*

What Is a Migraine?

A migraine headache is a cascade of electrical, chemical and inflammation-related blood vessel changes that occur in the brain, typically in distinct stages, but they can overlap…

• **Prodrome.** The warning stage. You may feel "off," irritable or moody…have amplified senses, such as a heightened sense of smell… and crave certain foods, such as sweets.

• **Aura.** Usually occurring five to 60 minutes before an attack, it involves visual disturbances such as flashing lights, zigzag lines or blind spots.

• **Headache.** Pain, mild to severe, often described as intense pounding or pressure, usually on one side of the head.

• **Postdrome.** The recovery period. You may feel fatigued over the next few hours or days.

• **Alcohol**—especially red wine, perhaps because of its high levels of histamine.

• **Nitrites.** Found in hot dogs, bacon, sausage and processed meats.

• **Monosodium glutamate (MSG).** A flavor enhancer that goes by many names, it is a powerful trigger for many people.

Taking the right steps at the first sign of a migraine coming on can lessen an attack—or avert it. *These natural remedies can help…*

• **Apply a cold pack to the site of the pain.** Cold may reduce blood vessel inflammation. A bag of frozen peas makes a good cold compress. It conforms to the shape of your head, and you can refreeze the bag for reuse. (Note: Don't eat thawed and refrozen peas—they can harbor unhealthy bacteria.)

• **Aromatherapy,** a popular migraine treatment in Europe, is not backed by strong scientific evidence, but some patients find it helps them relax and eases their headache pain. Tiger Balm—a mixture of camphor, menthol, cajuput oil and other herbals—is particularly effective and is available in supermarkets and pharmacies. Rub a small amount into your temples at the first sign of migraine. Other essential oils to try: Eucalyptus, lavender and peppermint.

• **Drink a caffeinated beverage**—but not more than 100 mg of caffeine (one cup of medium-roast coffee). Other options: Strong black tea (50 mg/cup)…green tea (25 mg/cup.) Warning: Caffeine triggers migraines for some people.

Regular tea and coffee drinkers: To avoid a caffeine-withdrawal headache—another migraine trigger—drink the caffeinated beverage at the same time each day.

VITAMINS AND HERBS THAT HELP

Certain supplements can reduce the frequency and/or intensity of migraines. *Try these one at a time for two or three months…*

• **Vitamin B-2 (riboflavin)** may reduce migraine frequency.

Try: 400 mg/day. Vitamin B-2 usually doesn't have adverse side effects.

• **Magnesium gluconate and magnesium taurate** may both prevent migraine.

Try: 500 mg to 600 mg/day of either one. Lower the dose if you have loose stools.

Option: 100 mg of either at the start of a migraine can reduce its intensity.

• **Feverfew has been used for centuries to prevent and relieve migraine.** Studies show that it can reduce migraine frequency and severity.

Try: A total of 50 mg to 125 mg/day (tablet or capsule) divided into three doses. Feverfew thins blood—don't take it if you are on aspirin therapy or take a blood thinner such as *warfarin* (Coumadin). Also avoid it if you are allergic to ragweed. Other side effects include joint aches and gastrointestinal disturbances.

NERVE STIMULATION

The FDA recently approved Cefaly, a noninvasive nerve stimulator that looks like a headband and is worn across the forehead. It delivers tiny, painless electrical pulses to the upper branch of the trigeminal nerve—the nerve responsible for sensations in your face and head. When inflamed, the trigeminal nerve overresponds to stimuli, possibly causing migraine pain.

Theory: Repeated pinging with electrical pulses might make the trigeminal nerve less sensitive to stimulation. In a recent Italian study, using Cefaly 20 minutes daily for four months reduced migraine frequency by more than 50%.

The device costs $349, plus $25 for three sets of electrodes (each set lasts about one month), and can be ordered online at Cefaly.us. It requires a prescription from your doctor and may not be covered by insurance. (Cefaly should not be used if you have a cardiac pacemaker, an implanted or wearable defibrillator, an implanted metallic or electronic device in your head or have pain of unknown origin.)

NEW HOPE FOR A CURE

New research shows that calcitonin gene-related peptide (CGRP), a strong vasodilator produced in neurons involved in the transmission of pain, could trigger and maintain migraines. During a migraine headache, CGRP binds to receptors in the trigeminal nerve. In recent clinical trials, an antibody treatment that blocks the activity of CGRP modestly reduced the number of days per month that patients were disabled by migraine and even eliminated migraines for up to 15% of patients. The treatment could become available as an injection later this year.

Headache When Bending Down...

Alan M. Rapoport, MD, clinical professor of neurology, David Geffen School of Medicine at UCLA, Los Angeles, and immediate past president of the International Headache Society.

Anytime someone has a headache or increased pressure in the head from bending, coughing or straining in some way, that person should be evaluated by a physician, who may recommend a neurological consultation and/or an MRI.

Although it is unlikely that there is any serious problem going on, especially if you have no other symptoms such as nausea, visual problems or severe pain, a doctor can assess whether there is some change in pressure in the brain upon changing head position.

Irregularities in cerebral spinal fluid pressure, lack of cerebral spinal fluid flow or structural abnormalities in the back of the brain all can be possible problems.

The good news is that most of the time nothing serious is found after a thorough evaluation from a doctor.

It is possible that the pain, pressure or lightheadedness you feel is due to a sinus problem. Or your symptoms might be a sign of high or low blood pressure, which can be easily treated with medication and lifestyle changes.

Go ahead and make an appointment to see your doctor so that you can find out what's going on.

What a Tender Temple Could Mean

Alan M. Rapoport, MD, clinical professor of neurology, David Geffen School of Medicine at UCLA, Los Angeles, and immediate past president of the International Headache Society.

Tenderness of the temple that's accompanied by symptoms such as headache, scalp tenderness, fever, pain in the jaw when chewing, fatigue, weight loss and vision loss can signal a condition known as giant cell arteritis (GCA)—sometimes referred to as temporal arteritis.

Most common in people over age 50, this inflammatory condition typically affects the temporal artery but can affect other medium- and large-sized arteries throughout the body as well, especially those within the brain and eye. The cause of this condition is inflammation in the lining of the arteries, but the reason for the inflammation is not known.

If GCA is untreated, it can lead to devastating, irreversible consequences including stroke, permanent vision loss, damage or rupture of the aorta and even death.

Important: You should see your doctor right away for a thorough evaluation. This exam typically includes a blood test to measure a marker of inflammation (erythrocyte sedimentation rate, or ESR), which may be followed by a biopsy from the temporal artery.

GCA is treated with corticosteroids. If it's treated promptly, most people with GCA recover fully, but relapses are common.

How to Relieve Shoulder Pain Without Surgery

Beth E. Shubin Stein, MD, associate attending orthopedic surgeon and a member of the Sports Medicine Service at Hospital for Special Surgery in New York City.

The shoulder is the most movable and complex joint in the human body. And it's basically unstable.

Imagine a golf ball perched on a tee. That's your shoulder. The humerus (upper arm bone) is the ball and the scapula (shoulder blade) is the tee. It doesn't take much to knock them apart.

So it's no wonder that as you get older, normal wear and tear often leads to shoulder pain. You might notice the discomfort while serving a tennis ball, reaching for a jar on a shelf, carrying a heavy suitcase or simply putting on a sweater or fastening a bra. The most likely culprits...

Impingement: The rotator cuff, a collection of muscles and tendons surrounding the humerus, gets pinched between that bone and the scapula.

Frozen shoulder: Tissue around the shoulder joint gets inflamed and stiff.

Tendinitis: Rotator cuff tendons become inflamed or irritated.

Bursitis: Tiny fluid-filled sacs (called bursa) that act as a gliding surface to reduce friction between shoulder tissues become inflamed.

Each condition is caused by inflammation, often as a response to tiny injuries that you didn't notice when they happened. Each can get so painful that surgery seems like a good idea. But why go through that discomfort, recuperation and expense if you can avoid it?

Surprising truth: With pain management and physical therapy, two-thirds of patients get better on their own.

But if your shoulder is bothering you, that doesn't mean you can just do nothing. Your pain will continue and even may intensify the next time you overstress the shoulder. Worse yet, you could get a rotator cuff tear, which definitely requires surgery and then four to six months of recovery.

To learn the best way to avoid shoulder surgery, we interviewed orthopedic surgeon Beth E. Shubin Stein, MD. *Her advice...*

If you feel pain in a shoulder and your movement is restricted, see an orthopedist right away to rule out a rotator cuff tear. As long as your rotator cuff is intact, you have a very good chance of making your shoulder feel better and avoiding surgery if you, in consultation with your doctor, follow these steps.

MANAGE YOUR PAIN

The first step is to manage your pain so that you can start physical therapy. Ice your shoulder for 20 minutes at a time, two or three times a day. Also, take a nonsteroidal anti-inflammatory drug (NSAID), either over-the-counter or prescription, to reduce inflammation and pain (don't exceed the recommended dosage).

If that's not enough to ease pain and allow exercise, your doctor can give you a cortisone shot. It's a potent anti-inflammatory, but repeated shots can limit a tendon's healing ability.

My protocol: If a first cortisone shot works for two months or more and you can exercise, I typically recommend a second shot and continuing physical therapy.

But if the first cortisone shot doesn't ease pain and allow exercise, I offer patients platelet-rich plasma (PRP) injections ($1,000 to $2,500). It's experimental and generally not covered by insurance. If PRP doesn't work, another option is to use donor stem cells from amniotic membranes to help regenerate tendon tissues. This can be about twice as expensive as PRP, and insurance most likely won't cover it either. These treatments don't work for everyone, but if they do, shoulder discomfort should subside within three days to a week.

Tip: You also may want to consider acupuncture as a complement to any of the above approaches.

Once pain isn't holding you back, it's time to get your shoulder moving. You can complete this stretching/strengthening program in 15 minutes. Do it twice a week. It's also great for anyone who wants to avoid shoulder problems.

Important: You should never feel pain when doing either stretching or strengthening exercises.

These exercises might sound like a lot of work, especially if you've become accustomed to avoiding using your shoulder because of pain. But take it from someone who both performs necessary shoulder surgery and does my best to help patients avoid it—it's well worth the effort to avoid the knife. I do these exercises myself two or three times a week—I've had shoulder pain in the past, but these exercises let me stay strong and pain-free.

EXERCISE STEP 1: GET LIMBER.

Much of the work of supporting the shoulder falls to the rotator cuff. *These stretches improve rotator cuff flexibility and support normal range of motion...*

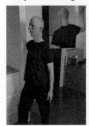

•**Wall crawl.** Stand facing a wall. Place the palm of one hand in front of your chest and "walk" it upward along the wall. Go as high as you can without feeling pain, hold for three to five seconds, and walk your hand back down. Do five to 10 repetitions. Switch hands and repeat.

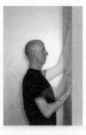

•**Doorway stretch.** Stand in an open doorway, and place your right hand flat against the wall next to the right side of the doorway frame at shoulder height, with your elbow bent. Keeping your right hand in place, step forward with your right foot, bending your right knee (as in a lunge), with your left leg stretched behind you. You should feel a stretch in your shoulder but not any pain. Hold for three to five seconds, and do five to 10 repetitions. Repeat with the left arm on the left side of the doorway and left foot stepping forward.

•**Side stretch.** Lie on your side on the floor (on an exercise mat or rug), your painful shoulder on the floor and your head supported on a pillow or bolster so that your spine is in a straight line. Bend the arm that's on the floor at the elbow, with the forearm and hand raised and palm facing your feet. Now use your other hand to gently push the wrist of the bent arm toward the floor. Hold for three seconds and release. Do a total of 10 reps. Repeat with your other arm.

STEP 2: STRENGTHEN THE RIGHT MUSCLES

While impingement, frozen shoulder, tendinitis, and bursitis often are referred to as overuse issues, I prefer to call them "understrength" issues. The problem isn't the 100 times you serve during a typical tennis match—it's that your muscles aren't strong enough to handle the stress you're placing on them. Even people who lift weights often focus on the biceps and triceps and ignore the rotator cuff.

Caution: Stay away from military presses and other exercises that require you to lift weights overhead—that can injure your shoulder. Skip kettle bells, too—they require swinging that can inflame your shoulder.

My recommendation: To build the strength of your rotator cuffs, use resistance bands, which do the job and are safer. *Try these three stability builders...*

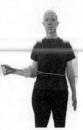

•**External rotation.** Loop a resistance band at waist height around a secure anchor such as the base of equipment at a gym or a strong door handle of a locked door at home. Standing sideways to the anchor, grab both ends of the band with one hand so it's taut. Keep your elbow bent and against your side and your hand near your stomach. Now pull the band away from your stomach, keeping your elbow against your side, until you feel light tension on the outside of the shoulder.

Hint: Your shoulder blade should move toward your spine. Hold for one second. Do a total of 10 reps. Repeat with your other arm.

•**Internal rotation.** This is the reverse of the external rotation. Keep the resistance band looped around a secure anchor, and stand in the same position as above. But this time, grab the band with the hand that is closest to where it's anchored. Keeping your elbow bent and at or near your side, pull the band across your torso toward your belly button. Hold for one second. Do a total of 10 reps. Repeat with your other arm.

•**Rowing.** With the elastic band securely anchored as above, grab one end of the band in each hand so it's taut. Pull both arms back, bending your elbows and keeping them close to your sides. Hold for one second. Do a total of 10 reps. Repeat with your other arm.

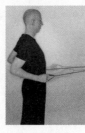

Is Your Back Pain an Imposter?

Stuart M. Goldman, DPM, a podiatrist in private practice in Baltimore who specializes in nonsurgical treatment of pain. Board-certified by the American Board of Foot and Ankle Surgery and a Fellow of the American College of Foot and Ankle Surgeons, he is author of *Walking Well Again: Neutralize the Hidden Causes of Pain.*

"**B**aby boomer back" is the nickname doctors have for lumbar spinal stenosis. That's because the condition mainly strikes adults over age 50. But even people in their 70s and up—or those only in their 20s—can be afflicted by spinal stenosis, a condition in which the spinal canal narrows and may compress the spinal cord or spinal nerves.

The symptoms are unpleasant, to say the least—low back, leg or foot pain that worsens when walking or standing, along with weakness, burning and/or tingling in the affected areas.

The first line of defense is usually pain medication—a nonsteroidal anti-inflammatory drug (NSAID), such as *ibuprofen* (Motrin), or nerve pain medication such as *gabapentin* (Neurontin). If that doesn't ratchet down the pain, the next step may be physical therapy, cortisone injections and/or back surgery to alleviate pressure on the spinal nerve roots.

The problem is, these treatments don't always work, and when they do, the relief may last only months, weeks or, in some cases, just days. Surgery can fail and, of course, it carries the risk for infection, blood clots and damage to structures, including nerves.

Surprising discovery: In many patients diagnosed with spinal stenosis, the symptoms are actually caused by pseudostenosis. This condition, in which the lower body structures (from feet to hip bones) are not functioning perfectly, can cause positional changes of the spine that exert pressure on bone structures or nerves, causing symptoms identical to those of spinal stenosis.

The tricky part is that an MRI may, in fact, reveal spinal stenosis—the two conditions often occur simultaneously. In my practice, I've found that pseudostenosis contributes to more than half of spinal stenosis cases.

Pseudostenosis is not a well-known concept—as a result, it is not considered by most doctors. Although the pain is coming through the spine, the actual cause is the poor function of the lower extremities. This is why standard treatments for spinal stenosis may be doomed to fail in these cases, even if they are done extremely well. Note: Pseudostenosis can also occur on its own, even if spinal imaging (such as an MRI or a CT scan) is negative.

Good news: Based on my clinical experience, 70% of patients with pseudostenosis experience near-complete relief of symptoms often within a day or two by making a few simple positional changes. If someone does not improve within two days, it means that the treatment did not properly address the true cause of pain.

DISCOVERING THE REAL CAUSE

Pseudostenosis has several causes. The most common are limb length discrepancy (one leg is shorter than the other) and flexible flat feet (the arch flattens when you step down). Other culprits may be any pain-inducing condition that affects the way a person walks. This may include arthritis of the feet, ankles, knees or hips…imperfect walking because of a nerve problem due to stroke or multiple sclerosis…tightness of the Achilles tendons…or a rigid flat foot.

Each of these conditions can affect your body in a way that mimics the effects of spinal stenosis, and more than one may be present at the same time, even if the patient is not aware of it. *Here's what you can do about the most common causes of pseudostenosis…*

•**Limb length discrepancy (LLD).** Either limb may be structurally shorter than the other, or one limb may function as if it is shorter, often because of an injury. Most people are unaware of the difference.

Red flags: With LLD, standing may cause more back and/or leg pain and leg tiredness than walking. To alleviate symptoms, people with LLD often feel the need to periodically "shake a leg" or shift their weight from side to side when standing. Even a mild LLD of 2 mm to 3 mm can cause symptoms.

Another sign of LLD: You have asymmetric wear-and-tear of your shoes. Often the wear is worse on the outer heel of your shoe worn on the shorter leg.

Quick test that may suggest LLD: Stand in front of a tall mirror, and look to see if your head tilts to one side and/or if your shoulders and hips are not horizontal. This asymmetry may be seen with either an LLD or scoliosis, which often occur together. (Wearing horizontal stripes and a belt makes the assessment easier.)

Next, put on a pair of shorts and stand in front of a long mirror to look at your legs. An LLD will often cause the foot of the longer leg to turn out more than the other. Then check your feet. Each leg may have different foot deformities, such as bunions, hammertoes, calluses or a flat foot.

How to treat LLD: A lift in the shoe of the shorter leg may quickly improve pseudostenosis symptoms. Don't go for the one-size-fits-all, shock-absorbing pharmacy inserts. A customized heel lift is critical in treating LLD. And no one will even notice that you're using it.

Websites such as GWHeelLift.com…and my site, WalkingWellAgain.com, offer solid heel lifts made of 1-mm to 12-mm durable plastic that can be stacked to achieve the perfect height.

Helpful: You can slip the heel lift under your shoe's insert to keep it in place.

•**Flexible flat feet.** Flexible flat feet are another common cause of pseudostenosis. This condition is usually easier to treat than rigid flat feet. If your foot has an arch when you're sitting but flattens out when standing, you have a flexible flat foot.

To test yourself for flexible flat feet: Take off your shoes and socks. If you have an arch when sitting, wet your foot and step on a brown grocery store bag. If the entire sole makes a print, that means that the arch has flattened, and you have a flexible flat foot.

How to treat flexible flat feet: Both orthotics and braces are available. Orthotics are custom-designed inserts that fit entirely inside a shoe. Ankle braces include a custom foot insert as well as an extension that goes above the ankle to increase stability.

To determine if orthotic control can help, a podiatrist may apply a tape strapping to your feet to control the foot function. If done well, it may simulate the effects of custom orthotics. The Unna Boot, a type of compression bandage that is embedded with zinc oxide paste to make it more supportive, can test for more aggressive control, such as a custom brace. Patients wanting to try self-taping may use Quick Tape, available at SupportTheFoot.com.

If symptoms improve with the tape strapping, podiatrist-fitted orthotics are the go-to treatment. Custom orthotics usually cost hundreds of dollars and are often not covered by insurance. If cost is a factor, excellent over-the-counter (OTC) orthotics are available from Vasyli Medical, at Amazon.com or from a distributor at VasyliMedical.com. Even though OTC orthotics are not necessarily as effective as custom devices, they sometimes do help and cost less than $100. Ankle braces are usually covered by health insurance.

With either heel lifts for LLD or supportive orthotics or braces for flexible flat feet, long-term treatment is often needed.

Takeaway: If you've been diagnosed with spinal stenosis, and your symptoms did not improve or returned after treatment, consider consulting a podiatrist to see whether pseudostenosis may be the real problem. To find a podiatrist near you, get a referral from your physician or check the website of the American Podiatric Medical Association, APMA.org.

Hidden Causes of Peripheral Neuropathy

Janice F. Wiesman, MD, FAAN, associate clinical professor of neurology at New York University School of Medicine and adjunct assistant professor of neurology at Boston University School of Medicine. She is also the author of *Peripheral Neuropathy: What It Is and What You Can Do to Feel Better.*

Tingling, burning, numbness and weakness. The symptoms of peripheral neuropathy are usually obvious, painful—and potentially debilitating. Yet the disorder is not always easy to diagnose.

About 20 million people in the US have peripheral neuropathy, a condition caused by damage to the peripheral nervous system. Most of these cases are linked to diabetes. But there are millions of other people who suffer from this condition and don't know why.

In fact, for about 30% of people with peripheral neuropathy, the cause remains mysterious. In these cases, it's diagnosed as "idiopathic" neuropathy—the same as saying "unknown cause."

The problem: Without identifying and treating the underlying cause of peripheral neuropathy, the symptoms will only get worse. At its most extreme, neuropathy can lead to difficulty standing or walking, as well as nonstop agony from dying nerves. While symptoms can be treated without knowing the cause, addressing the root of the problem is far more effective and may eliminate the neuropathy.

THE BASICS

Our peripheral nerves are in constant communication with our central nervous system (brain and spinal cord). Communication signals are transmitted to and from the central nervous system and all the distant (peripheral) parts of the body, such as the hands and feet.

Peripheral neuropathy occurs when the peripheral nerves become damaged—as a result of diabetes…or a less commonly recognized issue (see examples below). Those impaired nerves send pain or pins-and-needles tingling sensations…or they can fail to transmit physical signals, leading to numbness or muscle weakness. There's also the risk for injury when damaged nerves prevent you from feeling pain in dangerous situations.

THE BEST-KNOWN CULPRIT

Most people realize that neuropathy is commonly caused by diabetes (type 1 or type 2). It accounts for nearly two-thirds of all peripheral neuropathy cases. What happens: High blood sugar damages cells lining the blood vessels that transport nutrients and oxygen to body cells, which in turn harms nerves.

What you may not realize: When it comes to peripheral neuropathy, prediabetes (a precursor to diabetes) may be just as hazardous as full-blown diabetes. Nerve cell damage starts early. About 20% of patients newly diagnosed with diabetes already have neuropathy.

SURPRISING CAUSES

Besides diabetes, dozens of conditions can lead to neuropathy, including some that primary care physicians often don't consider, such as…

•**Celiac disease.** This autoimmune disorder causes the body to mount a powerful defense against gluten, a protein found in wheat, rye and barley. Eat a slice of wheat bread, and the body creates antibodies that attack the small intestine. The antibodies also cause general inflammation, which is thought to cause nerve damage.

Important: Neuropathy may be an early sign of celiac disease. And contrary to common belief, it can begin at any age. Celiac disease should always be considered when peripheral neuropathy is present. A blood test can be used to check for celiac antibodies. If tingling and numbness improve after going gluten-free, it's likely that celiac is the cause of the neuropathy.

•**Bariatric surgery.** Bariatric surgery for extreme weight loss is becoming more common, but it can cause a vitamin deficiency. This is partly because the surgery alters the digestive system in a way that can prevent nutrients from being properly absorbed. For example, some surgeries remove the part of the stomach responsible for creating a protein called intrinsic factor, which allows the body to absorb vitamin B-12. Severe B-12 deficiency leads to neuropathy.

Important: Neuropathy due to vitamin B-12 deficiency is also more common in people who follow a strict vegan or vegetarian diet. Long-term use of the medications metformin (for blood sugar control) or proton pump inhibitors (for acid reflux) also block B-12 absorption. A fasting blood test can determine your B-12 level. If it's less than 200 pg/mL, a B-12 deficiency may be causing your neuropathy.

•**Kidney disease.** If your kidneys can't properly filter toxins from your blood, the buildup of toxins can harm your nerves. Left untreated, even mild chronic kidney disease can result in peripheral neuropathy. Kidney disease is diagnosed with blood and urine tests.

•**Hepatitis C.** This virus causes white blood cells to create substances in the blood called cryoglobulins, abnormal proteins that damage nerve cells. A blood test can determine if you have hepatitis C.

•**Paraneoplastic syndrome.** When battling cancer, our bodies create antibodies to the cancer cells. Paraneoplastic neuropathy occurs when there is a cross-reaction between tumor cells and components of the nervous system. It can come on quickly, progress rapidly and is often extremely painful. Important: In some cases, neuropathy may be the first outward sign of cancer—and may be a vital diagnostic clue. This is especially true with lung cancer.

Since there are so many conditions that can cause neuropathy, in most cases your physician will determine the cause only after a thorough medical exam and after ruling out unlikely conditions.

WHAT YOU CAN DO

Neuropathy damage isn't necessarily permanent. Our bodies naturally repair our nerve cells all the time. However, the only way to halt the damage and repair your nerves is to get control over the original disease process. For diabetes, maintain tight control over blood sugar levels...for celiac disease, avoid gluten...seek care for kidney disease or hepatitis C...and get appropriate medical vitamin supplementation for a B-12 deficiency. Unfortunately, treating cancer with chemotherapy may cause neuropathy, which may improve if the chemotherapy regimen is changed.

If you smoke: Neuropathy is one more reason to quit. Nicotine constricts blood vessels, which can starve nerves of the oxygen they need and increase injury to nerves that are already damaged.

Also: Alcohol is one of the most common causes of neuropathy in the US. If you drink heavily or have neuropathy due to an underlying condition, cut down on alcohol use or stop drinking altogether.

The Right Moves to Fight Your Pain

Vicky Saliba Johnson, PT, FFFMT, FAAOMPT, cofounder of The Institute of Physical Art, an international post-professional continuing-education organization in Steamboat Springs, Colorado. She is a contributing author to *Orthopaedic Manual Physical Therapy: From Art to Evidence*.

If you have nagging joint pain in your hip or shoulder or suffer from mobility problems due to a neurological condition, such as Parkinson's disease or complications from a stroke, there is an approach used by physical therapists that you should know about...but probably don't.

Its official name, proprioceptive neuromuscular facilitation, is a bit of a mouthful, so it's known simply as PNF.

How PNF works: PNF-trained physical therapists use the brain and nervous system's complex feedback system to facilitate optimum patterns of movement and posture. The key to PNF is using the input from the skin, muscles and other sensory organs to influence the brain's ability to activate the right muscles and movement patterns, especially the proprioceptors, which tell the brain where your body is in space.

With PNF, practitioners observe and assess how problems in a patient's posture (such as a forward head position due to computer use) and/or movement such as walking without properly engaging the pelvis and trunk, may be causing or worsening an underlying condition. Performed repeatedly, such postures and movements not only place undue stress on our fascia (connective tissue) muscles and joints but also become ingrained in our "muscle memory." Eventually, these ingrained patterns can lead to pain and injury.

Once the problem is identified by the PNF-trained physical therapist, he/she designs a plan to retrain the patient's brain and body to move in safer, more effective ways.

This plan combines specific positioning with manual resistance and active stretching to remind the brain of the healthy alignment it used to know—before it was compromised by injury, disease or repetitive poor movements.

How PNF has evolved: The technique was originally developed in the 1940s by neurophysiologist and medical neurologist Dr. Herman Kabat and physical therapist Maggie Knott to address postural control and movement deficiencies in patients with neurological disorders. The practice later expanded to include head injuries, Parkinson's disease and more.

Over time, PNF has become an approach used for all patients, including orthopedic patients with knee, hip, neck, shoulder and ankle pain. More physical therapists are seeking this specialized training.

Scientific evidence: An important study published in the *Journal of Human Kinetics* found that PNF improves range of motion and increases muscle strength—both of which play a significant role in curbing pain and improving mobility.

How PNF may help you…

HANDS THAT HEAL

At the root of PNF theory is a principle called "overflow." When an area of the body has physical pressure applied to it with appropriate resistance and with proper manual contact, the brain responds by sending neurological impulses to the muscles of that area.

If the therapist continues to apply the appropriate amount of pressure over time, these impulses begin to overflow into the nerves that stimulate other muscles. PNF allows the therapist to direct this overflow to the weaker or inhibited muscles.

For example, a patient who has suffered a stroke or spinal cord injury may find it difficult to simply turn over in bed. In this case, the physical therapist might resist the hip flexors or shoulder extensors, which tend to be stronger, and direct the overflow toward the person's core muscles, which are probably weak as a result of the neurological event. Eventually, the brain will remember what it used to do to direct the body to roll over.

The length of treatment and the patient's ability to participate are dependent upon the injury and the patient's mental capacity. Most patients are given a home program for repetition to promote motor learning. An orthopedic patient with no neurological damage may need only a few treatment sessions. Patients who have neurological issues will require more sessions. Some insurance plans cover the cost of treatment.

IS PNF FOR YOU?

There are easy tests you can do on your own to help you determine whether you're a candidate for PNF. *For example, you can try the following if you are affected by…*

• **Low-back pain.** Try standing on one leg at a time. If you feel that you do not have good balance or your back arches while trying to stand on one leg, you are probably not using your pelvis to effectively connect your core to your legs. The low-back pain you are feeling is being aggravated with every step you take when your core is disconnected from your legs.

• **Shoulder pain.** Stand with your back against a wall. Press your lower back against the wall, then your middle and upper back. Now pull your shoulder blades together and rotate your palms forward. You should be able to keep your back flat against the wall.

If your back begins to arch as you do this, it indicates one of two things: Poor range of motion is compromising your ability to move the shoulder blade on the rib cage…or the brain cannot properly connect with the muscles needed to move the shoulder blade on the rib cage. In either case, a PNF-trained physical therapist will restore the brain's ability to connect with the muscles and create appropriate positioning of the shoulder blade.

• **Stroke.** If you have been discharged from medical care but everyday activities, such as getting out of bed or walking short distances, still feel challenging, PNF could help.

PNF is always done in conjunction with other physical therapy techniques. Depending on the problem, acupuncture and acupressure might also be appropriate.

To find a PNF clinician near you: Consult The Institute of Physical Art (InstituteofPhysical Art.com), which provides certification that ensures each certified therapist (CFMT) uses PNF in the most effective manner.

---

6 Common Stretching Mistakes That Can Hurt You

Karl Knopf, EdD, director of fitness therapy and senior fitness for the International Sports Sciences Association and retired director of adaptive fitness at Foothill College in Los Altos Hills, California. He is author of many fitness books including *Stretching for 50+* and a board member of Sit and Be Fit, a nonprofit organization dedicated to healthy aging.

W e now know that stretching is key to staying limber and flexible. But did you know that it also could be dangerous?

Many people stretch improperly, overstressing muscles and even tendons in ways that lead to strains and sprains. An injury can come on gradually as a result of cumulative "insults" from performing a stretch a certain way over and over again. You don't know you're hurting yourself…until you're really hurt.

Other people don't stretch wrong—they just don't stretch at all or only once in a while. Many people focus more on cardiovascular exercise and weight training, yet often neglect stretching—until they get hurt. To benefit from a flexibility program, you need to practice it regularly, ideally every day.

As we age, stretching becomes even more important. Our bodies undergo changes that result in lack of elasticity. Women tend to be more flexible than men, but starting in their 50s, both genders start to lose flexibility and range of motion, especially in the shoulders and low back, which can lead to shoulder and back issues. The good news is that this age-related decline can be slowed through a regular stretching program.

By learning to stretch properly, you'll maximize your mobility…greatly reduce the risk for pain and injury…perform better at any sport you engage in…and look younger. (One caution: If you've had a recent fracture, sprain, injury or surgery, or if you suspect that you have osteoporosis, speak to your doctor/physical therapist first.)

Here are common stretching mistakes that can hurt you—and how to steer clear of them…

HOLDING YOUR BREATH

One common stretching mistake is holding your breath as you hold a stretch. Muscles need oxygen throughout a stretch—plus, holding your breath can elevate your blood pressure. Breathe slowly and consistently throughout each phase of a stretch—especially when you're holding one.

Simple stretches, such as shoulder rolls (see "Safe, Effective Stretches You Can Do Anywhere" on the next page), don't require that you hold them. But most do. These stretches should be held for at least 20 seconds—and recent studies suggest that for older adults, 60 seconds is even better. Breathe throughout.

STRETCHING COLD

Not that long ago, we were instructed to stretch before playing sports when our muscles were "cold." Now we know that's a bad idea. Think of your muscles and tendons as taffy. Then imagine trying to stretch and bend cold taffy. It can snap. On a micro level, that's like stretching a cold, tight muscle. Ouch!

Much better: Warm up for five minutes or more first, before you do any stretch that you hold. Try light running…a few minutes in a steam room or sauna…or, if you're home, a warm bath.

GETTING INTENSE

Too many people follow the old paradigm that the more intense the exercise, the better. They overdo it with weights, aerobics—and stretching. In my opinion, no pain, no gain is…insane. If you feel sore a few hours after exercising, you overdid it.

Much better: When stretching, move slowly and gently, and stay within your comfort zone. You should feel mild tension in your muscles and joints. Don't push past it. Listen to your body, especially your neck, back, shoulders and knees. If you have tightness or joint pain, take some time off. If it continues, see your doctor or a physical therapist before it turns into a real issue.

GOING OLD SCHOOL—FAST AND BOUNCY

If you played a sport in high school, it's time to unlearn some things you learned, including bouncing toe touches. These moves weren't safe then, and they are even riskier now that you're older. Those neck circles you started every gym class with? Terrible! They strain supporting ligaments and can lead to pinched nerves.

That hurdler stretch where you sit with one leg out in front of you and the other bent behind you? It stresses the meniscus and the medial collateral ligament of your knee—an injury in the making. Windmill toe touches? No! Bending and rotating at the same time is a recipe for trouble.

Red flag: Avoid stretches such as the hurdler that make your knees twist or move in an unnatural position. Be careful about back bends that call for you to raise both hands over your head and lean back. That can pinch the facet joints of the spine.

Much better: Always keep knees "soft" (slightly bent) when stretching. When turning, move your body slowly, as a unit, and pivot your feet.

STRETCHING ONLY WHEN YOU EXERCISE

Chances are that if you stretch, you do so only before working out or playing a sport. Big mistake! To maintain flexibility, your muscles need to be worked just about every day.

Much better: Think of stretching as part of your daily routine, like brushing your teeth. You don't need a designated area or even to wear gym clothes. Spend a few minutes doing a body-flexibility session daily, especially in high-risk areas such as the hamstrings, shoulders and lower back.

NOT BEING WELL-BALANCED

The body is designed with opposing muscle groups, and each group needs to be worked equally. Weight training can unbalance muscles, so you need stretching to get you back into balance.

Example: If you do a movement such as a bench press that rolls your shoulders forward, you should do a stretch that pulls them back. My golden rule is, Do unto the front as you do unto the back, and do unto the left as you do unto the right.

Conversely, being too flexible can be a problem, especially if you don't have muscles that are strong enough to support your joints. I once taught a dancer who kept dislocating her shoulder joints because her muscles weren't strong enough to keep her shoulders in place. It's all about balance.

One final tip—enjoy your stretching session. It's a great time to integrate the mind and the body.

SAFE, EFFECTIVE STRETCHES YOU CAN DO ANYWHERE

Here are two different kinds of stretches—no-hold stretches that you can do anywhere anytime and standard stretches for which you warm up for five minutes and then hold for at least 20 seconds, ideally 60.

Together, these stretches work on your upper and lower body. Repeat each one at least three times.

Upper-body no-hold stretches…

•**Elbow touches (for the chest).** Place your hands on your shoulders (left on left, right on right), elbows pointing forward as much as possible. Slowly move your elbows out to the side as far as is comfortable, pinching the shoulder blades together, and hold for just a few seconds. Bring your elbows back to the starting position and repeat.

•**Shoulder rolls (for the upper back).** With your arms hanging down naturally, shrug your shoulders up and squeeze them back, as if attempting to touch them together…then relax them.

•**Apple pickers (for the shoulders).** Place your hands on your shoulders (left hand on left, right on right). Then slowly raise your right hand as high up as is comfortable—reach for that apple! Return to the start position, and repeat with the left hand. Keep good posture throughout.

These are standard "hold 'em" stretches…

•**Chest stretch (for the chest and shoulders).** Stand facing a corner. Place one hand on each side wall, with your elbows in a push-up position. Lean gently into the corner until you feel a stretch across your upper chest. Hold for at least 20 seconds.

●**Seated knee to chest (for the lower back and gluteal muscles/butt).** Sit on a stable chair with your feet flat on the floor. Clasp your hands beneath your left leg. Pull your left knee toward your chest with your hands and hold for at least 20 seconds, feeling the stretch in the gluteal and low-back area. Return to start position, and repeat with other leg.

●**Rear calf stretch (for your calves).** Stand facing a wall, with both hands on the wall at shoulder height. Your knees should be slightly bent. Keeping the heel down, slide your right leg back until you feel the stretch in the calf area. Hold for at least 20 seconds. Switch sides and repeat.

Joint-Friendly Advice

Anjum Lone, OTR/L, CHT, PM&R manager, occupational therapy, Phelps Memorial Hospital Center, Sleepy Hollow, New York.

I have arthritis in my hands. How can I avoid overusing my joints to minimize pain and stiffness?

Don't engage in exercise that involves your hands when the joints are inflamed. *Also helpful…*

●**Lift items with both hands** even if you're strong enough to use one.

●**Avoid carrying items with your fingers.**
Example: Loop handles of shopping bags over your forearm instead of carrying them with your fingers.

●**Opt for "joint-friendly" tools**—a brush for washing dishes (it's easier on hands than a dishcloth)…large nail clippers (easier to grip than small ones)…and spring-loaded scissors.

●**Rest your hands periodically when typing, working in the yard, etc.** Also, avoid repetitive motions and switch tasks often.

Skimping on Rehab Can Lead to Arthritis

Joseph M. Hart, PhD, associate professor of kinesiology at University of Virginia Curry School of Education in Charlottesville.

If you suffer a serious injury to a joint, there's a good chance that more bad news lies ahead—but you can avoid that if you know what researchers recently discovered about joint injuries.

Not only are joints that have been injured often later reinjured—these joints also face substantially increased risk for painful and potentially debilitating osteoarthritis. The new research found, for example, that people with a history of knee injuries are three to six times more likely to develop osteoarthritis in the injured knee than people with no history of knee problems. Osteoarthritis is especially likely if you rush back to your previous level of activity after an injury, short-circuiting the rehabilitation needed to allow the joint to heal fully. The knee is not the only trouble spot—injuries to hips, shoulders and ankles also have been linked to significantly increased risk for osteoarthritis.

Sustaining a serious injury to a joint can destabilize the joint…weaken the muscles surrounding it…and/or alter the way you use the joint during activity, leading to greatly accelerated cartilage wear. That's why adequate recovery, including a rehabilitation program to strengthen the muscles that support the injured joint, is crucial.

What to do: If you sustain an injury to a joint, ask your doctor about a physical therapy program and then stick with this physical therapy program for its entire recommended duration even if the joint has stopped hurting.

Ask your doctor or physical therapist what types of exercise are safe for the joint while it still is recovering, prior to returning to unrestricted physical activity.

Finally, if you have suffered a major knee-joint injury, have the joint and surrounding muscles reevaluated by a physical therapist, athletic trainer or sports medicine professional prior to returning to full activity levels and periodically in the years following your injury—even if it feels as good as new. There might be lingering issues such as muscle weakness or altered movement patterns that are too subtle for you to notice but that could increase your risk for osteoarthritis.

Knee Pain: 7 Things You're Doing That Make It Worse, Not Better

Nicholas A. Sgaglione, MD, director of the Northwell Health Orthopaedic Institute and chair and professor of orthopaedic surgery at the Donald and Barbara Zucker School of Medicine at Hofstra/Northwell, Hempstead, New York.

Sure, we put a lot of demand on our knees, but knee pain is not an inevitable part of aging.

Yes, over time, wear and tear can lead to arthritis or cartilage problems and, as it progresses, pain, but you can prevent a lot of damage to your knees by avoiding these common lifestyle mistakes, explained Nicholas Sgaglione, MD, director of the Northwell Health Orthopaedic Institute, who has spent 30 years caring for patients' knees.

1. Putting on pounds. With every step, skip and jump you take, your knees absorb the force of your body's weight. Each pound you gain adds exponentially to the amount of pressure exerted on your knees. In fact, each extra pound adds about four pounds of pressure. So if you've gained 20 pounds over the last few years, they feel more like 80 pounds to your knees.

There are three causes of knee problems—injuries, breakdown (of cartilage and other tissues) and deconditioning, the loss of strength in the muscles surrounding the joint. Being overweight puts you at risk for all three. As the obesity epidemic has increased in the US, so has the rate of knee problems. It's all about load on the knee. So the first mistake to avoid is putting on weight. And if you weigh more than you should, use diet and exercise to lose the extra pounds—it's never too late as far as your knees are concerned.

2. Getting weak in the knees. As important as your knee joints are, they depend on surrounding muscles for support. Deconditioning, which leaves knees weak and wobbly, is a setup for knee problems. Avoid this mistake by doing twice-weekly strengthening exercises that target the muscles in the fronts of your thighs (quadriceps), the backs of your thighs (hamstrings), your hips and your core.

Options include weight machines and resistance exercises. The best choice for you depends on your current fitness level and the health status of your knees. A physical therapist or orthopedist can tailor a program for you and show you how to do the exercises correctly so that you won't hurt yourself. Start slowly and progress slowly.

3. Letting your knees get stiff. Stiffness, or the lack of flexibility, does tend to come with age if you don't take steps to preserve it. Flexibility helps protect your knees from injury. Once you lose flexibility, it's hard to get it back. The answer is to stretch the muscles that support your knees through their range of motion. Just as with strengthening exercises, an exercise specialist can design a flexibility program for you and teach you the right way to stretch if you're unsure of where to start. Stretching incorrectly, such as not taking time to warm up (with light exercise) first, can cause damage. Also, avoid holding stretches for too long (no more than 30 to 40 seconds) and avoid bouncing. Make flexibility training a part of your daily workout.

4. Doing too much too soon. It's great to get started enthusiastically with exercise, but going from 0 to 60—trying to get into shape too fast or overtraining—is a recipe for an overload injury, particularly of the knees. This could happen if you've put on a few pounds and haven't been active in a while, yet go on vacation and play three hours of tennis or 36 holes of golf right off the bat. Don't exercise binge! Getting back into shape takes time. If you've planned an action vacation (or even one that involves a lot of walking), start scaling in right away. Don't wait until you're on vacation to start getting into shape.

5. Being a slave to shoe fashion. One way to help your knees is to add shock-absorbing cushioning to your footwear. Instead of seeing your shoes as a fashion statement, think of them as extra treads for your tires. This is especially important if you already have knee issues. If you need to wear dress shoes to work, go with styles that have cushioned foot beds. For women who feel that they must wear heels, wear sneakers to and from the office and change once you get there. (And limit heel height to no more than one to two inches.) Avoid hard-soled slippers or sandals on weekends—wear supportive sneakers instead. Also consider off-the-shelf orthotics, shoe inserts that add cushioning. Smart tip: Replace running shoes about every 300 miles. That's the average "life" of their shock-absorbing properties for a typical runner, depending on the type of shoe, the person's weight and other variables. Replace sooner if you start noticing pain anywhere in your body after a workout that typically doesn't cause a problem or if you notice pronounced wear on the heel.

6. Being set in your exercise routine. Doing only high-impact exercise or long-distance running may take a toll on your knees over time. Cross training will help preserve joints. Alternate between low-impact exercises and high-impact activities, mixing biking or swimming into a running program, for instance.

7. Relying on joint supplements to make up for bad habits. Glucosamine and chondroitin are among the most popular supplements taken by Americans, but it's important not to think of them as a shortcut to knee health or a substitute for the other recommendations here. There is very little evidence that these supplements will prevent knee damage or help relieve knee pain if you have knee damage. Even if you think they're helping, they can't compensate for a lack of exercise or the burden of carrying extra weight.

Need motivation to put a positive plan into action? Over time, overweight and inactive people with knee pain tend to need knee-replacement surgery while slim and active people tend to avoid it.

Your Knee Pain May Really Be a Hip Problem

Mitchell Yass, DPT, a specialist in diagnosing and resolving the cause of pain and creator of the Yass Method for treating chronic pain. He is the author of *Overpower Pain: The Strength Training Program That Stops Pain Without Drugs or Surgery* and *The Pain Cure Rx: The Yass Method for Diagnosing and Resolving Chronic Pain* and host of the PBS special *The Pain Prescription*.

If you're suffering from chronic knee pain and seek medical attention, the typical X-ray and/or MRI that's performed will show that you have arthritis or, worse, "bone on bone"… or maybe a meniscal tear.

As I've talked about in some of my other blogs, few doctors make any real attempt to understand the presentation of your symptoms—where in the knee region the pain is being experienced…what types of activities bring on your symptoms or which make them decrease. No attempt to determine if full range of motion is even present in the knee! The standard of care is pretty clear—the MRI or X-ray identified a structural variation so that must be causing your pain.

Here's what I do to determine the cause of knee pain.

First let's think about the knee joint. It is actually made of two joints—the first, between the two ends of the thigh bone and lower leg bone (the tibia) and the second, where the knee cap meets the thigh bone, ideally with a meniscus (cartilage) between them. If a structural variation like arthritis or a meniscal tear were to occur, it would alter the ability of the joint to achieve full range of motion. So, as I talked about in an earlier blog on joint pain, the first test is to check range of motion. Quite simply if you have full range of motion or the same range of motion at the affected knee as the unaffected knee, there is no possible way that a structural variation identified on a diagnostic test is causing your pain.

So let's assume you tested the range of motion of the knee joint and it is full or equal to the unaffected knee. We can conclude that the cause of the pain is muscular. (While it is possible that BOTH knees have a structural problem that needs aggressive intervention like surgery, it is highly unusual. Yet the diagnostic process holds true in a case like this as well—if this were causing pain, there should be a major loss of range of motion at both knees and at the end of range of motion it should feel like one bone is hitting another bone, stopping further motion from occurring.)

Now, when I say "muscular," I don't think most people have a good grasp of how a muscular deficit can cause joint pain. I'm going to give a lot of detail here, but it's important to fully understand just what is going on in your knee.

The positioning of the bones in the knee joint is based on the pulls of the muscles that attach to them. The joint functions optimally when the total surfaces of the ends of the bones that make up the joint are in perfect alignment. This means that 100% of the surface area of the joint will take 100% of the force running through the joint. This is the way that all joints are designed to work.

When muscles are strong and balanced, they are able to support the joint to sustain this optimal positioning of the bones. If there is muscle weakness or imbalance, the bones will shift position and less than 100% of the bone surface will be absorbing 100% of the force going through the joint. That type of contact can lead to a breakdown of the structures of the joint, leading to arthritic changes and degenerative tearing of the meniscus and, potentially, knee replacement surgery.

Of the two joints that make up the knee, the joint between the knee cap and the thigh bone has the greater force on it, and the muscles attached to this joint are more likely to become imbalanced. An imbalance between the quads (front thigh muscle) and hamstrings (posterior thigh muscle) can cause the quad to shorten, creating excessive upward force on the knee cap. This can lead to excessive compression of the knee cap in the joint, leading to pain around the knee cap. A strain of the quads can lead to a decrease in force applied to the knee cap, causing it to move laterally and create pain on the lateral border of the joint between the kneecap and thigh bone.

One of the indicators that the cause is muscular is when the pain seems to result from performing activities—but you have no pain when sitting or lying down. Sit to stand, negotiating stairs, kneeling, walking and prolonged standing are all activities that might bring on knee pain.

What I have been seeing more frequently is knee pain occurring after a hip replacement. In this case, a muscular deficit at the hip region causes knee pain. The gluteus medius muscle sits at the side of the pelvis above the hip joint. It is responsible for creating stability and balance, especially when single-leg standing, such as with walking. This muscle is also responsible for keeping the knee joint under the hip joint when standing.

Here are the red flags that your knee pain may be from a strained hip muscle…

• **Your knee pain** has occurred after getting hip surgery.

• **The thigh with the affected knee** seems more angled inward than the unaffected leg.

• **When you single leg stand,** your knee feels like it can't support you and that it might cave in.

• **Negotiating stairs** seems inhibited not only because of knee pain but a feeling that your leg won't support you.

• **Tenderness** when feeling the gluteus medius for knots or sensitivity.

These types of causes do not show up on diagnostic tests, and no medical specialty is educated or trained to identify or treat them. (This is why this blog is so important. You will get logic-based, symptom-based analysis to help you determine the cause of your symptoms. Without identifying the right cause, the symptoms will never be resolved and chronic pain will stay chronic.)

If it appears that the cause of the knee pain is due to a strained gluteus medius muscle, then perform hip abduction. *Here's how…*

• **Attach a resistance-band loop to the leg of a sturdy table or chair.** Stand with the affected leg's foot in the loop farther away from the structure than the unaffected leg. The feet should be close together to start. Turn the foot of the affected leg in so you lead to the side with the heel moving first. Step out so the outside of the ankle meets the line of the hip. Put all your weight on the leg you are stepping out with and then return to the start position. Do a total of three sets of 10 repetitions with a one-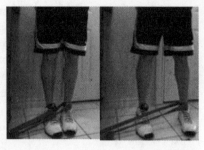minute rest between sets. As the resistance feels easier, either step farther away from the table/chair with both feet to increase the tension of the resistance band or use a more resistive band to continue to build the gluteus medius. Eventually the muscle will become so strong it will be able to support you and prevent the knee from losing alignment under the hip joint.

Best Treatments for Ankle Arthritis

Judith F. Baumhauer, MD, MPH, professor and associate chair of the department of orthopedics at University of Rochester School of Medicine, New York. Her research has been published in *The New England Journal of Medicine, Foot & Ankle International* and other leading medical journals. She is the recipient of the American Orthopaedic Foot & Ankle Society's Roger A. Mann Award for outstanding clinical study in 2017.

Remember that sprained ankle you suffered years ago? Or maybe it was an ankle fracture that left you hobbling around for weeks. Whatever the specific problem, be forewarned that ankle injuries can come back to haunt you—years or even decades later. *Here's how…*

SELF-CARE FOR ARTHRITIS

The ankle is vulnerable to the same types of arthritis that affect other joints. Post-traumatic arthritis is the most common form in the ankle, followed by age-related osteoarthritis and rheumatoid arthritis. For these forms of ankle arthritis, you might be able to manage discomfort with simple remedies.

But self-care is tricky. You can't "go easy" on the ankles in the same way that you would with certain other joints. People use their ankles all day, every day. *My advice for people with ankle arthritis…*

•**Choose activities that minimize ankle wear and tear.** To stay active and keep the muscles supporting the ankle strong, try biking, swimming, walking, rowing, elliptical workouts or other low-impact, weight-bearing exercises that don't cause relentless pounding.

•**Keep your weight down.** People with ankle arthritis tend to gain weight because they find it too painful to walk or exercise much… and the extra pounds accelerate joint damage by increasing the weight load on the ankles. Helpful: Losing even five pounds can reduce the ankle load by 20 pounds, which may be enough to minimize symptoms.

•**Exercise the ankles.** Ankle-specific exercises will build up the muscles surrounding the joint, keep the joint from getting stiff and reduce the bone-on-bone friction that occurs with arthritis.

Example: Several times a day, flex your foot upward (dorsiflexion) as far as it will go… hold for a few seconds…then flex it downward (plantarflexion). You can find dozens of ankle exercises on the Internet.

•**Wear shock-absorbing shoes.** Also known as "stability sneakers," they have a densely cushioned heel/sole that absorbs shocks when you walk, exercise, etc.

NOT READY FOR SURGERY

In addition to the steps above, some simple therapies can help slow the progression of arthritis. For example, it may help to wear an over-the-counter ankle brace that gives support and stability…apply cold packs when the ankle is hurting…and/or take as-needed doses of a nonsteroidal anti-inflammatory drug (NSAID), such as *ibuprofen* (Motrin) or *naproxen* (Aleve).* If you're lucky, these and other self-care therapies—including physical therapy—may be the only treatments you'll ever need.

Very helpful: A cortisone injection. Cortisone (sometimes combined with lidocaine) is a strong anti-inflammatory that can reduce or eliminate pain within a day. The shot is good for patients who are having moderate daily pain—

*Discuss the use of NSAIDs with your physician—they can cause side effects such as stomach upset, ulcers and high blood pressure.

and might be helpful for an upcoming vacation, for example, or when the pain is unusually severe. This shot won't stop the arthritis but can get you through a rough patch. In some cases, hyaluronic acid injections may be used but may not be covered by insurance.

WHEN SURGERY IS NEEDED

Even with the approaches described earlier, many people will eventually develop "end-stage" arthritis that does not improve and interferes with their daily activities. Once ankle arthritis progresses to that extent, it's serious business.

Until about 10 years ago, most patients with end-stage ankle arthritis were advised to have a procedure called ankle arthrodesis, commonly known as ankle fusion because affected bones are fused together to reduce pain and inflammation. Now, patients (based on their age and other factors) have a second option—a total ankle replacement.

Because long-term comprehensive studies haven't yet been done, there's still debate about which approach is better. Both procedures are effective...and both have downsides that patients need to know about. *Specifically...*

•**With ankle fusion,** the affected bones are locked together (with screws alone or plates and screws) and eventually fuse into a solid mass of bone. This eliminates the rubbing/friction that causes the pain and disability of ankle arthritis. Most patients will walk in a shoe (without a cast) in eight to 12 weeks. And unlike ankle replacement (discussed below), the procedure is permanent. You're unlikely to require an additional procedure unless it doesn't fuse.

Downside: Bone fusion eliminates ankle mobility. You might walk haltingly when you go up hills or down a flight of stairs. And because the ankle is locked in place, other structures in the foot assume more of the burden of daily movements—and could become more susceptible to arthritis.

Ankle fusion might not be the best choice if you have a highly active lifestyle that involves, for example, strenuous hiking, tennis, etc., and want your ankle to move "naturally"...or if you have other arthritic areas of your foot that couldn't take on more responsibility when the ankle is locked up.

•**With a total ankle replacement, the arthritic surfaces are replaced**—as also occurs with a knee or hip replacement—with an artificial joint. Surgeons advise patients that the implants might last for eight to 12 years. A recent study found that 73% were still working after 15 years.

The advantage of total ankle replacement is that the ankle will flex. Patients retain a greater degree of motion and experience less stress on surrounding joints.

Downside: The risk for additional procedures to repair/replace a damaged implant.

My take: I might recommend joint replacement for someone who's over age 60 and in good health but has other arthritis in the foot...or a person who is active with sports, such as tennis, that involve jumping and cutting. However, the choice between fusion and replacement is highly individualized.

Important: See a surgeon who's experienced in both procedures to get an unbiased opinion about the pros and cons of each. To find such a surgeon near you, consult the American Orthopaedic Foot & Ankle Society, AOFAS.org.

Insurance typically covers these procedures, but be sure to ask.

Avoid Repeated Steroid Shots

Timothy McAlindon, MD, chief of rheumatology, Tufts Medical Center, Boston.

A recent study of 140 patients with knee arthritis who got either steroid or saline shots every 12 weeks for two years showed no major difference in pain between the two groups... and those receiving steroids lost significantly more cartilage thickness, which could lead to increased pain and risk for joint replacement in the future.

Takeaway: An occasional shot (once a year or so) for a flare-up is probably fine, but consider alternatives such as exercise, topical nonsteroidal anti-inflammatory creams or knee braces for long-term pain relief.

A "Cinematic" Way to Beat Pain

Brennan Spiegel, MD, professor of medicine, director of Health Services Research and director of the master's degree program in health delivery science, all at Cedars-Sinai Health System in Los Angeles. He is also assistant dean at University of California, Los Angeles, David Geffen School of Medicine.

I *magine this:* You are lying in a hospital bed after surgery when you begin to feel a stabbing pain. Desperate for relief, you look for your daily dose of pain medication. Not so fast. Soon, you may reach instead for a set of virtual-reality goggles.

Using virtual reality (VR) for pain is not some sci-fi snake oil. This high-tech therapy, which immerses you in a three-dimensional, multisensory world of cinematic grandeur, is on the cutting-edge of pain relief approaches.

Scientific evidence: New research shows that VR significantly reduces many types of pain and may lessen (or, in some cases, replace) the need for pain medication—a well-timed breakthrough given the addiction epidemic that's being fueled by pain medicine such as opioids.

What you need to know about this exciting new advance…

VIRTUAL REALITY IN ACTION

So what's it like to experience VR? Once you slip on the somewhat clunky-looking headset or even a simpler pair of special goggles, you'll be ready to watch three-dimensional, 360-degree streaming video complete with sound that depicts a wide variety of vibrantly colored realistic scenes—either photographed or animated. You'll hear the sounds associated with that scene and even experience vibrations or other sensations for a completely immersive experience.

Depending on the purpose of the VR therapy—whether you need to focus your mind to distract yourself from pain, for example, or you need relief from anxiety—you may view scenes that give you the feeling of swimming with dolphins in the ocean…lobbing snowballs while hurtling through an animated snowscape…or relishing the splendor of a gushing waterfall.

VR therapy has been used successfully by scientists for years to help treat the symptoms of conditions such as stroke, post-traumatic stress disorder, social phobia and burns. In hospitals, VR therapy is used as needed with children to distract them from painful or scary procedures, such as getting blood drawn.

Until recently, however, VR therapy was too expensive and not widely available. That's now changing.

NEW SCIENTIFIC EVIDENCE

To learn more about the effects of VR, researchers at Cedars-Sinai Medical Center in Los Angeles recently studied 100 patients experiencing pain from many different causes, including cancer, bone breaks and other ailments. In this study, published in *JMIR Mental Health*, half of the study participants received 10 minutes of VR therapy once a day, and half watched a two-dimensional nature video with calming music on a high-definition computer screen.

Result: While both groups reported less pain, those undergoing VR experienced a significant 24% drop in pain compared with a 13% decrease in the relaxing video group. The period of pain relief varied but generally lasted at least an hour.

While this study did not identify the exact mechanism behind VR's effectiveness against pain, it is an example of the spotlight attention theory. According to this theory, the human mind is able to track only a certain amount of information at one time—the eyes focus on what is in a "spotlight" and not the areas in the background. With VR, the brain is overwhelmed with positive imagery that engages the mind so that other signals, such as pain, are not perceptible (or not as perceptible) at the same time.

REDUCING PAIN MEDICATION

Many people who use VR continue to have pain reduction even after discontinuing the therapy. Scientists theorize that VR may somehow reset the brain, making some people less susceptible to peripheral pain signals for a period of time.

Scientists are also investigating whether VR can reduce the use of painkillers after an acute injury, such as a broken leg, or postoperatively —for example, after hip- or knee-replacement surgery.

Sobering statistics: A one-day prescription of an opioid painkiller results in a 6% risk for use of the drug one year later. And when treated for at least 31 days with opioids, nearly 30% of patients were still taking the painkillers a year later.

VR EQUIPMENT

Cedars-Sinai and other medical centers use a VR kit provided by the company AppliedVR (go to AppliedVR.io). This kit consists of a Samsung headset and Galaxy phone at a cost of $800. A subscription to access the library of visualizations is extra.

But do not let that cost overwhelm you. You can use your own smartphone to access VR therapy by buying a headset (available on Amazon. com for about $20 to $100) and then streaming VR content by buying an app or going to You-Tube.com. Look online for lists of highly rated VR apps.

Important: The VR therapy used in hospitals is prescribed for specific conditions. When using VR therapy on your own, try it on a trial-and-error basis. For example, if you are looking to relax or alleviate anxiety, you can search "VR and beach" or "VR and relax," and try out different scenes. There may be minor side effects, such as dizziness. People with dementia, epilepsy, nausea and certain other conditions should not use VR therapy without checking with their doctors.

HOW TO ACCESS VT

Several hospitals across the country are conducting clinical trials on the use of VR therapy for pain management (including neuropathic pain and phantom limb pain) and other conditions such as attention deficit hyperactivity disorder (ADHD), traumatic brain injury, fear of heights and more.

To find a VR trial near you: Go to Clinical Trials.gov, type in "virtual reality" and choose your state or a nearby state.

Yoga as Good as PT for Back Pain

Robert B. Saper, MD, MPH, director of the program for integrative medicine and health disparities, Boston Medical Center.

Yoga works as well as physical therapy for back pain. When patients took yoga classes every week for three months, then attended more yoga sessions or practiced at home for nine months, they reported the same improvement in pain and activity limitation after one year as patients who had 15 visits with a physical therapist during the three-month period, then for the nine months had further sessions every two months or did prescribed home exercises.

The Posture Cure for Migraines and Other Chronic Headaches

Dr. Mitchell Yass, DPT, is the creator of The Yass Method, which uniquely diagnoses and treats the cause of chronic pain through the interpretation of the body's presentation of symptoms. Dr. Yass is author of *Overpower Pain: The Strength Training Program That Stops Pain Without Drugs or Surgery* and *The Pain Cure Rx: The Yass Method for Resolving The Cause of Chronic Pain*.

There are certain possible causes of headaches—like a cerebral bleed, meningitis, a tumor in the brain—that are very dangerous and can be life threatening. Most of these can be identified by the use of diagnostic tests like MRIs and CAT scans. And there is no question that these types of tests should be run in the case of severe headaches.

But what happens when all the tests come back negative? With no "cause" established, the goal simply becomes finding ways to reduce the intensity of the headaches. This leaves medical practitioners with little alternative but to prescribe pain medications or Botox injections. The problem here is that the side effects of most of these medications can be worse than the headaches they are intended to address…and Botox is only temporary. The headaches could continue indefinitely!

I have been able to resolve the headaches of many people—including those suffering with migraine headaches and cluster headaches—by addressing a postural deviation called "forward head and shoulder posture," where the head is forward and the shoulders rounded.

IT ALL STARTS WITH POSTURE

When standing with proper posture, your ears and shoulders should be directly aligned over the hips.

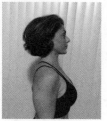

Proper   Forward head and shoulder

Forward head and shoulder posture is where these landmarks are in front of the hip when looking at a person from the side. The posture creates a hunching at the upper back.

This hunched posture is caused by a muscle imbalance between the chest muscles, front (anterior) shoulder and biceps versus the muscles between the shoulder blades, rear (posterior) shoulder and triceps. And it's this imbalance that could be the root of migraines and other chronic headaches.

THE SLOW TRAIN TO HEAD PAIN

If you just want to trust me and don't want all of the details, scroll down for the exercises that can relieve your headache pain...but my patients do better when they understand the mechanism they are working to correct. *Here's what happens, step-by-step, when headaches are caused by poor posture...*

•**The front set of muscles** (chest, front shoulder and biceps) tend to be excessively used because everything we do with our hands is done in front of us.

•**When this imbalance grows, the chest muscles can especially shorten.** Shortened chest muscles pull the shoulders forward, creating rounding of the upper back.

•**At the same time, the shoulder blades will be moving laterally farther away from the spine.** The muscles that support the head (called the levator scapulae and upper trapezius) attach from the shoulder blades to the upper cervical spine and skull. When the length of these muscles is increased, they can lose their ability to support the head.

•**These head-supporting muscles will strain,** which can create pain at the upper neck region and cause the head to move more forward.

•**As the head moves more forward, it increases the load on those supporting muscles** because the weight of the head is

MUSCLES OF THE UPPER BACK AND NECK

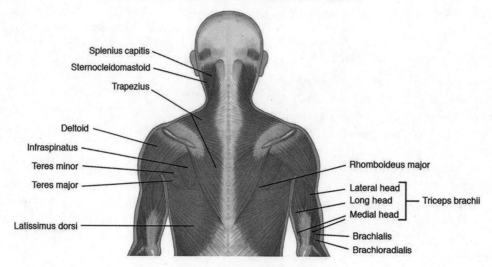

moving farther away from being properly supported over the cervical spine.

•**Since the upper trap muscles attach to the skull at its base,** the forward tilt of the head will begin to create an excessive pulling. Muscles don't actually attach to bones; they attach to the periosteum, connective tissue that surrounds bone. Connective tissue has a very high density of pain receptors in them. By pulling excessively on the periosteum, there is a good opportunity for the pain receptors to be ignited anywhere around the skull—causing headaches—because periosteum also surrounds the skull.

THE 4 EXERCISES FOR HEADACHE RELIEF

To resolve headaches generated by poor posture and the resulting muscle imbalance, you simply need to strengthen the weaker muscles. As these muscles are strengthened, you'll see improving posture and a reduction in headaches. Then you can say farewell to painkillers and bye-bye to Botox. Here are the four exercises—all you need is a resistance band, a door and a chair!

For each exercise, perform three sets of 10 repetitions with a minute rest in between each set. The series of exercises are performed three times a week with a day rest between. Resistance should be progressed to eventually get the muscles strong enough to perform all functional tasks without straining and eliciting symptoms.

1. Lat Pulldown (interscapular muscles: midtraps and rhomboids)

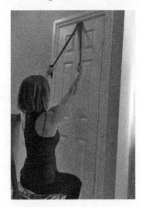 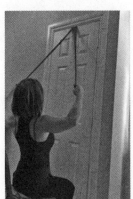

START   FINISH

Tie a knot in the center of a resistance band and secure it in place at the top of a closed door. Sit in a sturdy chair and lean back with an angle at the hip of about 30 degrees. Reach up for the ends of the band so that the start position begins with the arms nearly straight and the elbows just unlocked. Pull the band down, keeping your arms wide and bringing the elbows just below shoulder height and slightly behind the line of the shoulders. At this point, you should feel the shoulder blades squeeze together (the elbows will barely reach behind the line of the shoulders if performing this exercise correctly). Then return to the start position. Important: If the elbows start to drop so they are lower than the shoulders, you are using the incorrect muscles to perform the exercise.

2. Lower Trap Exercise (lower trapezius muscle)

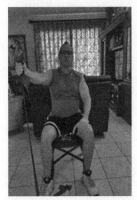 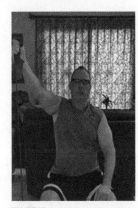

START   FINISH

Sit in a sturdy chair with a back and lean back slightly—about 10 degrees. This posture will prevent the resistance from pulling you forward. Step on one end of the resistance band to secure it and hold the other end in your working hand. Start with your arm halfway between pointing straight forward and pointing straight to the side, with your hand at shoulder height and your elbow just unlocked. Begin to raise the resistance until the arm reaches about 130 to 140 degrees (about the height of the ear). Then return to the start position at shoulder height.

3. Posterior Deltoids (posterior deltoids)
Stand with your feet more than shoulder width apart, knees slightly bent and your butt pushed behind you. Your weight should be mostly on your heels. Step evenly on the band

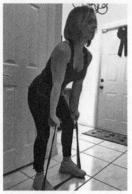

START   FINISH

and hold the ends in front of your thighs with your palms facing in and your elbows unlocked. Begin to move the resistance out to your side from the shoulders like a pendulum. Go out until you feel the shoulder blades start to move inward (about 60 degrees), and then return to the beginning position.

4. Skull Crushers (triceps, single and both arms)

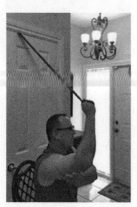

START   FINISH

There are a multitude of exercises that strengthen the triceps. This particular one is the most effective because it puts the long head of the triceps in the optimal position. The long head of the triceps is the only part of the triceps muscle that passes the shoulder joint. Therefore, it is the only part of the muscle that can affect the position of the arm bone in the shoulder joint. The exercise can be performed with one arm or both, depending on whether your pain is associated with one side or requires both arms to be strengthened to resolve it.

To perform the exercise, tie a knot in one end of a resistance band to secure it behind a closed door. Sit upright in a chair, back supported facing away from the door, with your legs comfortably open and feet firmly on floor. Start with your arm in front of you, upper arm just above parallel to the floor and elbow bent at 90 degrees. Keeping the upper arm in place (you can support with your other hand), begin to straighten the elbow, lowering the forearm until the elbow is just short of locked. Slowly return to the starting position.

Nerve Stimulation May Relieve RA

Study of 17 people with RA by researchers at Feinstein Institute for Medical Research, Manhasset, New York, published in *Proceedings of the National Academy of Sciences*.

Nerve stimulation may help RA patients. Electronic stimulation of the vagus nerve, which runs from the brain to the gut, improved joint swelling and other symptoms for some people with the painful autoimmune disease rheumatoid arthritis (RA), even in those for whom drugs had not worked well.

CHAPTER 18

Women's Health

9 Ways to Prevent Breast Cancer—Before and After Menopause

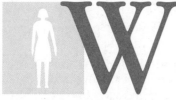

What are the most effective things women can do to avoid getting breast cancer? A team of researchers at the World Cancer Research Fund asked that question. Here's what they found.

Background: Every year, 315,000 American women are newly diagnosed with breast cancer. Although new treatments have improved survival, breast cancer remains the second-leading cause of cancer deaths in American women. Many known risk factors are hard to change—such as getting your first period before age 12…not ever having children or having your first child after age 30…hitting menopause after age 55…a family history of breast cancer…being exposed to high levels of radiation. But many lifestyle factors do make a difference—some, a big difference.

Study: The World Cancer Research Fund International and the American Institute for Cancer Research gathered an international panel of experts to review 119 scientific studies involving 12 million women about the ways diet, weight and physical activity affect a woman's risk of developing breast cancer. They then determined which of those factors protected women the most from getting the disease—both before and after menopause. (Since men account for only 1% of breast cancer cases, the panel limited its recommendations to women.)

Convincing evidence found that…

•**Physical activity and breastfeeding decrease the risk for breast cancer.**

Anne McTiernan, MD, PhD, research professor at Fred Hutchinson Cancer Research Center in Seattle, Washington, and author of *Starved: A Nutrition Doctor's Journey from Empty to Full*. She was a member of the World Cancer Research Fund International/American Institute for Cancer Research panel that issued the report titled "Continuous Update Project Report: Diet, Nutrition, Physical Activity and Breast Cancer 2017."

•**Drinking alcohol increases the risk.**

•**Eating certain kinds of vegetables and fruits reduces risk.**

Surprisingly, women who were overweight or obese between the ages of 18 and 30 were less likely to develop breast cancer, either before or after menopause, compared with women who were of normal weight between the ages of 18 and 30. The reasons aren't well understood. But while being overweight or obese throughout adulthood was still associated with less risk for premenopausal breast cancer, a pattern of adult weight gain—defined in different studies as after age 35 or age 50—was strongly associated with increased postmenopausal breast cancer risk.

Bottom line: These evidence-backed lifestyle habits can help prevent breast cancer…

BEFORE MENOPAUSE

•**If you have children,** breastfeed if you are able to. The longer you nurse and the more children you nurse, the more you reduce breast cancer risk thanks to the resulting hormonal changes that reduce estrogen exposure throughout your life.

•**Watch out for weight gain in your 30s,** 40s and 50s. Being overweight before age 30 is protective against breast cancer. But take steps to prevent the weight gain that tends to creep up after age 30.

AFTER MENOPAUSE

•**Redouble efforts to manage your weight.** Once through menopause, obesity increases breast cancer risk by a whopping 40%, according to some studies. Women who get and eliminate breast cancer have a higher chance of their cancer returning and a higher chance of dying of the disease if they are obese.

•**Whittle your waistline.** It's not just how much you weigh, but where weight lodges on your body. Extra fat around your middle can lead to inflammation, increased levels of estrogen (produced by the fat) and higher insulin levels—all of which can set the stage for breast cells to mutate and turn cancerous. It's tough to avoid turning apple-shaped after menopause. Try to keep your waist measurement less than

32 inches by eating healthy foods and staying active.

AT EVERY AGE

These lifestyle factors can help prevent breast cancer throughout life—and it's never too late to start them…

•**Curb your drinking.** Even one drink a day increases breast cancer risk by 5% if you're premenopausal—and by 9% if you're postmenopausal. Each additional daily drink increases risk, on average, by the same percentages. So if you like to have a glass of wine with a meal, do not pour more than five ounces—that is one drink.

•**Step up your activity level.** Any type of exercise reduces breast cancer risk. Aim for about 30 minutes at least five days a week. While moderately-intense activity such as brisk walking counts, exercising vigorously—running versus walking, kickboxing versus yoga—is particularly protective.

Higher-intensity workouts not only help you get rid of harmful belly fat but also boost the immune system so your body is better able to kill mutating cells before they form a tumor. (Exercise also can improve outcomes for people who have cancer, research finds.)

•**Get your calcium.** Diets rich in calcium protect against breast cancer both before and after menopause.

One reason: Calcium helps regulate cell growth, especially in breast tissue.

•**Load up on nonstarchy veggies.** There is evidence that eating nonstarchy vegetables—such as broccoli, leafy greens, summer squash, asparagus, tomatoes—is especially helpful in reducing the risk of estrogen-negative breast cancer, which tends to grow at a faster rate than hormone-positive cancers. Aim for at least one cup a day. (Starchy veggies such as potatoes don't count.)

•**Eat your carotenoids.** When choosing fruits and vegetables, go for color. Animal and test-tube studies have shown that carotenoids—fat-soluble pigments that give produce its coloring—have protective properties. Choose red, orange and yellow fruits and vegetables such as berries, beets, peppers and carrots.

How much can these healthy lifestyle habits help reduce breast cancer risk? By about one-third, the researchers estimate. That would be about 100,000 US women every year.

Home Test Warning

Anne McTiernan, MD, PhD, research professor at Fred Hutchinson Cancer Research Center, Seattle, and author of *Starved: A Nutrition Doctor's Journey from Empty to Full.*

The first-ever home test for breast cancer genes is inadequate—akin to performing a mammogram on just one part of the breast. The test, from the company 23AndMe, checks for only three of the many hundreds of mutations in two BRCA genes that increase risk. Doctor-ordered tests are much more extensive. Most breast cancer is not hereditary, but if the disease does run in your family, discuss genetic testing with your doctor.

Stop Dreading Your Mammogram!

Margarita Zuley, MD, FACR, chief of breast imaging and professor and vice chair of quality and strategic development for the University of Pittsburgh Medical Center department of radiology. A diagnostic radiologist specializing in breast imaging, she has been the principal investigator on multiple grants related to digital and 3-D mammography.

Not looking forward to your next mammogram? You're not alone. Many women experience anxiety in the days leading up to it.

In fact, the psychological distress surrounding mammograms (and the potential results) was a factor in the US Preventive Services Task Force's 2009 decision to change its recommendation to biennial (every other year), instead of annual, mammography screening for women of average risk, ages 50 to 74.

But mammograms do save lives. These X-rays help identify breast cancer in women with no signs or symptoms of the disease.

THE DISCOMFORT FACTOR

When researchers have studied mammogram pain or discomfort, their findings have varied wildly—based on numerous studies, anywhere from 1% to 77% of women report that the test was painful.

Meanwhile, an important study conducted at Beth Israel Deaconess Medical Center found that most women don't experience any pain or anxiety at all. Discomfort...perhaps. But pain is not a given—and quite subjective at that. Afterward, most women said the exam wasn't nearly as awful as they'd feared.

SIMPLE STEPS THAT HELP

Besides understanding that mammograms are often not nearly as uncomfortable or painful as many women fear, there are some simple things you can do to reduce pre-mammogram anxiety and to make the experience itself less unpleasant. *For example...*

•**Limit caffeine intake.** Caffeine can make your breasts more tender. Try decreasing your intake starting a few days before the exam. Don't eliminate caffeine, though, or you'll risk having a caffeine-withdrawal headache.

•**Try Tylenol.** Most women can safely use *acetaminophen* (Tylenol), taken at a standard dose within four hours of the exam, to minimize discomfort.

Bonus: It will reduce any soreness you might experience afterward. Avoid aspirin and other nonsteroidal anti-inflammatory drugs (NSAIDs) such as *ibuprofen* (Motrin, Advil), which can increase the risk for bruising.

•**Exercise before the test.** A recent study conducted by researchers at Barretos Cancer Hospital in São Paulo State, Brazil, found that women who exercised for 20 minutes just prior to their mammograms reported less pain after screening compared with women who didn't exercise—perhaps because the physical activity promoted the release of endorphins, hormones that have a pain-relieving effect. Exercises included warm-ups and stretching...then a series of 10 upper-body moves, such as arm and shoulder circles or interlocking the fingers behind the back and raising the arms.

•**Know what to expect.** Women who feel armed with information about the procedure experience less pain and discomfort from mammograms—likely because they feel less anxiety.

What helps: For first-timers, ask your doctor to walk you through the procedure when he/she prescribes your mammogram. A few days prior to the test, do a dry run to the facility so you know exactly how to get there and, if you're driving, where to find parking.

If possible, bring a friend or family member with you to your appointment for support. The less you have to worry about the day of your mammogram, the more relaxed—and therefore the less pain—you will feel.

WHAT WORSENS DISCOMFORT

Most women know that mammograms tend to be less uncomfortable during the first two weeks of the menstrual cycle when the breasts aren't as sensitive. Mammograms are also more accurate when performed on that schedule. This is likely because breast tissue is generally less dense at that time and more easily imaged.

What many women don't know: Certain health conditions can increase pain or discomfort during a mammogram. *What helps women affected by...*

•**Chronic pain.** When scheduling, alert the facility that you have chronic pain. There may be a technologist on staff who is trained in working with chronic pain patients. Continue taking any prescription medications as normal, and be sure to try the general tips above. Never be afraid to speak up if something hurts too much! The compression used for mammograms is based in part on the patient's tolerance.

•**Cold temperatures.** If you have trouble tolerating cold temperatures, ask the technologist for a robe or bring one from home. If your hands get cold, you can ask to wear surgical gloves.

•**Dense breasts.** Roughly 25% of postmenopausal women have dense breasts. This simply means that their breasts have denser, lumpier tissue. Dense breasts tend to be more sensitive to pain and are likely to benefit from a reduction in caffeine intake as described earlier.

•**A lumpectomy.** If you have had this procedure, which involves surgical removal of a suspected cancerous tumor and surrounding tissue, you should return to annual mammogram imaging after surgery.

Radiation and surgery can both cause changes in the breast tissue and skin that may make a mammogram less comfortable. The scar itself may be tender, and the skin may be more sensitive to the touch. Let your mammogram technologist know so that he/she can take any necessary precautions, such as making adjustments in position and compression.

•**Weight issues.** Obese women are nearly twice as likely to cite pain as a mammogram deterrent as nonobese women. The exact reasons are unknown, but being overweight has been associated with a lower pain threshold. Some obese patients also feel that having larger breasts or breast tissue that extends under the arms renders mammograms more painful. Be sure to try the general tips above.

DON'T LET A DISABILITY STOP YOU

Use of a wheelchair or scooter should not prevent you from getting screened for breast cancer.

What helps: When scheduling a mammogram, let the facility where you'll be tested know if you will need assistance undressing...standing...moving your arms...and/or transferring from your wheelchair or scooter. The technologist will work one-on-one with you to make the exam as comfortable as possible.

Breast Cancer Caution

Anne McTiernan, MD, PhD, research professor at Fred Hutchinson Cancer Research Center, Seattle, and author of *Starved: A Nutrition Doctor's Journey from Empty to Full.*

There's an increased risk for breast cancer in women who are using or have recently used birth control pills, implants, injections or intrauterine devices that release hormones. In a study of 1.8 million women, ages 15 to 49, breast cancer risk was increased by 20% among women who used hormonal birth control. Still, risk is low in these ages, so absolute risk was small—an extra 13 cases for every 100,000 women using hormonal contraceptives for one year. Women should balance breast cancer risk with the health risks of nonhormonal contraceptive methods, such as IUDs.

Women Are Skipping MRIs

Christoph I. Lee, MD, associate professor of radiology and health sciences (adjunct), University of Washington School of Medicine, Seattle.

Too many women are skipping breast MRIs. *Recent finding:* Among more than 422,000 women who got mammography at a screening facility that also offered magnetic resonance imaging (MRI), only 6.6% of those with a high lifetime risk for breast cancer got the additional screening. A woman is considered at high lifetime risk if she has risk factors such as a strong family history of breast cancer or inherited mutations to certain genes, such as BRCA1 or BRCA2.

Takeaway: Discuss your breast cancer risk level with your doctor and ask whether MRI is appropriate.

Exercise Eases Hot Flashes and More

JoAnn V. Pinkerton, MD, NCMP, executive director, North American Menopause Society, Pepper Pike, Ohio, and professor of obstetrics and gynecology and division director of Midlife Health at the University of Virginia Health System, Charlottesville.

A modest exercise program can help you to navigate the sometimes-turbulent waters of menopause. A recent study followed 166 postmenopausal sedentary women (none were using hormone therapy). Half of the women participated in a cardio/strength fitness program three hours per week for 20 weeks. They also received psychological counseling to help them set goals and deal with setbacks.

Results: Compared with the sedentary women, the active women had fewer hot flashes and better moods, lost weight, reduced blood pressure and increased flexibility.

Surprising Cancer Risk

Women who eat lots of high-calorie, low-nutrient foods, such as chips, fast food and candy, are 10% more likely, on average, to develop obesity-related breast, colon, ovarian, kidney or endometrial cancer.

The big surprise: The increased cancer risk was identified even among those of normal weight, according to the 15-year study that tracked 92,000 women.

Cynthia Thomson, PhD, RDN, professor, health promotion sciences, University of Arizona's Zuckerman College of Public Health, Tucson.

Teas for Menopause: Give Hot Flashes and Other Symptoms the Sip

Holly Lucille, ND, RN, a naturopathic doctor in private practice in West Hollywood, California, and author of *Creating and Maintaining Balance: A Woman's Guide to Safe, Natural Hormone Health*. She is a member of Bottom Line's Menopause Resource Center panel of experts. Her Bottom Line blog is *The Natural Side of Menopause*.

If you'd like to find a natural way to chill hot flashes, to get a decent night's sleep (finally!) and to ease other menopause symptoms, one answer is as close as your tea kettle. Many herbs that mitigate bothersome menopause symptoms contain active ingredients that are water-soluble—so they lend themselves to brewing in a tea.

With tea remedies for menopause symptoms, you'll be using pleasant and safe beverages as your medicine. In my practice as a naturopathic doctor, I often prescribe teas to my patients who are dealing with menopause symptoms. Sometimes they are enough on their own to help with symptoms. Other times, they are a wonderful addition to a comprehensive plan that may include supplements.

Here are some of my favorite teas for menopause symptoms.

One caveat: Some herbal teas can interact with medications, so if you are on a prescription medication, check in with your doctor before you start brewing. It's also important to check if you have a medical condition, such as a liver disorder. And because several of these teas affect hormones, including estrogen, it's particularly important to check with your doctor if you are taking hormone therapy.

HOLLY LUCILLE'S TOP TEAS FOR MENOPAUSE SYMPTOMS

•**For hot flashes: Black cohosh** (*Actaea racemosa, Cimicifuga racemosa*)

What it is: A perennial plant related to the buttercup and native to North America.

What it does: Puts the chill on hot flashes. Although studies looking at the effectiveness of black cohosh on alleviating hot flashes have had mixed results, many women report that it has helped them. In my experience with my patients, it's often very helpful.

How to use: Drink from one to three cups on days when your symptoms are bothering you.

Safety: Black cohosh is not estrogenic, as once believed, so it's safe for all women—even those with hormone-sensitive cancer such as certain breast cancers. Black cohosh has a good safety record, according to The North American Menopause Society.

•**For hot flashes and anxiety: Chasteberry** (*Vitex agnus-castus*)

What it is: The fruit of the chaste tree, which is native to central Asia and the Mediterranean region.

What it does: Helps boost levels of progesterone, a naturally calming hormone. It's wonderful especially in perimenopause, when progesterone levels start to decrease. It's helpful for myriad symptoms including hot flashes and moodiness.

How to use: Drink one to three cups on days when your symptoms are bothering you.

Safety: This tea has a very good safety record. Because it may affect hormones, however, check with your doctor if you have a hormone-sensitive cancer. Also, because it affects the brain chemical dopamine, avoid it if you're on a medication that affects dopamine such as one for Parkinson's disease.

•**For mood swings and brain fog: Ginkgo** (*Ginkgo biloba*)

What it is: The oldest living species of tree. The active ingredient is found in the leaf.

What it does: Improves blood flow, makes blood less "sticky" and is an antioxidant. It has been shown to improve circulation and enhance memory in people with Alzheimer's disease. But you don't have to have dementia to benefit from ginkgo! In my practice, I often recommend it to help women whose menopause symptoms include mood swings, irritableness and poor concentration, aka menopausal "brain fog."

How to use: Drink one to three cups on days when you're feeling a little brain foggy. If menopause-related cognitive issues are really bothering you, though, I would take an extract (standardized to contain 24% to 32% flavonoids and 6% to 12% terpenoids) as a supplement rather than a tea. Many studies that have shown cognitive benefits used 120 mg to 240 mg a day, in divided doses.

Safety: Ginkgo is a blood thinner, so talk to your doctor if you are taking a prescription blood thinner before drinking gingko tea or using it as a supplement. People with diabetes should also check with their doctors because gingko may reduce blood sugar levels.

•**For low libido: Maca root** (*Lepidium mayenii*)

What it is: A relative of the radish that grows in the Andes Mountains in central Peru. It's sometimes called Peruvian ginseng, although it is unrelated to "real" ginseng.

What it does: Reboot a subpar sex life! Research has shown that maca can improve mood and increase sexual desire. Exactly how isn't known, but it is rich in plant sterols, which may affect hormones, including estrogen. In my practice, I've found that maca root is one of the best teas to increase libido in women before and after menopause. It may also help ease hot flashes.

How to use: Start drinking up to three cups a day when you start to have perimenopausal symptoms—and continue drinking it regularly as long as you are symptomatic.

Safety: Maca root tea is safe to drink for most women. Because it may affect estrogen, though, talk to your doctor if you have a hormone-sensitive condition such as certain kinds of breast cancer.

THE HELPERS: LICORICE AND GINGER

Ginger tea and licorice tea each have properties that make them helpful for menopausal women. Ginger supports adrenal function, so it's great if you're feeling exhausted—it gives you energy. Licorice relieves pain and soothes indigestion, heartburn, gastritis and ulcerative colitis. It's fine to have a single-ingredient tea with either one, but they are also great ingredients in a tea blend.

Here's why: They add sweetness and flavor to make almost any other tea taste better. So look for tea blends that contain some licorice or ginger or both—or if you're making your own teas, try adding a little bit to make your own blends. You can grate a little fresh ginger into your tea or sprinkle in some dried ginger powder. The same with licorice—use fresh grated root or sprinkle on some powdered licorice root. (*Note*: Large amounts of licorice, such as half an ounce of dried root daily taken for more than two or three weeks, can increase blood pressure and interfere with some medications. The tiny amount in tea blends is safer, but check with your doctor if you have high blood pressure or take prescription medications.)

You don't need to use both ginger and licorice root—either one is good.

BEFORE YOU BREW

Whether you drink prepackaged herbal teas or brew your own from fresh or dried herbs—either is fine—you'll need to drink two or three cups a day of any given tea for best results. If you're having severe hot flashes, one cup of black cohosh tea won't do the job! *More tips…*

• **If hot flashes are bothering you,** avoid tea blends that contain caffeine, since it can exacerbate flashes.

• **Buy organic.** One online store I recommend is Mountain Rose Herbs.

• **To brew loose herbs,** use about one teaspoon of herb for each pint (16 ounces) of water.

• **Ice it!** Particularly if you're concerned about hot flashes, a steaming hot cup of tea may be the last thing you need. So brew your tea in advance, chill it in the fridge and serve it over ice—and use it to chill out at a moment's notice.

Got Hot Flashes? It Might Not Be Menopause

Julia Schlam Edelman, MD, a member of Bottom Line's Menopause Center Panel of Experts, is a board-certified gynecologist and a certified menopause practitioner in private practice in Massachusetts. She is author of *Menopause Matters: Your Guide to a Long and Healthy Life.* JuliaEdelmanMD.com

You're standing in line at the supermarket, and suddenly feel a whoosh of heat rise to the top of your head, leaving you flushed and sweaty and desperately fanning yourself. Yes—it's another hot flash.

This misery is a cliché of menopause, and these sweat-inducing menopausal heat surges can strike day or night—or both.

But what if those temperature spikes aren't menopause after all? As a gynecologist and menopause expert, I know that I have to check for other causes for these debilitating symptoms in my patients even if they're already going through menopause. Read on for the some of the other reasons you may be having hot flashes—and what actions to take.

These diseases can cause hot flashes…

THYROID DISEASE

The thyroid gland pumps out the hormones that control metabolism and body temperature, among other things. So it's no surprise that thyroid conditions can produce many of the temperature-related symptoms associated with menopause, including hot flashes, night sweats and a low tolerance for heat. Abnormal thyroid hormone levels can also mimic other common menopausal symptoms including brain fog, insomnia and irritability.

What to do: Since women are eight times more likely to develop a thyroid condition than men are, it makes sense to get your thyroid tested if you're experiencing hot flashes.

One key reason: Thyroid conditions require treatment to avoid potentially serious complications.

A simple blood test can measure your level of thyroid stimulating hormone (TSH), and if the level is abnormal, often the lab automatically will run extra tests to see whether you've developed a thyroid condition. Whether the thyroid gland is overactive (hyperthyroidism) or underactive (hypothyroidism), there are medications to correct the imbalance.

It takes time to ease thyroid-related hot flashes and night sweats, though. A doctor may have to adjust your medication several times, and even then it may take weeks or months to get complete relief.

Just be warned: If you're also going through menopause, you'll still suffer menopause-related hot flashes.

DIABETES

Low blood sugar can trigger hot flashes in people with diabetes. How can you tell? Your hot flashes not only leave you sweaty but shaky and weak.

What to do: Rule out diabetes by asking your doctor to check your blood glucose levels, especially if you have other signs such as extreme fatigue, blurred vision and tingling feet or hands. If you know you have diabetes, and your blood sugar hot flashes occur frequently, talk to your health-care provider about changing the dosage of your medication or switching medications.

CANCER

Certain cancers (and their treatments, see next page) can produce hot flashes and night sweats. Those cancers include leukemia and lymphomas as well as breast cancer.

What to do: Doctors will rule out cancer by checking for swollen glands, ordering a complete blood count or doing a biopsy (in the case of some lymphomas and breast cancer). If you do have cancer and debilitating hot flashes, check with your health-care provider to see whether hot-flash remedies such as creams, pills or patches delivering a low dose of hormones are safe for you to use. If they aren't, try nonhormonal medications.

ADRENAL GLAND DISORDERS

The adrenal glands, located above each kidney, produce more than 50 hormones, including estrogen and the stress hormone cortisol. If you have an adrenal gland disorder, you may experience not only extreme hot flashes and

night sweats but also other symptoms including fatigue, insomnia, moodiness and even depression. These are common menopausal symptoms, too, so it's easy to miss the adrenal gland diagnosis.

What to do: A blood test can rule out most adrenal gland disorders. If it turns out you do have an adrenal disorder, once it's treated, the hot flashes will stop—though you still could have menopause-related heat surges.

SARCOIDOSIS

Some researchers think bacteria causes sarcoidosis, which leads to inflammation in the lungs, eyes and lymph nodes. It's more common in women than in men, and one of the hallmark symptoms is night sweats.

What to do: Sarcoidosis usually begins in the lungs, so if in addition to night sweats, you feel short of breath and have a persistent cough or wheeze, ask your doctor about the possibility that it could be sarcoidosis. Doctors can diagnose the disease with an X-ray or a lung function test. If the X-ray catches a visible mass on the lungs, a doctor will perform a biopsy. Treatment with steroids or other medications will end night sweats caused by sarcoidosis.

TUBERCULOSIS

This bacterial infection usually attacks the lungs, but night sweats are a common symptom. Tuberculosis (TB) is rare in the US, but it does exist here, and you can more easily get it if you travel to many other countries.

What to do: If you work in a high-risk setting (such as a hospital, nursing home or prison) or have been traveling in an area where TB is common (such as South America, Eastern Europe or the Western Pacific region) and you have night sweats, ask for a skin test to rule out the disease. If you have TB, you'll need to take several drugs for six to nine months before you're cured. That should eliminate your TB-related night sweats.

These medical treatments can trigger hot flashes...

NIACIN

Niacin is a dietary supplement sometimes used to reduce LDL cholesterol levels. It can cause a flush that spreads from the neck to the face, though some women experience these surges as hot flashes.

What to do: If you take niacin, aren't perimenopausal and are having what feels like hot flashes, talk to your doctor about trying a time-release niacin capsule (less likely to cause flushing than other types) or switching to a lower dose of niacin and then increasing the dose to its desired level slowly.

STEROIDS

Doctors prescribe steroids to treat inflammation from a variety of conditions. Hot flashes can be a side effect of steroids—as can mood swings. If you are experiencing either of these potential steroid side effects, talk to your doctor about the possibility of lowering the dose.

TAMOXIFEN AND RALOXIFENE

The drugs *tamoxifen* and *raloxifene* are selective estrogen receptor modulators (SERMS) that mimic the effects of estrogen. Women who've had breast cancer take tamoxifen to reduce the risk of developing it again (or developing it in the other breast). Doctors prescribe raloxifene to strengthen bones for women with osteoporosis. Both can cause debilitating hot flashes and night sweats.

What to do: If night sweats are a problem, taking tamoxifen in the morning instead of at night may help. Medications such as *venlafaxine* (an antidepressant sold under the name Effexor) or *gabapentin* (an anticonvulsant) can ease hot flashes for women taking tamoxifen or raloxifene.

CHEMOTHERAPY

Chemotherapy can stop the body's production of estrogen and cause many side effects that mimic menopause, including trouble concentrating, mood changes, hot flashes and night sweats.

What to do: Hormone replacement therapy can help ease hot flashes and night sweats. But if you have breast cancer, you'll need to try a nonestrogen-based therapy. Some types of antidepressants as well as *clonidine* (Catapres), a drug typically used to treat high blood pressure, may help—as may hormone-free therapies generally recommended for menopausal

heat surges such as breathing techniques that cool down the body.

If you're middle-aged and are starting to experience hot flashes or night sweats, the mostly likely explanation is that you're in perimenopause. But make an appointment with your health-care provider to see whether something else might be causing your symptoms or making them worse.

Time Hormone Therapy Right

JoAnn V. Pinkerton, MD, NCMP, executive director, North American Menopause Society, Pepper Pike, Ohio.

Timing is important with hormone therapy (HT). When 8,000 women, ages 47 to 56, were studied for more than 20 years, those who began HT in their early 50s and continued for more than 10 years were half as likely to develop Alzheimer's disease as those who did not use HT.

Takeaway: If you're considering HT in your 50s for menopausal symptoms, there may be an added benefit for your brain…but until more research is done, HT is not recommended for the prevention of Alzheimer's.

Vaginal Hormone Therapy

Carolyn J. Crandall, MD, MS, professor of medicine, David Geffen School of Medicine at the University of California at Los Angeles.

The latest research on vaginal estrogen for menopausal symptoms shows that these creams, inserts or rings are safer than oral estrogen, which may increase stroke and breast cancer risk. A study of 45,663 women, followed for more than six years, found that those who used vaginal estrogen, compared with women who didn't use any hormonal product, had no greater risk for breast cancer, stroke, heart disease or hip fracture. Vaginal estrogen relieves symptoms including vaginal dryness, itching and urinary urgency.

Bad Hot Flashes? Watch Out for Pelvic Organ Prolapse

Angelo Cagnacci, MD, professor of gynecology and obstetrics, University of Udine, Italy, and lead author of the study "Association Between Pelvic Organ Prolapse and Climacteric Symptoms in Postmenopausal Women," published in *Maturitas, the European Menopause Journal.*

The "pelvic floor" is a network of muscles, ligaments and other tissue that acts like a sling to support a woman's pelvic organs. The bowel and bladder are controlled by contracting and relaxing these muscles and tissues. When the pelvic floor becomes weak, the organs above it can bulge toward your vaginal opening and even push out of it. The medical name for this hernia of the pelvic organs is pelvic organ prolapse.

Risk factors for it include menopause, age, obesity, repeated heavy lifting and traumatic injury—as may happen during childbirth, for example, or from a hip or back injury. But there's been little research into whether menopausal symptoms themselves are linked to prolapse risk.

New study: Italian researchers analyzed data on 1,382 postmenopausal women attending an outpatient service for menopause at a university hospital. The women were asked 21 questions to rate the severity of menopausal symptoms such as hot flashes, night sweats, fast heartbeats and sleep problems. The incidence of prolapse was also tracked.

Results: Women with a higher degree of menopausal symptoms were more likely to suffer pelvic organ prolapse—specifically, a prolapsed bladder. This study wasn't designed to show how it might happen, but the researchers note that high levels of the stress hormone cortisol—which often rise in the menopausal transition—can impair collagen tissue that's a key component of the pelvic floor.

Bottom line: If you have severe menopausal symptoms, explore ways to ease them—including mind-body approaches. But now is also a good time to check with your doctor to see whether you also have pelvic floor weakness that may lead to prolapse. You may be able to prevent this condition by losing weight and practicing Kegel exercises, which strengthen the pelvic floor muscles. Even if you already have prolapse but it's not causing significant symptoms, such lifestyle approaches may be enough to keep it from getting worse. Treatment options include the use of a pessary—a medical device that provides structural support—or surgery.

Ovarian Cancer Deaths Down

Study by researchers at University of Milan, Italy, published in *Annals of Oncology.*

US ovarian cancer deaths are down 16%. The decline is from 2002 to 2012 (latest data available).

Reasons: Long-term use of oral contraceptives, which are known to protect against ovarian cancer...and reduced use of menopausal hormone therapy, which can raise cancer risk.

Where Ovary Cancer Starts

Victor Velculescu, MD, PhD, codirector of cancer biology, Johns Hopkins Kimmel Cancer Center, Baltimore, and leader of a study published in *Nature Communications.*

Ovarian cancer may not start in the ovaries. *Recent finding:* The most common type of ovarian cancer—high-grade serous carcinoma—begins in the fallopian tubes. If the early research is confirmed, it could make earlier treatment possible.

Experience Is Contagious

Tasleem Padamsee, PhD, assistant professor of health services management and policy, The Ohio State University, Columbus.

Loved one's cancer experience impacts prevention decisions.

New Breast Cancer Care

A device that treats early-stage breast cancer tumors by targeting them with precisely focused beams of radiation, minimizing damage to surrounding tissue, received FDA clearance in December 2017. The Gamma Pod is expected to shorten the standard three-to-six-week radiation treatment and may eliminate the need for surgery. To find a hospital using GammaPod, go to Xcision. com and click on "patients."

William F. Regine, MD, Isadore and Fannie Schneider Foxman Endowed Professor and Chair of Radiation Oncology, University of Maryland School of Medicine, Baltimore, and GammaPod coinventor.

New study: Half the women at high risk for breast cancer who had experienced the death of a loved one from any type of cancer were likely to choose aggressive measures—such as mastectomy—to prevent their own cancer. By comparison, just 3% of women with a loved one who survived cancer chose aggressive measures.

If you have risk factors for breast cancer: Make sure your doctor fully explains all preventive treatments before you choose which is best for you.

To Enhance Sexual Desire, Women Need "Just Right" Testosterone

James A. Simon, MD, professor of obstetrics and gynecology, George Washington University School of Medicine, Washington, DC, and coauthor with Jill M. Krapf, MD, of an article titled "A Sex-Specific Dose-Response Curve for Testosterone: Could Excessive Testosterone Limit Sexual Interaction in Women?" published in *Menopause*.

When it comes to testosterone, women share a few things with men. Like men, they produce the hormone, although in much smaller amounts. Like men, they make less as they get older. And like men,

women with low libidos who get testosterone treatments often experience a boost in sexual desire and enjoyment. No wonder millions of American women turn to their doctors to get testosterone prescriptions to enhance their sex lives—even though it's not FDA-approved for women.

Yet, when it comes to testosterone and libido, women aren't really like men—at all. For women, unlike men, just a little extra "T" can backfire in the bedroom.

Background: "Hypoactive sexual desire disorder" (HSDD)—the medical term for low libido—affects both men and women, but it's particularly common in postmenopausal women. While there are many factors, including vaginal dryness, that can affect sexual comfort, low levels of testosterone may play a role, too.

Women make small amounts of testosterone in their adrenal glands, ovaries (even after menopause) and in cells with testosterone receptors, but levels start declining in their 20s and are often quite low by the 50s and beyond.

In women with HSDD, testosterone treatment can be an effective treatment, studies show. But there are sometimes side effects, including hair growth, acne and even mood changes.

Study: My colleague and I reviewed existing studies, including animal research, to identify whether women respond to testosterone treatment for HSDD differently from men—and why. One reason the FDA has approved dozens of testosterone products for men but none for women, they suggest, is that the proper dose for each individual woman isn't understood yet.

Results: Men taking testosterone have a linear dose-related response when it comes to libido. At higher doses of testosterone, men have a bigger increase in libido than they do when taking a smaller dose.

In women, more testosterone may actually mean less desire.

Example: 318 postmenopausal women with HSDD were treated with different doses of testosterone or a placebo for 24 weeks. Those who got the lowest daily doses—150 micrograms (mcg)—didn't have any sexual benefit. Those who got 300 mcg had more sexual desire and more frequent "sexually satisfying" events. But increasing doses up to 450 mcg not only didn't increase those benefits, it was actually associated with lower levels of desire. Plus, unpleasant side effects were a little higher in these women.

Women, it appears, don't have a linear response to testosterone treatment—their response is more like a bell curve. You might call it the "Goldilocks effect"—the amount of testosterone that is just right for them.

Surprising finding: To dig deeper into what's behind this phenomenon, we reviewed animal as well as human studies. One possible reason for the bell curve—while increasing concentrations of testosterone in women increase sexual function, at a certain point the "masculine" effects get in the way. These physical effects include deepening of the voice, hair loss where there should be hair, excessive hair where there shouldn't be and acne. Not exactly turn-ons. Psychological effects of too much testosterone treatment may also include aggression, anxiety and depression.

Any of these features may affect a woman's sexual desire and function—and she may become less sexually attractive to her partner. That's true in animals. Human sexuality is a lot harder to study, we admit, so it's just a thought experiment for now.

Bottom line: Discuss with your doctor whether this is the best approach for you—depending on your issues, there are many libido-boosting options.

Because there is no FDA-approved testosterone treatment for women, there is no approved dosage, either. If you do decide to be treated using testosterone, work with your doctor, who should be a hormone expert, to determine the dose that seems best for you…and then pay close attention to how the dose you're taking is affecting you—body and mind. Just a little too much might actually dampen desire. In women, testosterone appears to work best in moderation.

Hidden Dangers of Feminine Hygiene Products

Kieran C. O'Doherty, PhD, associate professor, department of psychology, and researcher on the human microbiome, University of Guelph, Ontario, Canada. He is lead author of the study "Vaginal Health and Hygiene Practices and Product Use in Canada: A National Cross-Sectional Survey," published in *BMC Women's Health.*

Women, listen up! You may love those feminine creams, lubricants and wipes, but are these products doing more harm than good? Perhaps so, according to new research.

Background: It's been known for some time that douching can disrupt the vaginal flora—the balance of "friendly" and "unfriendly" bacteria in the vagina. When this occurs, it increases a woman's risk for bacterial vaginosis, a mild vaginal infection that commonly results in a fishy-smelling discharge.

To learn more about other vaginal health practices, researchers from University of Guelph in Ontario asked 1,500 Canadian women about their use of vaginal hygiene (aka "feminine hygiene") products, such as anti-itch creams, sanitizing gels, moisturizers/lubricants and feminine wipes, during their lifetimes and in the last three months. These over-the-counter (OTC) products are used for everything from vaginal dryness to smelly female parts.

Study results: A whopping 95% of the women surveyed reported that they had used vaginal hygiene products. The study, published in *BMC Women's Health*, further revealed big differences in the rates of infection between users and nonusers of vaginal hygiene products.

Biggest offender: Women who applied vaginal gel sanitizers (sometimes known as "vaginal deodorizers") reported having eight times as many yeast infections and almost 20 times as many bacterial infections as those who didn't "sanitize."

The use of feminine washes or gels was associated with three-and-a-half times higher odds of having bacterial vaginosis compared with nonusers. Among women who used these products, there was two-and-a-half times higher odds of having a urinary tract infection (UTI).

There were similar findings among those who used feminine wipes and lubricants/moisturizers. Women who used these products reported having a UTI twice as often and a yeast infection two-and-a-half times as often, respectively.

Even though the researchers can't say for sure that these products caused any of the infections, the study results do provide a reason to further investigate whether these gels, creams, wipes, etc., disrupt the natural vaginal environment and inhibit the growth of healthy bacteria.

Without enough healthy bacteria, a woman's body is less capable of fighting off infections. In addition to UTIs and yeast infections, this could theoretically mean that women are also increasing their risk for other conditions linked to unhealthy vaginal flora—such as pelvic inflammatory disease, cervical cancer and sexually transmitted diseases. If additional research supports the findings, these products could indeed be doing more harm than good.

Bottom line: The body naturally produces secretions that clean the vagina from the inside. To play it safe, it's best for women to limit their cleansing and freshening routine to a once-a-day wash (maybe more than once if you're menstruating) with warm water and perhaps a mild, unscented soap.

Your vagina doesn't need to smell like lavender or jasmine or a tropical rainstorm to be healthy. In fact, those added scents may just add to your problems. It's seems that this part of a woman's body can take care of itself just fine—thank you very much!

Acupressure for Menstrual Cramps

Claudia M. Witt, MD, of the Institute for Complementary and Integrative Medicine at University Zurich and University Hospital Zurich in Switzerland and the Center for Integrative Medicine at University of Maryland School of Medicine in Baltimore and coauthor of the study "Effectiveness of App-based Self-acupressure for Women with Menstrual Pain Compared to Usual Care: A Randomized Pragmatic Trial," published in *American Journal of Obstetrics & Gynecology*.

Are you suffering with menstrual pain? Relief may literally be at your fingertips. No meds needed.

In a pilot study, women who also used acupressure—pressing their fingers on their skin at certain points—to ease menstrual pain experienced more relief than women using only their usual care methods of pain medicine and oral contraceptives.

Participants followed instructions from an acupressure app called Luna.Selfcare.

The app told them how to press on three key acupressure points: SP6 on the inside of the leg just above the ankle bone, LI4 is at the highest spot of the muscle of your hand when your thumb and index finger are brought close together, and LR3 is where the skin of your big toe and the second toe joint.

Women using the app applied pressure to each site on both sides of the body for one minute each at the same time every day beginning five days before they expected their periods to begin and continuing until their periods ended. The app included reminders, a diary and feedback questionnaires, and the study lasted for six menstrual cycles. Another group of women in the study, the control group, had no acupressure and continued to follow their typical care plan, such as taking pain medication.

The results: 37% of the women who did self-acupressure reported that the intensity of their pain during their periods had decreased by half or more after three months. After six months, 58% of the women found that level of relief. In contrast, only 25% of the women in the non-acupressure group reported a similar reduction in pain intensity at either three or six months.

A few women in the self-acupressure group had a negative reaction to the treatment, such as greater pain or bruising. But the number of instances declined over the first three months of the study.

The app, developed in Germany for the study, was not yet available in the US as we were writing this, but the good news is, you don't need an app to practice self-acupressure and get similar benefits. Claudia M. Witt, MD, the lead author of the study, said that while features of the app are helpful, acupressure could also be applied without an app if you can commit to making the change in behavior required—often the most "difficult" part of any self-care initiative.

Applying acupressure without the app: Schedule a session with an experienced acupressure professional in your area to show you exactly where the SP6, LI4 and LR3 points are located and how to properly apply pressure to them. And then follow the system used in the study and described above (once a day at the same time each day starting five days before your anticipated period and continuing until it ends). Also, be patient, as the study results showed that the effect of acupressure increased over time.

Caution: If your menstrual pain tends to be very severe, talk to your doctor because that level of pain could be a symptom of a serious condition such as endometriosis or adenomyosis, said Dr. Witt.

Resource: You can find an acupressure therapist by searching the National Certification Board for Therapeutic Massage & Bodywork.

The Health Risks of Iron After Menopause

Study titled "Serum Ferritin Level Is Positively Associated with Insulin Resistance and Metabolic Syndrome in Postmenopausal Women: A Nationwide Population-based Study" by researchers at Yonsei University College of Medicine in Seoul, Republic of Korea, published in *Maturitas.*

After menopause, a woman's risk for diabetes and heart disease goes up. One likely culprit is the loss of estrogen because of menopause. But another factor also may play an important role—excess iron.

Background: After menopause, women are at higher risk for metabolic syndrome, a cluster of symptoms including abdominal obesity and high blood sugar, often due to insulin resistance. The syndrome increases the risk of developing diabetes and heart disease.

Why does the risk go up after menopause? It's true that the loss of estrogen is known to negatively affect the lining of blood vessels in ways that increase many of these risk factors. But another line of evidence points to excess iron as an additional risk factor. Because iron in blood is no longer lost with each menstrual cycle, iron levels generally increase after menopause. Korean researchers set out to determine whether there was a statistical link between high iron levels, insulin resistance and metabolic syndrome.

Study: 2,734 postmenopausal women in a large health database all had extensive exams that included blood samples, so the researchers could sort them into four groups based on blood levels of ferritin, a protein that's a marker for body levels of iron. They then analyzed ferritin levels against rates of insulin resistance and metabolic syndrome.

Results: After the researchers adjusted for other known factors (age, smoking, drinking and amount of exercise), it was evident that women with the highest levels of ferritin, compared to women with the lowest levels, were...

•**More than twice as likely to have insulin resistance**

•**Almost twice as likely to have metabolic syndrome.**

What's so bad about excess iron? It promotes oxidation (think: rust), which can lead to body-wide inflammation—and that in turns increases all the above risk factors. Plus, there is evidence that too much iron may interfere with normal glucose and insulin activity in muscles. Because this is an observational study, however, it can't determine whether high ferritin levels cause insulin resistance/metabolic syndrome—or are simply a marker for these risk factors.

Bottom line: The authors advise that getting your iron level checked—it's part of a regular checkup anyway—could be an early tip-off to these risk factors. Then you can take lifestyle steps, including weight loss if needed, that can independently reduce your risks.

You may also want to talk with a nutritionist about your diet. After menopause, a woman's daily iron requirement goes from 18 mg to 8 mg. However, recent research has found that some postmenopausal women may still be at risk for iron deficiency anemia—an issue best dealt with by eating more iron-rich foods.

In particular, be cautious about your vitamin/mineral supplement(s). According to the National Institutes of Health, postmenopausal women should not take a supplement that includes iron unless they have been diagnosed with iron deficiency. If you are concerned about anemia, get tested and discuss with your doctor whether supplementing with iron is appropriate for you.

Good Sleep Solutions for Menopause

Michael J. Breus, PhD, a clinical psychologist, diplomate of the American Board of Sleep Medicine and fellow of the American Academy of Sleep Medicine. He is the coauthor of *The Power of When*. TheSleepDoctor.com

---

If you put 100 women going through the menopausal transition into a room and asked each one if she has trouble sleeping, roughly half would tell you, "Yes, I do!"

Why are sleep problems so common during this time? You're probably thinking—hot flashes! And it's true that waking up in the middle of the night drenched in sweat counts as "trouble sleeping." But there are many other triggers of sleep problems around the time of menopause. One large 14-year study of sleep and menopause found that while hot flashes were strongly linked with sleep problems for some women, a large percentage of poor sleep happened to women in the absence of hot flashes. Other research has found that some women self-report that hot flashes are the cause of their sleep problems, but when their hot flashes and sleep are monitored in a sleep lab, that link just isn't there.

This research is important because it suggests that the sleep problems experienced by midlife women may be connected to other causes that may be going unnoticed...and unaddressed. To learn more, we spoke with Michael Breus, PhD, a clinical psychologist and an expert on sleep problems.

MENOPAUSE AND SLEEP

If hot flashes aren't alone on the hot seat for menopausal sleep problems, what other issues are linked to both menopause and poor sleep? One may simply be a coincidence—age. Just getting older is, unfortunately, often a game-changer when it comes to sleep. Brain levels of melatonin, a hormone that helps control sleep and wake cycles, decline with age in both genders. Diagnoses of chronic insomnia—defined as problems falling asleep and/or staying asleep that happen at least three times a week and continue for at least three months—may just happen coincidentally around the time of menopause symptoms.

While there isn't much you can do about age, there are a few other health issues that you can actively address...

•**Sleep apnea.** This condition, in which breathing pauses or stops multiple times during the night, causing multiple awakenings, may play an important role in menopause-related sleep disorders. Before menopause, women are only half as likely as men to have sleep apnea, but the rate rises steadily after menopause. Why isn't clear, but a leading suspect is menopausal weight gain. It's well-established that being overweight or obese greatly increases the risk of having sleep apnea. (Oddly enough, one symptom of sleep apnea in postmenopausal women is nocturnal enuresis...bed-wetting.) What do to: If you suspect you may have sleep apnea, ask your doctor about getting a sleep study—or get a referral to a sleep center (see page 327).

•**Restless leg syndrome (RLS).** This often-overlooked problem affects up to 10% of the population, mostly women. RLS sufferers describe creeping, crawling sensations in their legs that occur at rest and at night. Sometimes RLS causes involuntarily movements of the legs that can wake up someone from a sound sleep. In one study of 100 perimenopausal and postmenopausal women with poor sleep who underwent a sleep study in which their hot flashes, leg movements, breathing and sleep quality were measured, more than half were found to have either sleep apnea, RLS—or both. And interestingly, laboratory-measured hot flashes were not found to be major predictors of the subjects' sleep efficiency (how well they slept according to scientific measurements). What to do: If you suspect RLS, ask your doctor to give you a ferritin test to see if you're anemic. If you are, your doctor will likely recommend iron supplementation, which can be quite helpful for relieving restless leg syndrome. If iron is not the issue, seek out a neurologist who is certified in sleep medicine.

•**Stress.** It may be a ubiquitous catchall, blamed for everything from heart disease to cancer to obesity, but stress is a major contributor to poor sleep. When we perceive danger or a threat, our bodies produce the so-called stress hormone cortisol. This substance floods our bodies with extra energy and heightens awareness. Not exactly a great state for restful sleep! Falling levels of estrogen may also make the brain less resilient to stress. During the transition to menopause, levels of both hormones fluctuate to an unusual degree, often over a period of several years. This state of hormonal flux can make good sleep harder to get.

And let's be honest…menopause itself can be psychologically stressful. Anxiety and emotional issues surrounding the menopause transition can feed into these physiological processes, making stress worse…and sleep more elusive.

What to do: One of the best ways to learn new ways to handle stress during menopause is cognitive behavioral therapy. (*Bonus*: It also helps with hot flashes and night sweats.)

SLEEPING THROUGH MENOPAUSE

It's all well and good that researchers are investigating the causes of sleep difficulties that plague women at midlife, but if you're staring at the ceiling at night and nodding off during the day, what you really need are solutions. If you've ruled out a medical condition such as sleep apnea or RLS, the first step is to get to the basics of good sleep hygiene…using your bed only for sleep and sex…banishing noise…turning down lights and turning off TV and other screens (phones, laptops, tablets) an hour before bedtime…and keeping to a consistent bedtime/wake-up schedule.

Next, practice these tips, based on the latest research, that zero in on the sleep issues that women in menopause and perimenopause are most likely to experience…

•**Keep your bedroom cool.** This is a good idea for everyone, but it's especially important if you are prone to hot flashes—or their midnight cousins, night sweats. As you sleep, your core body temperature drops a few degrees, which helps trigger your body to fall asleep. Help this process along by keeping your bedroom temperature between 60°F and 67°F. There are also special chilling pillows, blankets and mattress pads that can help keep you cool. I like the Chillow pillow and the ChiliPad Cube.

•**Practice deep breathing.** If you wake up in the middle of the night, what you do in the next few minutes can make the difference between drifting back to sleep or remaining wide-eyed until morning. Just like your body temperature, your heart rate decreases when you're asleep. If you wake and immediately succumb to being frustrated and angry at your wakefulness and probably allowing worries about the next day to creep in, your heart rate inevitably rises. That makes it harder to fall back to sleep. Since menopause is a time when stress levels rise, it's particularly important to learn ways to bring your heart rate down quickly—like deep breathing.

My favorite: The "4-7-8 method." To do it, slowly breathe in for four seconds, hold for seven seconds, and slowly breathe out for eight seconds. Repeat this exercise five to 10 times or as long as necessary until you feel more relaxed and drowsy.

•**Become a quick-change artist.** If you're having hot flashes and waking up soaked to the skin, keep an extra set of PJs by your bed so that you can quickly change without rousing yourself much. It's not just about getting into dry sleep clothes—you also want, again, to keep your heart rate from climbing, which it might do if you had to get up, flip on the light and rummage through your dresser or closet. The idea is to limit the amount your heart rate climbs.

If all else fails, get up! If your deep-breathing exercises don't work and you've been lying awake in bed for more than 30 minutes, it's time to get out of bed. Why? You don't want to train your body into the idea that lying awake for long periods is a normal part of your sleep pattern. You can sit in a chair and read a book (no screen!). I often suggest to my patients that they create a gratitude list—with a pad and pen or pencil, write down a few things or people that you're glad are in your life. It's a positive thing to reflect on until you feel tired enough to go back to sleep.

•**Time your caffeine and alcohol.** If you're experiencing problems with sleep, you probably know that you should avoid having a latte at 6 pm—or even 3 pm. After all, it takes up to five hours for the body to get rid of half the caffeine that you consume. But what about alcohol? Although a drink may make you drowsy at first, a few hours later, as your body processes the alcohol, it can increase your heart rate and body temperature, waking you up from a sound sleep. I ask women to stop drinking alcoholic beverages about three hours before bedtime. (Caffeine and alcohol can also be hot flash triggers for some women.)

•**Watch out for antianxiety medications.** *Benzodiazepines* (such as Valium and Xanax) are prescribed for anxiety—which menopause can sometimes bring on—and it can be tempting to use them for sleep. While these pills can reduce anxiety, however, they don't actually help you sleep better…and they're habit-forming. If you have been prescribed a benzodiaz-epine for an anxiety disorder, that's one thing, but don't use it for the sole purpose of helping you sleep.

IF SELF-HELP ISN'T ENOUGH…

•**Investigate a sleep center.** If you have sleep problems that last longer than three months, consult a sleep expert—if you can, at a sleep center. These centers, sometimes located at large academic medical institutions, are stocked with the latest diagnostic equipment and can help determine what is keeping you from a good night's sleep. You can find a sleep center near you by putting "find a sleep center" into any search engine. (You may also be interested in my recent blog post, "When is it time for a sleep study?")

•**Try cognitive behavioral therapy.** This specialized form of therapy focuses on changing our cognitive processes (how we structure our thoughts) and our behavior (how we act). Increasingly, sleep experts advocate this approach as a way to tackle many common sleep problems without the use of drugs. CBTI—the "I" stands for insomnia—is specifically designed to help treat insomnia. Finding a therapist who practices CBTI can be challenging, but there are online programs (like Sleepio and SHUTi) that allow you to take a self-guided course.

Getting a good night's sleep on a regular basis is one of the best things you can do to feel better and stay healthier—even protect against menopause-related depression. Want even more motivation? Good sleep may be the key to a better sex life, too.

Index